Handbook of Nephrology and Hypertension

Seventh Edition

Christopher S. Wilcox, MD, PhD, FRCP (UK), FACP
Editor-in-Chief
Department of Medicine
Division of Nephrology and Hypertension
Georgetown University
Washington, DC

Michael Choi, MD
Department of Medicine
Division of Nephrology and Hypertension
Georgetown University
Washington, DC

Mark S. Segal, MD, PhD
Division of Nephrology
College of Medicine
University of Florida
Gainesville, Florida

Limeng Chen, MD, PhD
Division of Nephrology
Peking Union Medical College Hospital
Beijing, China

Winfred W. Williams, MD
Division of Nephrology
Harvard Medical School
Massachusetts General Hospital
Boston, Massachusetts

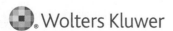
Wolters Kluwer

Philadelphia • Baltimore • New York • London
Buenos Aires • Hong Kong • Sydney • Tokyo

Acquisitions Editor: James Sherman
Senior Development Editor: Ariel S. Winter
Editorial Coordinator: Christopher Rodgers
Marketing Manager: Kirsten Watrud
Production Project Manager: Frances Gunning
Manager, Graphic Arts & Design: Stephen Druding
Manufacturing Coordinator: Beth Welsh
Prepress Vendor: Aptara, Inc.

7th Edition
Copyright © 2023 Wolters Kluwer.
6th edition © 2009 by Lippincott Williams & Wilkins, a Wolters Kluwer business
© 2005, 1999 by Lippincott Williams & Wilkins
© 1995, 1993 by JB Lippincott

9 8 7 6 5 4 3 2 1

Printed in Singapore

Library of Congress Cataloging-in-Publication Data available upon request

978-1-9751-6572-7

---

shop.lww.com

To our past and present fellows, residents, students, and trainees.
May you provide your patients compassionate care guided
by science and scholarship.

I demand of my students the passion of science and
the patience of poetry.
Vladimir Nabokov (Strong Opinions, Interviews, 1962)

In memorium
Stuart and Imogen Wilcox
Francis Wilcox
Elizabeth Wilcox
Alex and Petra Wilcox

Mohammed A. Alshehri, MD

ABIM in internal medicine and Nephrology
Assistant Professor, Internal Medicine
    Department
College of Medicine
King Khalid University
Abha, Saudi Arabia

Jeanette M. Andrade, PhD

Assistant Professor, Food Science and
    Human Nutrition
University of Florida
Gainesville, Florida

Afia Ashraf, MD

Nephrology Fellow, Nephrology
MedStar Georgetown University Hospital
Washington, DC

Danielle F. Aycart, MS

Doctoral Student, Nutritional Sciences
Food Science and Human Nutrition
University of Florida
Gainesville, Florida

Azra Bihorac, MD, MS, FCCM, FASN

Senior Associate Dean for Research
MD-Nephrology
University of Florida
Gainesville, Florida

Benjamin K. Canales, MD, MPH

Associate Professor
Department of Urology
University of Florida
Gainesville, Florida

Muna T. Canales, MD, MS

Assistant Professor of Medicine and Staff
    Physician Medicine
University of Florida and the Malcom
    Randall VA Medical Center
Gainesville, Florida

Gajapathiraju Chamarthi, MD

Clinical Assistant Professor
Department of Medicine
Division of Nephology
University of Florida
Gainesville, Florida

Steven Gabardi, PharmD

Transplant Clinical Specialist
Department of Transplant Surgery
Brigham and Women's Hospital
Boston, Massachusetts

Saraswathi Gopal, MD

Clinical Assistant Professor
Department of Medicine
Division of Nephrology, Hypertension and
    Renal Transplantation
University of Florida
Gainesville, Florida

Judit Gordon-Cappitelli, MD

Assistant Professor of Medicine
Department of Nephrology and Hypertension
MedStar Georgetown University Hospital
Washington, DC

Keiko I. Greenberg, MD, MHS

Assistant Professor of Medicine
Department of Nephrology and Hypertension
MedStar Georgetown University Hospital
Washington, DC

Behnaz Haddadi-Sahneh, MD

Nephrologist
Private Practice
Fairfax, Virginia

Mohammad A. Hashmi, MD

Transplant Nephrologist
Virtua Health
Camden, New Jersey

Amir Kazory, MD, FASN, FACC
Professor and Chief
Division of Nephrology, Hypertension, and
  Renal Transplantation
University of Florida
Gainesville, Florida

Abhilash Koratala, MD, FASN
Assistant Professor of Medicine
Nephrology, Medical College of Wisconsin
Milwaukee, Wisconsin

Wai Lang Lau, MD
Assistant professor
Division of nephrology, hypertension, and
  renal transplantation
University of Florida
Gainesville, Florida

Michael Lipkowitz, MD
Assistant Professor of Medicine
Department of Nephrology and Hypertension
MedStar Georgetown University Hospital
Washington, DC

Rajesh Mohandas, MD, MPH
Associate Professor of Medicine
Division of Nephrology Hypertension and
  Transplantation
University of Florida
Gainesville, Florida

Chanigan Nilubol, MD
General Nephrology
MedStar Georgetown University Hospital
Washington, DC

Olanrewaju A. Olaoye, MD
Assistant Professor of Medicine
Department of Medicine and Nephrology
University of Florida
Gainesville, Florida

Negiin Pourafshar, MD
Assistant Professor
Department of Nephrology
MedStar Georgetown University Hospital
Washington, DC

Robert J. Rubin, MD
Distinguished Professor of Medicine
Georgetown University
Washington, DC

Rupam Ruchi, MD, FASN
Associate Professor of Medicine
Program Director, Nephrology Fellowship
  Program
University of Florida
Gainesville, Florida

Chintan V. Shah, MD
Assistant Professor of Medicine
Division of Nephrology, Hypertension & Renal
  Transplantation
University of Florida College of Medicine
Gainesville, Florida

Wen Shen, MD
Nephrology
MedStar Georgetown University Hospital
Washington, DC

Ashutosh M. Shukla, MD
Professor in Medicine
Director of Advanced CKD and Home
  Dialysis Services
University of Florida
Faculty in Nephrology
North Florida/South Georgia VHS
Gainesville, Florida

Jogiraju V. Tantravahi, MD, PhD
Division of Nephrology
Department of Medicine
University of Florida College of Medicine
Gainesville, Florida

I. David Weiner, MD
Professor of Medicine, Renal Division
University of Florida and Chief Nephrology and
  Hypertension Section, GVAMC
Gainesville, Florida

Charles S. Wingo, MD
Professor of Medicine and Physiology
Department of Medicine
University of Florida
Gainesville, Florida

PREFACE

Each of the previous editions of this *Handbook of Nephrology and Hypertension* have refined the text and discussion and added new topics to cover developments in the field. We have striven throughout to provide a concise and reliable overview of the subject up to the level required for the American Board of Internal Medicine in Nephrology or the Hypertension Specialist of the American Society of Hypertension. Its primary target readership remains Nephrology fellows and trainees but it should also be of value for practicing physicians, nurses and paramedical personnel, including pharmacists and those working in the pharmaceutical industry requiring an up-to-date overview of a topic in nephrology or hypertension. To maintain this focus, all chapters are written by practicing nephrologists and several are co-authored by nephrology trainees. This ensures that the topics covered are those most in need of discussion or explanation. Most chapter authors also are clinical investigators who bring special insights from their fields of research. All are faculty members at Georgetown University, the University of Florida, Harvard Medical School or the Medical College of Peking.

The seventh edition is rewritten with several new chapters. An important improvement is to provide all those who purchase a copy of this edition with the opportunity to upload it to the Internet to provide a readily accessible source of reference during clinical encounters. This edition is co-authored by practicing nephrologists with special expertise in physiology and hypertension (Christopher Wilcox), clinical nephrology and glomerulonephritis (Michael Choi and Mark Segal), human genetics and molecular biology (Limeng Chen), and renal transplantation and immunology (Winfred Williams). Despite its widened scope, the present edition retains a concise format with only a modest increase in page numbers

We hope that those who read this book will find it informative, enjoyable and, at times, provocative.

Christopher S. Wilcox, MD, PhD, FRCP (UK), FACP

ACKNOWLEDGMENTS

C. Craig Tisher, MD, first proposed a *Handbook of Nephrology and Hypertension*. He generously invited me to co-author the first and subsequent editions. Dr. Tisher was the chief of the Division on Nephrology, Hypertension and Transplantation of the Shands Hospital and I was chief of Nephrology and Hypertension of the Veterans Administration Hospital and Director of the Hypertension Center at the University of Florida. After his retirement, I have assumed authorship of this edition. I am fortunate to have been able to maintain the strong ties with the University of Florida and its faculty. I have included Mark Segal, MD, their chief of nephrology for 11 years, as co-author and many of their excellent faculty as chapter authors. I have had the pleasure of writing and lecturing at the Peking Union Medical College in Beijing where I developed an admiration and friendship with Limeng Chen, MD, their chief of nephrology. I was delighted to invite her to be a co-author of this new edition and thereby to introduce it to a new Chinese readership. I developed a strong appreciation for the knowledge and clinical skills of Winfred Williams, MD while at the Brigham and Women's Hospital in Boston. I consider his new chapters on renal transplantation to have strengthened this new edition greatly. Most importantly, I am delighted to welcome Michael Choi, MD as co-author. He is the past president of the American Kidney Foundation and my successor as chief of the Division of Nephrology and Hypertension at Georgetown University Medical Center. He brings many of our excellent faculty and fellows as chapter authors. Dr. Choi has an unparalleled reputation as a clinical nephrologist and has made a major contribution to this edition.

CONTENTS

Evaluation of the Patient
with Renal Disease

1

Clinical and Laboratory Evaluation of Kidney Disease and Fluid Status

Mohammed A. Alshehri, Chanigan Nilubol

I. **HISTORY AND PHYSICAL EXAMINATION.** Kidney disease may be part of a systemic, inherited, or drug-induced disease process. A comprehensive history, including questions about over-the-counter medications, and a physical examination is essential. The physical examination is unreliable in complex intensive care unit situations where invasive procedures may be required to assess a patient's volume status. Whenever possible, an evaluation should include the measurements of blood pressure and heart rate while the patient is lying down quietly and after 2 minutes of standing, a fundoscopic examination and a urinalysis.

A. **Clinical Assessment of Volume Status.** Orthopnea is a sensitive symptom of volume overload. Distention of the internal or external jugular vein >3 cm above the sternal angle is an abnormal jugular venous distention, which is confirmed if there is hepatojugular reflux or Kussmaul sign. Jugular venous distention from congestive heart failure (CHF) must be differentiated from pure right-sided heart failure, which accompanies pulmonary hypertension or pulmonary emboli. These patients have an accentuated pulmonary second heart sound. An echocardiogram is helpful for diagnosis. A third heart sound is a normal finding in persons <45 years or may indicate CHF with fluid overload or hypertrophic obstructive cardiomyopathy. A worsening of hypertension is a valuable clue to the presence of fluid overload in patients with chronic kidney disease (CKD) or end-stage kidney disease (ESKD). The discovery of fine rales at the end of inspiration suggests pulmonary edema, fibrosis, or atelectasis. Peripheral edema implies fluid retention or fluid redistribution. It suggests CHF, nephrotic syndrome, cirrhosis, cor pulmonale, malnutrition, or a complication of calcium channel blockade. Postural hypotension (a fall in systolic blood pressure >20 mm Hg or >10 mm Hg in diastolic blood pressure) with reflex tachycardia indicates intravascular volume depletion. More severe volume depletion reduces skin turgor and axillary sweating. Postural hypotension without an increase in heart rate indicates autonomic insufficiency, old age, or beta-blocker therapy. Increased plasma levels of brain natriuretic peptide suggest volume overload, but they become unreliable in renal insufficiency unless serial measurements can be obtained. Point-of-care ultrasound is a promising tool for volume status assessment.

B. **Clinical Diagnosis of Uremia.** Initial symptoms of CKD are often nonspecific. Nocturia suggests a failure to concentrate the urine or orthostatic hypotension. Shortness of breath can indicate CHF, anemia, or metabolic acidosis. Anorexia, dysgeusia, nausea, vomiting, and confusion in the presence of established

CKD point to uremia. Uremic encephalopathy alters mental status and may cause grand mal seizures. Uremic pericarditis causes a pericardial friction rub and may increase pericardial fluid accumulation that can be detected by an echocardiogram.

II. BIOCHEMICAL TESTS

A. Blood Urea Nitrogen. The normal blood urea nitrogen (BUN) is 7 to 18 mg/dL or 2.5 to 6.4 mmol/L. Urea is freely filtered at the glomerulus but up to 50% is reabsorbed. The reabsorbed fraction and the production of urea are increased by volume depletion or in any prerenal state, which accounts for an elevated BUN level or an increased BUN:creatinine ratio. However, the utility of this ratio to guide the diagnosis is questionable. Urea clearance is an imprecise estimate of glomerular filtration rate (GFR). Moreover, many conditions may affect BUN independent of the GFR:

- Increased BUN: High-protein diet or increased protein catabolism from gastrointestinal bleeding, corticosteroids, tissue trauma, burns, or tetracyclines
- Decreased BUN: Low-protein diet or decreased protein catabolism from liver disease or cachexia

B. Serum Creatinine. The upper limit of serum creatinine (S_{Cr}) is 1.2 to 1.5 mg/dL or 106 to 133 mmol/L. Creatinine is freely filtered at the glomerulus. It is secreted at the proximal tubule, and some are also reabsorbed. However, S_{Cr} normally provides a better estimate of the GFR than does BUN because the degree of creatinine reabsorption and secretion is relatively small compared with filtration. Thus, a rise in S_{Cr} from 1.0 to 2.0 mg/dL normally indicates a decrease in GFR of approximately 50%. However, several factors can affect S_{Cr} independent of the GFR:

- Increased S_{Cr}: Increased intake of creatine or creatinine from a recent high animal protein meal or creatine supplements; decreased secretion because of competition from ketoacids, organic anions (in uremia), or drugs (e.g., cimetidine, trimethoprim, acetylsalicylic acid)
- Decreased S_{Cr}: Decreased creatine intake or generation from diminished muscle mass associated with cachexia, aging, a low-protein diet, or corticosteroid use
- Variation in S_{Cr}: Poor standardization between laboratories in the calibration of S_{Cr}

C. Creatinine Clearance. Creatinine clearance (C_{Cr}) can be measured directly from a timed urine collection (usually a 24-hour sample):

$$C_{Cr} \text{ (mL/min)} = \text{(Urine creatinine [mg/dL]} \times \text{Urine volume [mL/24 h])}/(S_{Cr} \text{ [mg/dL]} \times 1{,}440 \text{ [min/24 h])}$$

The normal ranges for adults aged 20 to 50 years are 97 to 137 mL/min/1.73 m^2 for men and 88 to 128 mL/min/1.73 m^2 for women. Normally, creatinine excretion should be 15 to 25 mg/kg/day in men and 12.5 to 20 mg/kg/day in women. These values decrease with advancing age and decreased muscle mass. A creatinine excretion outside the normal range raises suspicion for improper collection.

Tubular secretion of creatinine normally accounts for 10% to 40% of that excreted, but this percentage increases in those with CKD. Thus, C_{Cr} systematically overestimates the GFR, particularly in CKD. Cimetidine blocks the tubular secretion of creatinine. Loading with cimetidine before a 24-hour urine collection has been suggested as a more reliable estimate of the true GFR.

D. Cystatin C. Cystatin C is produced in all nucleated cells. It is freely filtered, and 99% reabsorbed in the proximal tubule where it is degraded. As cystatin C is less affected by muscle mass and diet compared to creatinine, it is more accurate than creatinine for estimating GFR. The assay is more costly. It is routinely measured in some countries in addition to creatinine. Kidney disease improving global outcomes (KDIGO) 2012 clinical practice guidelines for the evaluation and management of CKD suggest cystatin-based estimated GFR (eGFR) measurement in certain situations when creatinine-based eGFR is less accurate. It should be noted that thyroid disorders and corticosteroid use can affect cystatin generation.

E. Estimation of GFR. Values obtained in a 24-hour urine sample are often unreliable due to improper collection and variable tubular handling of creatinine. An alternative is to utilize validated mathematical formulas. An eGFR is useful for assessing the overall functional capacity of the kidneys, as a predictor of the time to the onset of ESKD, and for dosing medications appropriately. The Modification of Diet in Renal Disease (MDRD), Chronic Kidney Disease Epidemiology Collaboration (CKD-EPI), and Cockcroft–Gault (C-G) formulas are the three most common equations.

- The MDRD abbreviated equation:

$$eGFR = 186 \times (S_{Cr})^{-1.154} \times (Age)^{-0.203} \times (0.742 \text{ if female})$$

- The CKD-EPI abbreviated equation:

  $eGFR = A \times (S_{Cr}/B)^{C} \times 0.993^{age}$, where A, B, and C are the following: A:144, B:0.7, and C:−1.209 if female. A:141, B:0.9, and C:−1.209 if male. (Given a $S_{Cr} > 0.7$ in females and >0.9 in males.)

- The C-G formula:

  $$eGFR = ([140 - age] \times \text{Lean body weight [kg]})/(S_{Cr} \times 72) \times 0.85 \text{ in women}$$

The CKD-EPI equation (2009) is considered as the most accurate creatinine-based method for estimating GFR. It has less risk of bias and higher precision throughout the GFR ranges. As such, C-G equation should no longer be used as a standard for estimation of the GFR.

F. Assessment of Tubular Function. A decline in GFR is normally matched by a proportionate decline in tubular function. This is apparent as a diminished ability to concentrate or dilute the urine or to conserve or eliminate H+, Na+, K+, and other electrolytes. Therefore, patients with kidney disease are at special risk for developing disorders of water, electrolyte, or acid–base status.

Some patients have a more selective defect in tubular function, for example, a renal tubular acidosis. The specialized tests of urine concentration or dilution and of acid excretion are described in Chapters 13 and 15.

III. NUCLEAR MEDICINE TESTS

A. Renogram. The renogram is used primarily to assess renal function although gamma camera pictures provide some information about renal size and shape. Several radionuclides are available:

  i. **Technetium-99m diethylenetriamine penta-acetic acid (^{99m}Tc-DTPA):** Is freely filtered by the glomerulus and is not reabsorbed. It delineates the contours of functional renal tissue. It can be used to assess cortical scarring from pyelonephritis or vesicoureteral reflux or to diagnose a renal infarct.

   ii. **Radio-iodinated orthoiodohippurate (Hippuran):** Is secreted into the tubules and used to assess renal blood flow.

   iii. **Tc99m Mercaptoacetyltriglycine (Tc99m MAG):** Combines the benefits of Tc99m scanning with many of the characteristics of Hippuran. Currently, it is the agent of choice in most units.

   A renogram is obtained by scanning over each kidney for 15 to 25 minutes after an intravenous (IV) injection of a radiotracer. The counts normally rise to a peak, reflecting filtration and secretion of the marker, and decline, reflecting elimination of the marker from the nephron. A delay in the time to peak and in the time for elimination occurs in patients with renal parenchymal disease, renal artery stenosis (RAS), or outflow obstruction. In the latter case, IV furosemide, given halfway through the scan, fails to enhance elimination. This "furosemide renogram" is a sensitive index of outflow obstruction.

   The delays in peak and decline in patients with functionally important renovascular hypertension are accentuated after an angiotensin-converting enzyme inhibitor (ACEI). This results from the withdrawal of angiotensin II–dependent tone in the efferent arterioles. The resultant sharp decrease in GFR reduces the rate of uptake and excretion of the marker. However, the use of ACEI renogram to diagnose RAS is controversial but can help provide functional information for unilateral or asymmetrical RAS. (See Chapter 20.)

B. Nuclear Medicine Studies of Renal Function. The renal blood flow is quantified by Hippuran, and the GFR by DTPA. Both agents are eliminated only by the kidneys. After IV injection, their plasma levels decline exponentially with a slope that is proportional to their clearances. The combination of plasma disappearance with scanning over the kidneys can estimate the single kidney GFR or renal blood flow. This is useful to predict the effects of a planned nephrectomy on overall kidney function. The indications for renography are summarized in Table 1.1. There are also several other agents available.

IV. EXAMINATION OF THE URINE. A complete urinalysis is a vital part of the assessment of kidney disease. It can be used as a "biomarker" in a number of acute kidney diseases, an early indicator to alert providers of the presence of kidney disease as well as to guide therapy and provide prognosis.

A. Color. Urine is normally clear and yellow. A dark brown color suggests bilirubinuria. A red color suggests hemoglobinuria, myoglobinuria, porphyria, or drugs

TABLE 1.1 Indications for a renogram

Renogram type	Use
Furosemide renogram	Detects outflow obstruction
Angiotensin-converting enzyme inhibitor renogram	Detects functional renovascular hypertension
99mTc-DTPA	Detects cortical scarring or infarct
Hippuran or diethylenetriamine penta-acetic acid	Measures renal blood flow or glomerular filtration rate

such as rifampin or phenazopyridine (Pyridium). A turbid white color suggests pyuria or crystalluria.

B. Specific Gravity. The normal range is 1.005 to 1.030. A specific gravity of 1.010 is isosthenuric and corresponds normally to a urine osmolality of approximately 300 mOsm/kg. Radiocontrast agents, protein, and glucose increase the specific gravity more than the osmolality because they are large, dense molecules. Otherwise, a high specific gravity suggests a volume-depleted state with a preserved concentrating function.

C. pH. The normal urine pH is 4.5 to 7.0. A persistent acidic pH is a normal finding. A persistent alkaline pH is found in vegetarians, in patients with classic distal renal tubular acidosis, in urinary tract infection with urea-splitting organisms, after administration of alkali or acetazolamide, in severe potassium depletion with excessive excretion of ammonia, in respiratory alkalosis, or during correction of metabolic alkalosis.

D. Glucose. Normal urine should contain no glucose. Urine glucose suggests either diabetes mellitus or decreased glucose reabsorption from the proximal tubule (renal glycosuria, Fanconi syndrome, proximal renal tubular acidosis, or sodium-glucose linked transporter 2 inhibitors (SGLT2i) use). Pregnancy reduces the renal glucose threshold and can lead to glycosuria in otherwise normal women.

E. Leukocyte Esterase and Nitrite. A positive reaction for leukocyte esterase indicates pyuria. Nitrite suggests gram-negative bacteriuria. Both lack sensitivity.

F. Protein. Normal urine contains no more than a trace of protein. A positive test should be followed by either a 24-hour urine collection for protein and albumin or a random urine for a spot protein or albumin to creatinine ratio. Excretion of >150 mg/24 h of protein (urine protein:creatinine ratio >150 mg/g) or >30 mg/24 h of albumin (urine albumin:creatinine ratio >30 mg/g) is abnormal. Pure tubular dysfunction should not result in proteinuria >1.5 g/24 h. Greater quantities of proteinuria indicate glomerulopathy. Proteinuria >3.5 g/24 h is termed nephrotic range. The dipstick test does not detect Bence Jones protein, which requires testing with sulfosalicylic acid and estimation by urine protein electrophoresis. A false-positive test for protein occurs with phenazopyridine, gross hematuria, or a very high pH.

G. Blood. A positive dipstick for blood can indicate the presence of hemoglobin or myoglobin. A positive blood on dipstick without true hematuria is highly suggestive of myoglobinuria or rhabdomyolysis-related acute kidney injury. See Chapter 4 for approach to hematuria.

V. EXAMINATION OF URINARY SEDIMENTS. A urine specimen obtained within the last 2 hours should be tested first with a dipstick. A 10-mL sample should be centrifuged at 3,000 revolutions/min for 3 to 5 minutes, the supernatant should be visually inspected, then removed. The sediment should be resuspended and placed on a slide under a coverslip and examined under the microscope. It is often helpful to add one drop of methylene blue dye to the spun sediment.

The slide should then be examined under light microscopy or phase-contrast microscopy starting with 10× lens for low-power field followed by 40× for high-power field as needed.

A. Cells. Dysmorphic red blood cells indicate glomerular pathology. See Chapter 4 for discussion of hematuria. Polymorphonuclear white blood cells often indicate bacterial urinary tract infection while mononuclear cells may indicate interstitial disease or nonbacterial urinary tract infection. Occasionally, they

TABLE 1.2	Urine casts

Type	Description and clinical relevance
Hyaline	Mucoprotein matrix without cellular elements; does not indicate renal disease
Red cell	Indicates glomerular bleeding
Leukocyte	Occurs in pyelonephritis, interstitial nephritis, and glomerulonephritis
Renal tubular epithelial	Occurs in acute tubular necrosis, glomerulonephritis, and tubulointerstitial disease
Granular, waxy	Represents degenerative cellular elements
Broad	Characteristic of chronic kidney failure

can appear as clumps or casts in the more severe cases of infection. Renal tubular epithelial cells are slightly larger than white blood cells with more cytoplasmic area. Renal tubular cells are pathognomonic finding for acute tubular injury or necrosis as they indicate the "sloughing off" tubular cells into renal tubules. In the more severe cases, renal tubular cells can be seen connected to each other to form a row (as opposed to white blood cells in a clump). Squamous epithelial cells usually indicate contaminated sample from the skin area and often invalidate a diagnosis of urinary tract infection.

B. **Casts.** Casts comprise the base mucoprotein and cellular or cell degradation product components. The base mucoprotein "Tamm–Horsfall protein" is excreted into urinary space and is not pathologic. Table 1.2 details the types of casts. Figure 1.1 demonstrates various types of casts.

C. **Crystals.** It is not uncommon to see various types of crystals in the urine. They may be classified as common, pathologic, or crystals caused by drugs. Crystal examination should be performed on a fresh urine sample as some compounds can precipitate even in healthy individual's sample that has been left stand for a long period of time. Table 1.3 details various types of crystals.

D. **Organisms.** Various microorganisms can be seen on spun urine examination from bacteria (gram-negative rods, etc.), fungus (budding yeast or hyphae in cases with vaginitis), or parasites (Schistosomiasis).

VI. BIOCHEMICAL ANALYSIS OF URINE

A. **Urinary Sodium Concentration.** A urinary sodium concentration $(U_{Na}) < 10$ mEq/L in a patient with oliguric azotemia indicates a prerenal physiology which includes cardiorenal and hepatorenal syndromes. A $U_{Na} > 40$ mEq/L in an azotemic patient indicates acute tubular necrosis, diuretic use, or adrenal insufficiency (Table 1.3). Intermediate levels require the calculation of the fractional excretion of sodium (FE_{Na}):

$$FE_{Na} (\%) = (U_{Na}/S_{Na}) \times (S_{Cr}/U_{Cr}) \times 100$$

where S_{Na} and S_{Cr} indicate the serum sodium and creatinine concentrations, respectively, and the U_{Na} and U_{Cr} the urinary sodium and creatinine concentrations, respectively. FE_{Na} should be interrupted with caution since it can be affected by several factors and the diagnosis should be made based on the whole clinical picture.

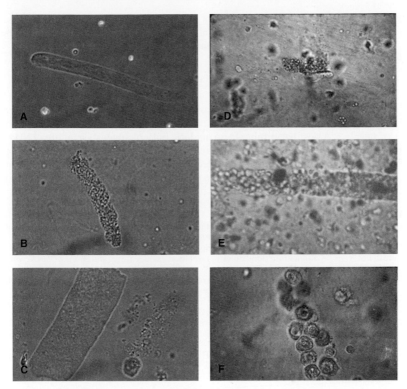

FIGURE 1.1: Urine Casts. A: Hyaline cast. **B:** Granular cast. **C:** Broad cast. **D:** Red blood cell cast. **E:** White blood cell cast. **F:** Renal tubular epithelial cell cast.

B. Urinary Chloride Concentration. This is valuable to diagnose the cause of metabolic alkalosis. A urinary chloride concentration (U_{Cl}) < 15 mEq/L suggests chloride-responsive metabolic alkalosis. This is characteristic of extrarenal Cl^- loss, prior diuretic use, or severe volume depletion leading to contraction

T A B L E **1.3**	Common crystals

Crystal	Appearance
Monohydrated calcium oxalate	Ovoid, dumbbells, biconcave discs
Bihydrated calcium oxalate	Bipyramidal or "envelope"
Calcium phosphate	Prism, star-like particles, or needles of various sizes
Triple phosphate	"Coffin lids"
Cystine	Hexagonal plates with irregular sides
Acyclovir	Birefringent fine needles
Indinavir	Birefringent plate-like rectangles, star-like forms, irregular plates
Sulfadiazine	Birefringent "shocks" of wheat

alkalosis. A $U_{Cl} > 15$ mEq/L indicates chloride-resistant metabolic alkalosis. This is characteristic of Bartter or Gitelman syndrome, primary hyperaldosteronism, or current diuretic use (see Chapter 15).

C. Urinary Anion Gap

$$\text{Urinary anion gap (UAG)} = (U_{Na} + U_K) - U_{Cl}$$

The UAG represents unmeasured anions (mainly phosphate, sulfate, or bicarbonate) in excess of unmeasured cations (mainly $NH4^+$). A normal gap is zero or negative. A positive number in an acidotic patient suggests a failure of $NH4^+$ excretion because of renal tubular acidosis or administration of a carbonic anhydrase inhibitor. A strongly negative number suggests extrarenal losses of bicarbonate, which occurs in diarrhea or pancreatic drainage, and a preserved ability to generate and excrete $NH4^+$.

VII. SUGGESTED READINGS

Cavanaugh C, Perazella MA. Urine sediment examination in the diagnosis and management of kidney disease: core curriculum 2019. *Am J Kidney Dis*. 2019;73(2):258–272.

Cohen RA, Brown RS. Clinical practice. Microscopic hematuria. *N Engl J Med*. 2003;348:2330–2338.

Coresh J, Stevens LA. Kidney function estimating equations: where do we stand? *Curr Opin Nephrol Hypertens*. 2006;15(3):276–284.

Feehally J, Floege J, Tonelli M, et al. Investigation of renal disease. In: Feehally J, Floege J, Tonelli M, et al., eds. *Comprehensive Clinical Nephrology*. Elsevier; 2019.

Hsu C. Clinical evaluation of renal function. In: Greenberg A, Cheung AK, Coffman TM, et al., eds. *Primer on Kidney Diseases*. 4th ed. Saunders; 2005:20–25.

Levin A, Stevens PE, Bilous RW, et al. Kidney disease: improving global outcomes (KDIGO) CKD work group. KDIGO 2012 clinical practice guideline for the evaluation and management of chronic kidney disease. *Kidney Int Suppl*. 2013;3(1):1–150.

Simerville JA, Maxted WC, Pahira JJ. Urinalysis: a comprehensive review. *Am Fam Physician*. 2005;71(6):1153–1162.

2 Evaluation of Kidney Structure: Radiology and Biopsy

Michael Choi

The patient with kidney disease often presents with nonspecific signs and symptoms that include nausea, anorexia, lethargy, edema, dyspnea, and diminished urine output. Consequently, the physician must rely on laboratory studies to assist in the evaluation and diagnosis of kidney disease. This chapter reviews the use of radiologic procedures and kidney biopsy to aid in this evaluation.

I. RADIOLOGIC ASSESSMENT

A. Ultrasonography. Ultrasound is useful in the assessment of renal location, size, and contour. It also can be used to identify the cortex, medulla, renal pyramids, and a distended collecting system or ureter (Table 2.1). A kidney length of <9.5 to 10 cm or a size difference of >1.5 to 2 cm between the two kidneys is abnormal in an adult. Simple cysts are easily identified, are common, and are uniformly benign. They contain no internal echoes, have a sharply defined smooth internal wall, and have increased through transmission of posterior sound energy. Other hypoechoic renal mass lesions to consider include lymphoma, infarct, hematoma, and xanthogranulomatous pyelonephritis. Complex cysts or solid lesions require further investigation with contrast computed tomography (CT), magnetic resonance imaging (MRI), or, possibly, angiography. Ultrasound has become the procedure of choice in the early diagnosis of or screening for autosomal dominant polycystic kidney disease. Hydronephrosis appears as a multiloculated fluid collection within the renal sinus; however, ultrasound does not assess the functional importance of obstruction. An apparent obstruction can occur with anatomic variants such as an extrarenal pelvis, vesicoureteral reflux, and pregnancy. Hydronephrosis may persist after the obstruction has been relieved. A furosemide renogram may document functional obstruction as contrast will be excreted from the dilated collecting system after furosemide administration. Investigation of the renal vasculature is possible using color Doppler but lacks the sensitivity of power Doppler. Ultrasound examination of the kidneys should be the initial imaging procedure in the clinical setting of acute kidney injury (AKI) of unknown cause/chronic kidney disease (CKD) (Table 2.2). Small, echogenic kidneys with thin cortices may indicate that the patient has CKD.

B. Intravenous Pyelography. The intravenous pyelogram (IVP) provides an overview of the kidneys, ureters, and bladder. The nephrogram is formed by the opacification of the renal parenchyma; its density depends on the glomerular filtration rate (GFR), rate of tubular fluid reabsorption, type and dose of radiographic contrast agent, and rate of intravenous injection. Renal insufficiency (serum

T A B L E 2.1	Indications for renal ultrasound

To quantify kidney size
To screen for hydronephrosis
To identify and characterize kidney mass lesions
To evaluate perirenal space for abscess or hematoma
To screen for autosomal dominant polycystic kidney disease
To localize kidney for invasive procedures
To assess residual bladder volume in excess of 100 mL
To evaluate for renal vein thrombosis (Doppler)
To assess renal blood flow (Doppler)

creatinine >2 to 3 mg/dL) decreases the diagnostic value of the IVP and greatly increases the danger of causing AKI. IVP use has decreased significantly because of the availability and diagnostic advantages of ultrasound, CT, and MRI.

C. **Computed Tomography.** CT is useful for the further investigation of abnormalities discovered on ultrasound or IVP, and is now used with increasing frequency as the initial diagnostic imaging technique for a host of renal and collecting system abnormalities (see Table 2.3). CT without contrast may detect kidney stones with thin slices to image the kidneys, ureters, and bladder. Noncontrast CT can detect hydronephrosis but is limited for evaluation of renal masses. Intravenous contrast is filtered by the glomeruli and concentrated in the tubules, thus allowing parenchymal enhancement and visualization of neoplasms or cysts. Renal vessels and ureters can be identified, and CT also is useful in the evaluation of mass lesions or fluid collections in the kidney or retroperitoneal space, particularly when ultrasound examination is hindered by intra-abdominal gas or obesity (Table 2.4). CT angiography is a noninvasive procedure that is useful in screening evaluation of renal artery stenosis. CT urogram allows for the assessment of kidney parenchyma and collecting system. It is often used now in lieu of the IVP. Combined with a noncontrast CT done first, it is useful in the radiologic evaluation of hematuria.

T A B L E 2.2	Initial choice of imaging techniques in kidney disease

AKI/CKD	Ultrasound
Obstruction	Ultrasound
Kidney stones	Ultrasound, stone protocol CT without contrast
Hematuria	Nonenhanced CT scan followed by CT urogram
Renal infection/inflammation	CT
Renal artery stenosis	Doppler ultrasound
Nephrocalcinosis	Nonenhanced CT
Papillary necrosis	CT urogram
Renal infarction	Contrast CT
Renal vein thrombosis	Contrast CT
Retroperitoneal fibrosis	Contrast CT

AKI, acute kidney injury; CKD, chronic kidney disease; CT, computed tomography.
Note: Modified with permission from Parsons RB, Simpson WL Jr. *Imaging.* In: Fehally J, Floege J, Johnson RJ, eds. *Comprehensive Clinical Nephrology.* 3rd ed. Mosby; 2007:51–67.

TABLE 2.3	Indications for computed tomography

To further evaluate a kidney mass
To investigate the cause of isolated hematuria
To display calcification patterns in a renal mass
To detect retroperitoneal fibrosis
To evaluate a nonfunctioning kidney
To delineate the extent of kidney trauma
To detect renal infection, renal infarction, and papillary necrosis
To diagnose adrenal causes for hypertension
To detect renal vein thrombosis

D. Magnetic Resonance Imaging. MRI is useful in the identification of the boundary between the cortex and the medulla. The loss of the corticomedullary demarcation, when observed with MRI, is a nonspecific but helpful feature of renal disease. Renal cysts are well visualized but, unlike CT, MRI cannot accurately define the foci of calcification. In the staging of solid renal lesions, MRI may be superior to CT because it can detect tumor thrombus in major vessels and can distinguish hilar collateral vessels from lymph nodes. However, some renal neoplasms appear homogeneous with the surrounding normal renal parenchyma, and therefore may be missed with noncontrast MRI. MRI can help in differentiating adrenal mass lesions because characteristic images often occur in pheochromocytoma; it is also useful in diagnosing renal vein thrombosis (Table 2.4). MR angiography, especially when performed with intravenous contrast administration, has been used more commonly to evaluate renal arteries for the presence of stenosis. This procedure is especially useful in patients with an allergy to iodine because it relies on the use of gadolinium, an iodine-free, paramagnetic contrast agent. MR angiography may be superior to intra-arterial digital subtraction angiography for the detection of renal artery stenosis and is less invasive. Nephrogenic systemic fibrosis (NSF), a progressive irreversible skin thickening that can affect other organs, was linked to contrast MRI studies given to patients with stage 4 to 5 CKD or severe AKI. Linear gadolinium contrast has a much higher risk with NSF than macrocyclic compounds and the latter compounds should be used for patients with stage 4 and 5 CKD if gadolinium is required. Initiation of hemodialysis for the sole purpose of removing macrocyclic gadolinium is not recommended.

E. Arteriography and Venography. Contrast imaging of the arterial and venous vasculature is useful to assess renal artery stenosis, renal vein thrombosis, renal

TABLE 2.4	Indications for magnetic resonance imaging

To serve as an adjunct to CT in evaluating kidney masses
To serve as an alternative to CT in patients who are intolerant of radiographic contrast agents
To evaluate suspected pheochromocytoma
To detect renal vein thrombosis

CT, computed tomography.

TABLE 2.5	Indications for scintigraphy

To measure renal blood flow and glomerular filtration rate
To detect outflow obstruction
To detect renovascular hypertension
To detect cortical scarring or infarct

infarction, or a renal mass. It is performed by the percutaneous cannulation of femoral vessels and sometimes aided by digital subtraction techniques. Arteriography is useful in the evaluation of atherosclerotic or fibrodysplastic stenotic lesions of the renal arteries, aneurysms, arteriovenous fistulas, large-vessel vasculitis, renal infarction, and renal mass lesions. It can be combined with selective renal vein renin sampling for evaluation of renovascular hypertension, percutaneous transluminal balloon angioplasty or stent placement, or renal ablation. Venography is performed to diagnose renal vein thrombosis.

F. **Radionuclide Evaluation.** Scintigraphy represents a noninvasive method to examine kidney structure and function and provide both qualitative and quantitative information (Table 2.5). As mentioned in Chapter 1, the choice of radiotracers determines the specific data that is provided by the technique. For instance, radiotracers such as ^{99}Technetium (^{99}Tc)-labeled diethylenetriamine pentaacetic acid (DTPA) that is cleared primarily by glomerular filtration can be used for imaging and to measure GFR. Those that are secreted by the renal tubule, such as o-iodohippurate, [^{131}I]OIH (Hippuran), can provide a measure of effective renal plasma flow. Agents that can also be useful for renal imaging because they are retained by the tubules include ^{99}Tc-labeled glucoheptonate and ^{99}Tc-labeled dimercaptosuccinic acid (DMSA). DMSA is used to evaluate for kidney scarring such as in reflux nephropathy where scarring can be seen in upper and lower poles of the kidney.

1. **Renal Function.** GFR can be quantified using ^{99}Tc-DPTA and renal blood flow by Hippuran because these agents are eliminated exclusively by the kidneys. Following intravenous administration, their plasma levels decline exponentially, yielding a slope that is proportional to their clearance. Single-kidney GFR or renal blood flow, or both, can be determined by combining a kidney scan with the plasma disappearance method.

2. **Renogram.** A renogram is obtained by scanning repeatedly over each kidney with a gamma camera following an intravenous radiotracer injection.
   Normally, counts rise to a peak, which reflects either filtration or secretion of the marker, followed by a decline in activity, which denotes elimination of the radiotracer from the nephron. Either a delay in the time to peak or in the elimination, or both, is observed in patients with renal artery stenosis, renal parenchymal disease, or obstruction of the urinary tract. With outflow obstruction, the administration of intravenous furosemide (Lasix) midway through the procedure fails to enhance elimination, thus providing a very sensitive measurement of obstruction. Likewise, administration of an angiotensin-converting enzyme inhibitor in patients with suspected renovascular hypertension and elevated angiotensin II levels will markedly reduce the rate of uptake and excretion of the radiotracer, thus theoretically identifying patients with a functionally important lesion. However, this is rarely used for screening for renal artery

stenosis because test results do no correlate well with benefit from intervention (see Chapter 20).

G. **Summary.** Radiologic tests can be very valuable diagnostic tools; however, they are expensive and carry a risk of adverse reactions. Proper patient selection and preparation can increase the value of the procedure and diminish toxicity. Most intravenous contrast studies are now performed using low-osmolar nonionic agents, reducing nephrotoxicity. It is now felt that much of the AKI associated with IV contrast use is due to clinical factors (infection, hypotension) that would have caused AKI independent of contrast. Contrast-induced AKI, where the contrast is thought to be the cause of the AKI, occurs in a much smaller subset of patients, such as those with severely impaired GFR (<30 mL/min/ 1.73 m^2) who may be volume depleted. Prevention and management of radiocontrast-induced renal damage are discussed in Chapter 35. Consultation with a radiologist before selecting the test is often very helpful. A guide for the preferred use of various radiologic tests is provided in Table 2.2.

II. **KIDNEY BIOPSY.** Percutaneous needle biopsy of the kidney can be useful for establishing a diagnosis, assessing prognosis, monitoring disease progression, or selecting a rational therapy.

A. **Indications**

1. **Acute Kidney Injury.** When the underlying cause of AKI is not evident initially, or recovery of renal function has not occurred after what might be expected from supportive therapy, biopsy may be necessary to distinguish acute tubular necrosis from a host of other kidney diseases that may require alternative management (see Chapter 35).

2. **Chronic Kidney Disease.** In those patients with unexplained CKD with near normal–sized kidneys, a biopsy may be helpful in determining the etiology. In contrast, biopsy is seldom useful in small kidneys because of extensive renal parenchymal damage, including tubulointerstitial fibrosis and glomerulosclerosis (see Chapter 36).

3. **Nephrotic Syndrome.** A kidney biopsy is usually performed in infants less than 1 year of age and in the adult nephrotic patient without evidence of systemic disease to diagnose primary glomerular diseases. In adults, the most frequently encountered entities include membranous glomerulopathy, focal segmental glomerulosclerosis, membranoproliferative glomerulonephritis, immunoglobulin A nephropathy, amyloidosis, and minimal change disease (see Chapters 3, 7, and 8).

4. **Proteinuria.** In the setting of persistent proteinuria, or when associated with an abnormal urine sediment or with documented functional deterioration, a kidney biopsy may detect underlying renal disease. Patients with orthostatic proteinuria do not require biopsy (see Chapter 3). Those with proteinuria less than 0.5 to 1 g/day without hematuria or systemic disease who have normal renal function may not need a kidney biopsy.

5. **Hematuria.** A kidney biopsy may be helpful in patients with microscopic hematuria persisting longer than 6 months or in those with episodic gross hematuria or a family history of hematuria, particularly when there is an associated abnormal urine sediment or proteinuria. Secondary causes of hematuria must be excluded. If a glomerular disease is diagnosed on biopsy, likely pathologic findings include Alport syndrome, thin basement membrane disease, and immunoglobulin A nephropathy. Usually, biopsy is not

helpful in the clinical setting of short-term, isolated microscopic hematuria (see Chapter 3). However, those with systemic lupus erythematosus (SLE) and >500 mg/day of proteinuria and hematuria have been found to have diffuse proliferative glomerulonephritis and should undergo kidney biopsy.

6. **Systemic Disease.** Various systemic disorders may have associated kidney involvement. These include diabetes mellitus, SLE, IgA vasculitis, polyarteritis nodosa, anti-GBM disease/syndrome, ANCA-associated vasculitis thrombotic microangiopathies, and certain dysproteinemias. Biopsy is often performed to confirm the diagnosis, establish the extent of kidney involvement, and guide management (see Chapters 7 to 9).

7. **Transplant Allograft.** Biopsy of the allograft helps differentiate various forms of rejection from acute tubular necrosis, drug-induced tubulointerstitial nephritis or nephrotoxicity, hemorrhagic infarction, and de novo or recurrent glomerulonephritis (see Chapter 35).

B. **Contraindications.** Commonly accepted contraindications to percutaneous needle biopsy include the presence of an uncorrected bleeding disorder, recent antiplatelet or anticoagulant therapy or severe thrombocytopenia, severe uncontrolled hypertension, small kidneys (usually indicative of chronic irreversible renal disease), CKD with GFR <30 mL/min/1.73 m^2, renal infection or skin infection overlying the biopsy site, renal neoplasm, hydronephrosis, and an uncooperative patient. A solitary kidney can be biopsied if the patient is otherwise at low risk for bleeding. Transjugular biopsy is the preferred method for a horseshoe kidney.

C. **Patient Preparation and Complications.** Routine laboratory tests before biopsy should include a prothrombin time, partial thromboplastin time, complete blood count, platelet count, blood type, an antibody screen for possible cross-matching should the need for transfusion arise, and urinalysis to exclude a urinary tract infection. If coagulation parameters are abnormal, a bleeding time should be obtained. Patients should avoid ingestion of nonsteroidal anti-inflammatory agents, aspirin, or fish oil in the week preceding biopsy.

The percutaneous biopsy is usually performed with ultrasound or CT guidance. After biopsy, the patient should remain on bed rest for 6 to 8 hours. Frequent vital signs are recorded to monitor evidence of hypovolemia as a result of hemorrhage. Hematocrits may be obtained 4 hours after the biopsy, and again the next morning if the patient is admitted. Aliquots of each voided urine are saved to observe for gross hematuria. Increasingly, percutaneous needle biopsy of the kidney is being performed in the outpatient setting.

The most frequent complication of a kidney biopsy is bleeding, but that is usually self-limited. Significant bleeding requiring transfusion (0.9% to 5%), percutaneous arterial embolization of a bleeding vessel (<0.5%), or nephrectomy (0.01% to <0.5%) are uncommon. The mortality rate of 0.02% to 0.007% is very low. When percutaneous needle biopsy is technically not feasible and a histologic diagnosis is imperative, an open biopsy or a laparoscopic biopsy should be considered.

The tissue specimen should be submitted for light, immunofluorescence, and electron microscopy and evaluated by a pathologist experienced in the interpretation of kidney biopsies.

III. SUGGESTED READINGS

Croker BP, Tisher CC. Indications for and interpretation of the renal biopsy: evaluation by light, electron and immunohistologic microscopy. In: Schrier RW, ed. *Diseases of the Kidney and Urinary Tract.* 8th ed. Lippincott Williams & Wilkins; 2007:420–447.

Fried JG, Morgan MA. Renal imaging: core curriculum 2019. *Am J Kidney Dis.* 2019;73(4):552–565.

Hogan JJ, Mocanu M, Berns JS. The native kidney biopsy: update and evidence for best practice. *Clin J Am Soc Nephrol.* 2016;11(2):354–362.

Parsons RB, Simpson WL Jr. Imaging. In: Fehally J, Floege J, Johnson RJ, eds. *Comprehensive Clinical Nephrology.* 3rd ed. Mosby; 2007:51–67.

Whittier WL, Korbet SM. Timing of complications in percutaneous renal biopsy. *J Am Soc Nephrol.* 2004;15(1):142–147.

3 Proteinuria and the Nephrotic Syndrome

Wen Shen

A healthy adult excretes less than 150 mg of protein per day in the urine. Excessive amounts of urine protein may denote the presence of a benign condition, but may indicate a serious underlying disorder. If proteinuria is present, one must be careful not to label a patient with a serious disorder because the prevalence of transient proteinuria in healthy subjects can be as high as 25%. Yet, only a small percentage of these patients will have underlying kidney disease.

I. **PATHOPHYSIOLOGY.** The kidney processes about 150 L/day of filtrate containing 60 to 80 g/L of protein. However, the majority of the filtered protein is reabsorbed by renal tubules. This results in less than 150 mg/day of protein excreted in the urine. Therefore, proteinuria formation is determined by two factors: first, the glomerular filtration barrier, which comprises the fenestrated endothelial cell, the basement membrane, and the epithelial cell foot processes, restricts the filtration of most proteins; second, the proximal tubule, which reabsorbs and degrades most of the filtered protein.

A. **Glomerular Proteinuria.** The glomerulus is a highly efficient filter that restricts the passage of molecules based on size and charge. Neutral dextrans with a radius less than 1.8 nm (18 A) are freely filtered, while those that are 4.2 nm (42 A) or greater are restricted by the glomerular capillary wall. Molecules within these limits have clearance rates that decrease progressively as their size increases. The glomerular capillary wall also carries a negative charge. This anionic state of the filtration barrier limits the filtration of molecules with a negative charge, while molecules carrying a more positive charge have a higher fractional excretion. This explains why albumin (5.5 nm or 55 A), an anionic molecule, is not filtered across the glomerulus. In certain conditions, such as minimal change disease, the charge-selective barrier is lost, resulting in a selective proteinuria that is predominantly albuminuria. The disruption of the glomerular filtration barrier is the common pathway shared by different glomerular diseases. Damage to podocyte, the cellular structure that stabilizes glomerular filtration barrier and maintains its integrity, can lead to increased cell motility and effacement of foot processes which play a central role in glomerular filtration barrier dysfunction and glomerular proteinuria formation.

B. **Tubular Proteinuria.** Many low–molecular-weight proteins that are filtered by the glomerulus are reabsorbed and degraded by the renal tubules, predominantly the proximal tubule. If the proximal tubule is damaged, as in tubulointerstitial disease, tubular proteinuria can occur, but it is rarely greater than 1,500 mg/24 h unless accompanied by glomerular injury.

C. **Overflow Proteinuria.** This is usually seen in patients with no apparent kidney disease but occurs due to the overproduction of immunoglobulin light chains and heavy chains or other small proteins. The overflow occurs because the amount of filtered protein exceeds the resorptive capacity of the tubules, for example, in multiple myeloma.

II. INTERPRETATION OF PROTEINURIA. Measurement of urine albumin and total urine protein can help determine the type of proteinuria. A positive dipstick suggests albuminuria, and hence glomerular proteinuria. A negative dipstick in the presence of proteinuria suggests tubular or overflow proteinuria. Proteinuria can be further subdivided into several patterns.

A. Transient Proteinuria. This is usually seen in patients with a febrile illness, congestive heart failure, stress, or following heavy exercise. There is no long-term risk of developing renal insufficiency.

B. Orthostatic Proteinuria. This denotes the presence of proteinuria only in the erect position. Protein excretion rarely exceeds 1 g/24 h. Measuring urine protein excretion separately on upright and supine collections helps the diagnosis. There is no increased risk of developing renal insufficiency or hypertension. It is relatively commonly seen in adolescence, but not in adults older than 30 years.

C. Persistent Proteinuria. This pattern of proteinuria usually indicates underlying kidney disease, even with a normal glomerular filtration rate (GFR). The kidney disease may be due to a primary glomerular disorder or to a renal process secondary to a systemic disease.

III. NEPHROTIC SYNDROME. The presence of nephrotic-range proteinuria with clinical and other laboratory abnormalities defines nephrotic syndrome. Diagnostic features include proteinuria >3.5 g/day, hypoalbuminemia <3.0 g/dL, edema, and hyperlipidemia. The common causes of nephrotic syndrome are listed in Table 3.1.

 TABLE 3.1 Common causes of persistent proteinuria or nephrotic syndrome

Primary glomerular disorders
Membranous glomerulonephritis
Membranoproliferative glomerulonephritis
Focal segmental glomerulosclerosis
Immunoglobulin A nephropathy
Minimal change disease
Mesangial proliferative glomerulonephritis
Fibrillary glomerulonephritis

Secondary disorders
Hereditary-familial: Alport syndrome; sickle cell disease; Fabry disease
Metabolic: Diabetes mellitus; obesity
Autoimmune: Systemic lupus erythematosus; antiglomerular basement membrane disease (Goodpasture syndrome); microscopic polyangiitis; granulomatosis with polyangiitis; eosinophilic granulomatosis with polyangiitis
Infectious: Postinfectious glomerulonephritis; endocarditis; hepatitis B and C; human immunodeficiency virus
Drug-induced: Nonsteroidal anti-inflammatory agents; heroin; gold; mercury; D-penicillamine
Neoplastic: Hodgkin disease; lymphomas; leukemia; multiple myeloma
Miscellaneous: Amyloidosis; preeclampsia–eclampsia; interstitial nephritis

Complications of nephrotic syndrome include increased risk of thrombosis, infections, severe edema, hyperlipidemia, hyponatremia, and acute kidney injury. Thrombosis can occur in both the arterial and venous circulations with a predilection for renal veins. Disorders associated with a higher risk for thrombosis include membranous nephropathy, lupus nephritis, and amyloidosis. A sudden increase in the degree of proteinuria, flank pain, hematuria, or worsening renal function in patients with nephrotic syndrome due to the above causes should raise a clinical suspicion of renal vein thrombosis. One should suspect pulmonary emboli if there is shortness of breath.

IV. INVESTIGATIONS. The presence of persistent proteinuria warrants a further workup. A 24-hour urine collection is a gold standard to quantify the protein excretion. To ensure an adequate urine collection, the creatinine excretion should also be measured. Men normally excrete 20 to 25 mg/kg of creatinine per day, and women excrete 15 to 20 mg/kg/day. The calculated and measured creatinine excretion should be compared to ensure a complete collection.

The ratio of spot urine protein to creatinine in an early morning urine sample has largely replaced 24-hour urine sample measurements to obviate problems including overcollection and undercollection of samples, patient inconvenience, and lack of immediate results with 24-hour collections. The ratio of urine protein concentration (mg/dL) to urine creatinine concentration (mg/dL) is roughly equivalent to the total number of grams of protein excreted during a 24-hour period (e.g., 200 mg/dL protein/100 mg/dL creatinine ~2 g of protein/24 h). Larger individuals who have higher urine creatinine excretions per day will have higher urine protein excretions per day. If the spot urine protein to creatinine ratio is 1 g/g of creatinine in a patient with a large muscle mass with 2 g/d of urine creatinine excretion per day, the 24-hour urine protein value is 2 g/day.

A microscopic analysis of the urine sediment should be undertaken. The presence of hematuria and red cell casts suggests a glomerulonephritis. A renal ultrasound can be performed to assess the size of the kidneys and the degree of parenchymal echogenicity, as well as to evaluate for the presence of anatomical abnormalities. Renal vein Doppler studies should be performed if renal vein thrombosis is suspected, which usually occurs in nephrotic syndrome. Basic blood chemistries such as creatinine, blood urea nitrogen, albumin, and cholesterol should be obtained. In selected patients, one may also obtain complement levels, antinuclear antibody pattern and titer, human immunodeficiency virus and hepatitis B and C serology, cryoglobulins, serum and urine electrophoresis, antineutrophil cytoplasmic antibodies, and antistreptolysin O. In adults, a kidney biopsy is generally performed in patients with nephrotic range proteinuria, or non-nephrotic proteinuria with active urine sediment or worsening renal function to reach histologic diagnosis and guide management. A schematic approach to the clinical evaluation of proteinuria is shown in Figure 3.1.

V. SUPPORTIVE MANAGEMENT. Patients may need immunosuppression and this is discussed in other chapters.

A. Renin–Angiotensin–Aldosterone System Blockade. Proteinuria is an independent risk factor for the progression of chronic kidney disease (CKD). Studies suggest that significant and prolonged proteinuria is associated with a proinflammatory state leading to the progression of CKD. Reduction of proteinuria has

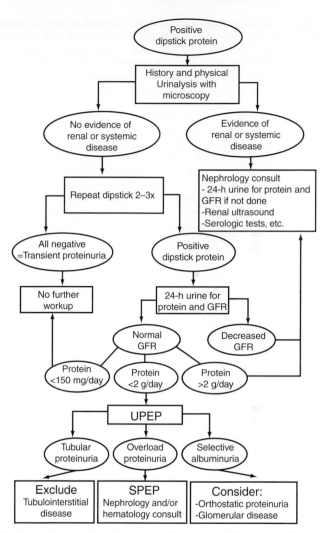

FIGURE 3.1: Approach to the clinical evaluation of proteinuria. GFR, glomerular filtration rate; SPEP, serum protein electrophoresis; UPEP, urine protein electrophoresis. (Modified from Ibrahim H, Rosenberg M, Hostetter T. Proteinuria. In: Seldin DW, Giebisch G, eds. *The Kidney: Physiology and Pathophysiology.* 3rd ed. Lippincott Williams & Wilkins; 2000:2269–2294.)

been recognized as the treatment target to delay the progression of CKD. The presence of proteinuria is also associated with a higher risk for cardiovascular mortality and morbidity, as reported in the Framingham study.

The approaches to reduce proteinuria include treating the underlying disease process with corticosteroids and/or cytotoxic agents and inhibiting renin-angiotensin-aldosterone system (RAAS) by angiotensin-converting enzyme (ACE) inhibitors or angiotensin receptor blockers (ARBs). ACE inhibitors and ARBs reduce proteinuria through lowering intraglomerular pressure.

ACE inhibitors reduce proteinuria significantly by 30% to 35% in both diabetic and nondiabetic renal diseases. ARBs are as effective as ACE inhibitors. The combination of ACE inhibitor and ARB is not recommended due to increased risks of hyperkalemia, acute kidney injury, and hypotension without benefits in reducing mortality. Mineralocorticoid receptor antagonists, spironolactone and eplerenone, have shown favorable results in proteinuria reduction and renoprotection.

The role of dietary protein restriction in management of proteinuria is still uncertain. In the presence of normal kidney function, daily dietary protein intake should not exceed 0.8 g/kg body weight. With renal insufficiency, intake should be further reduced to 0.6 to 0.8 g of high–biologic-value protein/kg body weight. Low-protein diet <0.6 g/kg/day is not recommended.

B. Edema. Treatment consists of dietary salt and fluid restriction, and the judicious use of diuretic agents. Rapid correction of edema should be avoided because some patients with hypoalbuminemia and edema are intravascularly volume contracted. Diuretics in this setting may cause prerenal azotemia and worsen kidney function. The combination of a loop diuretic (e.g., furosemide) with a thiazide diuretic (e.g., metolazone) has additive effects and can be used in patients not responding to loop diuretics alone. Patients receiving these agents need to be monitored for hypokalemia. If this problem occurs, supplementation of potassium or addition of potassium-sparing diuretics (amiloride or spironolactone) may be necessary.

C. Hyperlipidemia. Hyperlipidemia increases the risk for atherosclerosis and is associated with cardiovascular disease in the nephrotic patient. There is also evidence that hyperlipidemia may promote progressive kidney injury. Hence, it is important to treat this condition. A diet low in saturated fat and cholesterol should be initiated, as well as discouraging smoking and encouraging exercise. Statins are the treatment of choice to manage hyperlipidemia.

D. Hypercoagulability. The presence of thrombotic complications such as acute renal vein thrombosis in patients with nephrotic syndrome requires immediate hospitalization and heparin anticoagulation. Oral anticoagulation with warfarin should be continued for at least 6 months after initial heparin therapy. Membranous nephropathy has the highest risk of thromboembolism. Prophylaxis with anticoagulation in patients with membranous nephropathy is recommended if serum albumin level is <2.5 g/dL and if the risk of bleeding is low. The treatment of other complications mentioned earlier can be found in the list of Suggested Readings that follows.

VI. SUGGESTED READINGS

Bernard DB, Salant DJ. Clinical approach to the patient with proteinuria and the nephrotic syndrome. In: Jacobson HR, Striker GE, Klahr S, eds. *The Principles and Practice of Nephrology.* 2nd ed. Mosby; 1995:110–121.

Fried LF, Emanuele N, Zhang JH, et al. Combined angiotensin inhibition for the treatment of diabetic nephropathy. *N Engl J Med.* 2013;369:1892.

Glassock RJ. Prophylactic anticoagulation in nephrotic syndrome: a clinical conundrum. *J Am Soc Nephrol.* 2007;18:2221–2225.

Ibrahim H, Rosenberg M, Hostetter T. Proteinuria. In: Seldin DW, Giebisch G, eds. *The Kidney: Physiology and Pathophysiology.* 3rd ed. Lippincott Williams & Wilkins; 2000:2269–2294.

Johnson RJ, Floege J, Rennke HG, et al. Introduction to glomerular disease. In: Feehally J, Floege, J, Johnson RJ, eds. *Comprehensive Clinical Nephrology.* 3rd ed. Mosby Elsevier; 2007:181–192.

Schrier RW, Abraham WT. The nephrotic syndrome. In: Schrier RW, ed. *Diseases of the Kidney and Urinary Tract.* 8th ed. Lippincott Williams & Wilkins; 2007:2206–2213.

4 Hematuria

Mohammed A. Alshehri, Chanigan Nilubol

I. HEMATURIA

A. Definition and Classification. Hematuria can be classified by type (e.g., gross vs. microscopic), cause (e.g., glomerular vs. nonglomerular), or by recurrence (e.g., transient vs. persistent). Gross hematuria is indicated by red, pink, or brown urine. Microscopic hematuria is defined as three or more red blood cells (RBCs) per high-power field (HPF) on the spun urine sediment. This is usually performed after an abnormal dipstick test that utilizes the reaction between ortho-toluidine and hemoglobin or myoglobin. Transient microscopic hematuria is relatively common. Up to 39% of adults between the ages of 18 and 33 may have microscopic hematuria at least once, and up to 16% on two or more occasions. Therefore, an extensive workup is not warranted except in intermediate and high-risk patients.

B. Risk Stratification. Patients are considered at high risk if they meet one of the following criteria: age >60, smoking history with >30 pack-years, >25 RBC/HPF on urinalysis (UA), having a history of gross hematuria, and individuals looking to become a living kidney donor. However, urine microscopy should be repeated to confirm the resolution of the hematuria even in low-risk patients.

C. Clinical Evaluation

1. **Glomerular Hematuria.** Glomerular hematuria is characterized by dysmorphic RBCs on the urine sediment examination. A combination of dysmorphic RBCs, particularly acanthocytes (abnormal RBCs with spikes of different lengths and widths unevenly positioned on the cell surface), and significant proteinuria, is highly indicative of glomerular pathology. The differential diagnosis for glomerular hematuria is extensive and requires a comprehensive clinical evaluation. A kidney biopsy is usually required to reach an accurate diagnosis. Figure 4.1 summarizes a diagnostic approach to hematuria.

2. **Nonglomerular Hematuria.** The assessment of nonglomerular causes often includes specific imaging studies to support the clinical history and presentation. Renal vein thrombosis, which may complicate nephrotic syndrome, may be detected with renal venography, ultrasound with duplex Doppler velocimetry, or magnetic resonance venography. Renal infarction may be detected with renal angiography or magnetic resonance angiography. Polycystic kidney disease may be diagnosed by the radiologic imaging of multiple cysts and large kidneys in an appropriate clinical setting (see Chapter 14). Renal cell carcinoma, transitional cell carcinoma, and other malignancies can present with hematuria. These malignancies can be diagnosed with imaging and cystoscopy. Renal stone disease (nephrolithiasis) can easily be identified by helical computed tomography. When stones contain calcium, a plain abdominal film may be sufficient (see Chapter 21).

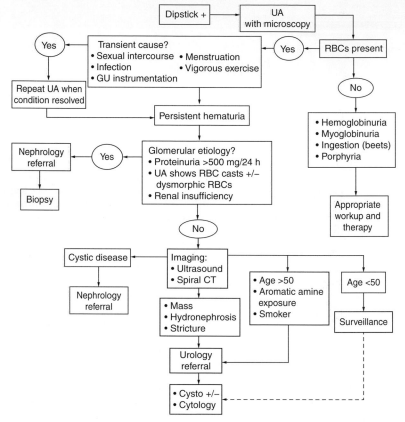

FIGURE 4.1: Evaluation of hematuria. CT, computed tomography; GU, genitourinary; RBCs, red blood cells; UA, urinalysis.

Other miscellaneous causes of hematuria also need to be considered. Papillary necrosis can complicate analgesic nephropathy, sickle cell disease, or diabetes mellitus. It can cause gross hematuria, but microscopic hematuria is frequent. Urinary tract infection often is associated with transient hematuria that may become persistent if complicated by pyelonephritis or abscess formation (see Chapter 22). Hematuria due to anticoagulation is usually accompanied by abnormal bleeding from other sites. Therefore, isolated hematuria in such cases raises the possibility of an underlying disease that should be investigated. Severe hematuria may accompany cystitis, especially when caused by cyclophosphamide toxicity.

II. SUGGESTED READINGS

Barocas DA, Boorjian SA, Alvarez RD, et al. Microhematuria: AUA/SUFU guideline. *J Urol.* 2020; 204(4):778–786.

Cavanaugh C, Perazella MA. Urine sediment examination in the diagnosis and management of kidney disease: core curriculum 2019. *Am J Kidney Dis.* 2019;73(2):258–272.

Krishnan A, Adeera L. Laboratory assessment of kidney disease: glomerular filtration rate, urinalysis, and proteinuria. In: Yu A, ed. *Brenner and Rector's The Kidney.* 11th ed. Elsevier; 2020.

Glomerular and Tubulointerstitial Diseases and Vasculitis

5 Diabetic Kidney Disease

Jogiraju V. Tantravahi

I. INTRODUCTION. Diabetic kidney disease (DKD) affects patients with both type I and type II (T1 or TII) diabetes mellitus (DM). The early hallmarks of diabetic nephropathy (DN) include hyperfiltration and low-grade proteinuria (microalbuminuria) that, if left untreated, progress to overt proteinuria and loss of renal function. Currently, DKD is the commonest cause of end-stage renal disease (ESRD). This chapter reviews the epidemiology and pathogenesis of DN and outlines current prevention and treatment strategies.

II. EPIDEMIOLOGY. Of the prevalent 724,075 patients with ESRD in the United States, 38% have DKD as their primary renal diagnosis. There are more than 13 million patients with DKD in the United States and more than 125 million worldwide.

Albuminuria and a reduced glomerular filtration rate (GFR) are infrequent within 10 years of diagnosing T1DM. However, after 15 years patients with T1DM begin to develop macroalbuminuria. Effective glycemic and BP control can modify the natural history of DN but about one-half of the patients with microalbuminuria eventually progress to ESRD. The United Kingdom Prospective Diabetes Study (UKPDS) reported that, after 10 years of follow-up, 25% of the patients with TIIDM had microalbuminuria, 5% had overt proteinuria, and 0.8% had developed ESRD. There is an increased prevalence of DN in African Americans and Native American Pima Indians. However, even among Pima Indians, the development of DN can be reduced with medical therapy.

The importance of genetic susceptibility to DN is unclear. Among Pima Indians with TIIDM, the risk of developing proteinuria is highest among those in whom both parents have proteinuria. Patients with T1DM who have a first-degree relative with nephropathy have an 83% risk of developing DN. The gene polymorphisms implicated in DN include those for the angiotensin-converting enzyme (ACE), angiotensin-II type 2 receptor (AT2), and aldolase reductase.

III. PATHOGENESIS AND PATHOLOGY. Mogensen and Christensen's five-stage schema of the natural history of T1 and TIIDN is outlined in Table 5.1. Stages I and II are subclinical but patients at stage III develop hypertension and microalbuminuria (30- to 300-mg protein per 24 hours) and the GFR begins to decline. Patients at stage IV have overt proteinuria (>300 mg per 24 hours) and a further loss of GFR ending in ESRD.

Hyperglycemia induces renal hypertrophy by activation of insulin-like growth factor I (IGF-I) and transforming growth factor β (TGF-β). IGF-I is implicated in afferent arteriolar dilatation resulting in glomerular hypertension and hyperfiltration. Restoration of glomerular hemodynamics can mitigate further renal damage. Hyperglycemia also induces mesangial expansion and increased deposition of type IV collagen with thickening of the glomerular basement

TABLE 5.1 Mogensen and Christensen schema for the progression of renal disease in IDDM

Stage I. Renal hypertrophy with hyperfiltration (increase in eGFR by 20–50%) with no pathologic lesions or alteration in renal function.
Stage II. Persistent hyperfiltration with early DN on a renal biopsy.
Stage III. Incipient DN with microalbuminura and hypertension without loss of renal function.
Stage IV. Overt proteinuria (>0.5 g/24 h), hypertension, and loss of renal function with histologic evidence of nodular intercapillary glomerulosclerosis.
Stage V. ESRD with other microvascular complications, including retinopathy, cardiovascular disease, and peripheral arterial disease.

membrane (GBM). The loss of negatively charged heparin sulfate proteoglycans permits the negatively charged albumin to pass into the glomerular filtrate. Untreated, hyperglycemia leads to the deposition of advanced glycation end products (AGEs) in the kidney that further exacerbate the mesangial expansion. Finally, excess generation of angiotensin II increases the inflammatory cytokine TGF-β. The combined effects of mesangial expansion, altered GBM, glomerular hyperfiltration, and glomerular and tubular inflammation and fibrosis culminate in overt proteinuria and a rapid loss of renal function.

The histopathologic findings in DN are reviewed in Table 5.2. Nodular intercapillary glomerulosclerosis (or the Kimmelstiel–Wilson lesion) is associated with DN but occurs also in membranoproliferative glomerulonephritis, light-chain deposition disease, and amyloidosis. Hypertensive changes, vascular disease, tubular atrophy, and glomerulosclerosis are also observed.

The Heart Outcome Prevention Evaluation (HOPE) and the Diabetes Control and Complication Trial (DCCT) studies reported that microalbuminuria in patients with DM increased the risk for all-cause mortality and cardiovascular events. Patients with DN require careful management of glycemia and BP, and reduction of albuminuria to forestall a progressive loss of GFR.

TABLE 5.2 Histologic features of diabetic renal disease

Glomerular lesions
    Diffuse intercapillary glomerulosclerosis
    Nodular intercapillary glomerulosclerosis
    Capsular drop lesion
    Fibrin cap lesion
    Glomerular basement membrane thickening
Vascular lesions
    Subintimal hyaline arteriosclerosis
    Benign arteriosclerosis
Tubular and interstitial lesions
    Hyaline droplets in proximal tubules
    Glycogen deposits (Armanni–Ebstein lesion)
    Tubular atrophy
    Interstitial fibrosis

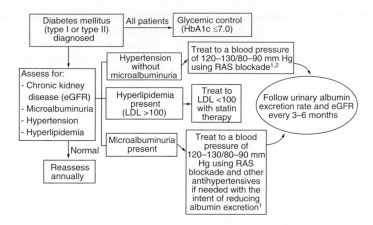

[1]Assuming no contraindication to RAS blockade, such as pregnancy, hyperkalemia, or angioedema.
[2]Based on the BENEDICT study results. See Suggested Readings.

FIGURE 5.1: An algorithm for the management of DN.

IV. DIFFERENTIAL DIAGNOSIS. Microalbuminuria and a progressive decline in renal function in a patient with long-standing DM strongly suggest DKD. In patients with T1DM, there is a strong correlation between diabetic retinopathy and DN but retinopathy occurs in only 50% of patients with T1IDM. Patients with DN have a decline in GFR with increasing proteinuria over several years. The urinary sediment is bland and markers of inflammation are minimal. A kidney biopsy can establish the diagnosis.

V. TREATMENT AND PREVENTION. Optimal management of DKD requires strict glycemic, BP, and lipid control (Fig. 5.1). Sodium-glucose cotransporter-2 (SGLT2) inhibitors and nonsteroidal mineralocorticoid receptor antagonists recently have shown beneficial effects for the treatment of DKD.

A. Glycemic Control. The 1993 DCCT trial reported that patients randomized to intensive glycemic control who achieved an HbA1c of <7% had a 35% to 45% decreased risk of developing microalbuminuria while the UKPDS study reported that patients randomized to intensive glycemic control had a decrease in proteinuria and in the risk for doubling of the serum creatinine. The American Diabetes Association suggests controlling the HbA1c to 7% or less in patients with T1 and T1IDM.

Insulin and glipizide are cleared by the kidney and require dosage reduction in patients with stage IIIa CKD or below. Metformin should be dosed carefully in patients with CKD.

B. Hypertension, Reduction of Proteinuria, and the Renin–angiotensin System. Parving et al. reported that treating 11 hypertensive patients with T1DM to a mean BP of 143/96 to 129/84 mm Hg reduced the monthly loss of GFR over 6 years from 0.89 to 0.22 mL/min/mo and the reduced albuminuria by 50%. They concluded that good BP control could slow the natural history of DN.

Patients with T1DM develop systemic and intraglomerular hypertension with renal fibrosis driven by the renin–angiotensin–aldosterone system (RAAS). The Collaborative Study Group randomized 400 patients with T1DM and >500-mg proteinuria and a creatinine <2.5 mg/dL to treatment with capto-pril versus placebo over 3 years. Despite a similar BP, there was a 43% reduction in the doubling of the serum creatinine and a significant reduction in time to death, dialysis, or need for transplantation in those randomized to captopril. This study established that ACE inhibitor therapy for T1DN is the standard of care.

Two large studies demonstrated the effectiveness of angiotensin recep-tor blockers (ARBs) in the treatment of TIIDN. The Reduction in Endpoints in NIDDM with the Angiotensin II Antagonist Losartan (RENAAL) study and the Irbesartan in DN Trial (IDNT) study both reported that therapy with an ARB in TIIDM decreased the rate doubling of the serum creatinine and the risk of devel-oping ESRD or death from all causes. Subsequent analysis reported that the risk of death or dialysis increased 7% for every 10 mm Hg rise in the baseline systolic BP (SBP) while CV risk decreased by 18% for every 50% decrease in albuminuria. Although the risk of renal failure decreases with BP up to an SBP of 120 mm Hg, all-cause mortality increases with a reduction in SBP below 120 mm Hg (J-curve phenomenon). Hence, the target SBP should be 120 to 130 mm Hg.

The Bergamo Nephrologic Diabetes Complications Trial (BENEDICT) ran-domized patients with TIIDM and hypertension but without microalbuminuria to an ACE inhibitor, a calcium channel blocker (CCB), both, or a placebo. After 3.6 years, those randomized to an ACE inhibitor had a 50% reduction in microal-buminuria. Thus, RAAS blockade should be initiated in hypertensive patients with DM regardless of proteinuria.

C. **Special Considerations in the Treatment of Hypertension in DN**. Most patients with DKD require several medications for BP control in addition to RAAS blockade. Non-dihydropyridine CCBs (diltiazem and verapamil) decrease BP and albu-minuria. The ONTARGET and VA-NEPHRON D trials reported that dual therapy with an ACE inhibitor and an ARB worsen renal function and increase hyper-kalemia, and death and therefore cannot be recommended.

Spironolactone can decrease proteinuria beyond that achieved with an ACE inhibitor or an ARB in T1 or TIIDN but can worsen hyperkalemia. Patients with DKD receiving an ACE inhibitor or ARB randomized in the FIDELIO-DKD trial to the nonsteroidal mineralocorticosteroid receptor antagonist (MRA) finerenone had a reduced rate of loss of GFR or death from renal or CV causes. This trial of patients with high-grade proteinuria and stage IIIb CKD was fol-lowed by the FIGARO trial that reported that patients at an earlier stage of CKD randomized to finerenone had a lower incidence of CV events. Hyperkalemia was the commonest renal-related adverse event but appeared to be less fre-quent than with spironolactone. The addition of finerenone to RAAS blockade has the greatest benefit in those at highest risk with high-grade proteinuria and stage IIIb or worse CKD but this group has a high incidence of hyperkalemia.

D. **Hyperlipidemia**. Patients with DN have increased CV events associated with hyperlipidemia. Although lipid lowering has not been demonstrated to decrease the loss of their GFR, hyperlipidemia should be managed aggressively to a target LDL of 100 mg/dL or less to avoid CV events.

E. **Newer Therapies for TIIDM**. Therapy has been extended beyond insulin, sulfon-ylureas, metformin, and thiazolidinediones to include dipeptidyl peptidase-4 (DPP-4) inhibitors, glucagon-like peptide 1 (GLP-1) agonists, and SGLT2 inhibi-tors. Studies of DPP-4 inhibitors or GLP-1 agonists have reported improvement in albuminuria but not in the rate of loss of GFR. In contrast, several studies have reported that patients randomized to SGLT2 inhibitors have a survival benefit in heart failure. Post hoc analyses of the trials of all three current SGLT2 inhibitors (empagliflozin, canagliflozin, dapagliflozin) have demonstrated reduced risk of worsening nephropathy, progression to macroalbuminuria, doubling of the serum creatinine, or ESRD in patients with DM. The DAPA-CKD trial reported that therapy with dapagliflozin reduced the risk of a 50% decline in the eGFR or of ESRD, or death from a renal or CV cause in patients with CKD both with and without DM.

F. **Advanced Chronic Kidney Disease and ESRD.** Patients with DM and ESRD have an increased risk of CV complications. They require particular attention to the management of hyperglycemia, hypertension, hyperlipidemia, anemia, and bone disease. Kidney transplantation is the preferred mode of renal replacement. Patients with T1DM can also be offered pancreas transplantation. However, the lesions of DN can recur in the renal allograft and eventually progress to ESRD.

VI. **MANAGEMENT RECOMMENDATIONS.** Management of DKD should include strict glycemic and BP control with RAAS blockade. The addition of an SGLT2 inhibitor can slow the loss of GFR beyond that with RAAS alone. The 2020 Kidney Disease Improving Global Outcomes (KDIGO) clinical practice guideline recommends treatment with an SGLT2 inhibitor in all patients with an eGFR ≥30 mL/min but this can be complicated occasionally by genitourinary infections including Fournier gangrene, euglycemic ketoacidosis especially in T1DM, and volume depletion. While combined treatment with an ACE inhibitor and an ARB has been associated with worse renal outcomes, the use of a nonsteroidal MRA with RAAS blockade can improve renal outcomes particularly in DKD patients with high-grade proteinuria but the serum potassium concentration should be monitored closely. Future management of DKD will require multidrug therapy to preserve renal function.

VII. **SUGGESTED READINGS**
Bakris GL, Agarwal R, Anker SD, et al. Effect of finerenone on chronic kidney disease outcomes in type 2 diabetes. *N Engl J Med.* 2020;383(23):2219–2229.

Brenner BM, Cooper ME, de Zeeuw D, et al. Effects of losartan on renal and cardiovascular outcomes in patients with type 2 diabetes and nephropathy. *N Engl J Med.* 2001;345(12):861–869.

Heerspink HJL, Stefánsson BV, Correa-Rotter R, et al. Dapaglifozin in patients with chronic kidney disease. *N Engl J Med.* 2020;383(15):1436–1446.

Pitt B, Filippatos G, Agarwal R, et al. Cardiovascular events with finerenone in kidney disease and type 2 diabetes. *N Engl J Med.* 2021;385(24):2252–2263.

Wanner C, Inzucchi SE, Lachin JM, et al. Empagliflozin and progression of kidney disease in type 2 diabetes. *N Engl J Med.* 2016;375(4):323–334.

6 Nephrosclerosis

Christopher S. Wilcox

I. **DEFINITION AND PATHOPHYSIOLOGY.** Nephrosclerosis is ideally diagnosed on renal biopsy with a pattern of global glomerulosclerosis, arteriosclerosis, interstitial fibrosis, and tubular atrophy. It is a complication of hypertension but also an expected finding in kidneys from hypertensive but otherwise healthy elderly subjects. The pathophysiology is uncertain but likely entails an initial microvascular change of arteriosclerosis that causes ischemic glomerular damage leading to thickening of glomerular capillary basement membranes, podocyte detachment, a modest increase in glomerular permeability, proteinaceous accumulation in Bowman space and peritubular fibrosis. This terminates in collapse and sclerosis of glomerular tufts with atrophy of downstream tubules and accumulation of surrounding interstitial fibrosis. This underlies the age-dependent loss of renal size.

II. **CLINICAL FEATURES.** Nephrosclerosis progresses slowly, but usually relentlessly. It can terminate in end-stage renal disease (ESRD). It is usually diagnosed in hypertensives with CKD and minimal proteinuria. Nephrosclerosis is commoner in those of African American descent where it is frequently accompanied by abnormal apolipoprotein E1 gene alleles that are almost absent in Caucasians. About one-half of the increased incidence of ESRD among African Americans may be related to the adverse influences of APOL1 and much of the remainder to socioeconomic factors that lead to lesser healthcare delivery.

III. **THERAPY.** The effect of antihypertensive therapy on the progression of hypertensive nephrosclerosis in African Americans remains controversial. Slowing of the loss of kidney function by antihypertensive treatment with diuretics or beta-blockers in African American men was not reported in the Multiple Risk Factor Intervention Trial (MRFIT). Likewise, slowing of the loss of GFR in African American hypertensives in the African American Study of Kidney Disease and Hypertension (AASK) trial was not observed at a lower BP goal of 130/80 mm Hg versus 140/90 mm Hg. However, use of a calcium channel blocker (amlodipine) was associated with more rapid loss of GFR than the use of an ACEI (ramipril) or a beta-blocker (metoprolol). However, a post-trial follow-up noted a slow, but progressive, increase in proteinuria and, among proteinuric patients, use of an ACEI reduced progression to ESRD.

Nephrosclerosis is less common in Caucasians. The Systolic Blood Pressure Intervention Trial (SPRINT), randomized hypertensive subjects with one or more cardiovascular risk factors to intensive or standard BP control with goals of systolic BP <120 mm Hg or <140 mm Hg, respectively. CKD and diabetes were exclusion criteria but more than 2,500 patients had CKD at baseline.

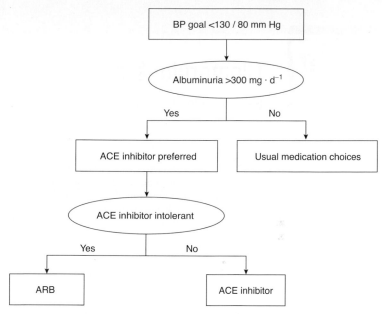

FIGURE 6.1: Treatment of hypertension in patients with CKD.

It is likely, but unknown, that many had nephrosclerosis. An outcome of a 50% fall in eGFR or development of ESRD was not reduced in those in the intensive treatment group although this group did derive significant benefit from reduced cardiovascular outcomes and all-cause mortality.

IV. MANAGEMENT. In the present state of uncertainty, it is reasonable to assume that an African American hypertensive patient with CKD and low-grade proteinuria without a suggestive history of other causes likely suffers from nephrosclerosis and may have an underlying abnormal APOL1 genotype. Calcium channel blockers should be avoided as first-line, single-agent treatment that should probably include an ACEI or an ARB. Even less certainty surrounds the management of similar Caucasian patients. However, the use of an ACEI or ARB becomes beneficial in those developing more than 1 to 3 g of proteinuria daily. This is summarized in Figure 6.1. In all, irrespective of racial background or age, an SBP goal of <130 mm Hg is advised (see Chapter 23).

V. SUGGESTED READINGS

Cohen E, Nardi Y, Krause I, et al. A longitudinal assessment of the natural rate of decline in renal function with age. *J Nephrol.* 2014;27(6):635–641.

Glassock RJ, Rule AD. The implications of anatomical and functional changes of the aging kidney: with an emphasis on the glomeruli. *Kidney Int.* 2012;82(3):270–277.

Lipkowitz MS, Freedman BI, Langefeld CD, et al. Apolipoprotein L1 gene variants associated with hypertension—attributed nephropathy and the rate of kidney function decline in African Americans. *Kidney Int.* 2013;83(1):114–120.

Glomerular Diseases

Behnaz Haddadi-Sahneh, Michael Choi

Glomerular diseases may present clinically as acute glomerulonephritis (GN), nephrotic syndrome, or asymptomatic proteinuria and/or hematuria (Table 7.1). Some glomerular diseases appear limited to the kidney (so-called "primary" glomerular diseases), whereas others may be part of a systemic process ("secondary" glomerular diseases). Diagnosis of the glomerular disease may be suggested by the type of clinical presentation, the presence or absence of systemic symptoms, and the laboratory findings. A "definitive" diagnosis usually requires a kidney biopsy, which will define the disease based on its histologic pattern which may have more than one etiology, and this may affect management. Clinical syndromes associated with the various glomerular diseases are shown in Table 7.1 and are discussed in detail below. Some of the common systemic causes of glomerular disease are discussed in later chapters (see Chapters 8 to 11).

I. **CLINICAL PRESENTATION AND LABORATORY EVALUATION.** Patients with acute GN usually present with a "nephritic urinary sediment" characterized by hematuria, red +/− white blood cells and granular casts, and varying degrees of proteinuria, often accompanied by hypertension, edema, and some degree of renal dysfunction. When the presentation is severe with acute kidney injury (AKI), often with oliguria, the clinical syndrome is called rapidly progressive glomerulonephritis (RPGN) and requires immediate hospitalization.

A second major presentation of glomerular disease is the *nephrotic syndrome* (see Chapter 3), in which patients manifest marked proteinuria (>3.5 g/day) with pitting edema of the lower extremities, hypoalbuminemia, hyperlipidemia, and fatty casts in the urine. The most common cause is diabetic nephropathy, but there are also many diseases that appear to be specific to the kidney that can cause this syndrome. In contrast to the acute inflammatory or "nephritic urinary sediment" associated with acute GN, the sediment in subjects with nephrotic syndrome may contain casts containing refractile fat bodies that demonstrate a characteristic "maltese cross" under polarized light. A slight degree of microscopic hematuria may be detected on urinalysis.

Finally, some subjects with glomerular disease may manifest *asymptomatic micro- or macroscopic hematuria,* especially those with immunoglobulin (Ig) A nephropathy, or *low-grade (<2 g/day) proteinuria.* Patients with asymptomatic hematuria and an absence of other findings suggestive of the presence of glomerular disease usually require a workup to rule out other causes of bleeding in the urinary tract (see Chapter 3). Similarly, the spectrum of diseases associated with low-grade proteinuria is wide and can include glomerular (membranous nephropathy [MN], Alport syndrome), tubular (chronic tubulointerstitial disease), or other (e.g., monoclonal gammopathies) causes (see Chapter 4).

TABLE 7.1	Definition and categorization of glomerular diseases

Clinical syndrome	Manifestations	Major etiologies
GN	RBC, RBC casts, proteinuria, hypertension, renal dysfunction	Postinfectious glomerulonephritis (PIGN, *Staphylococcus aureus*, *Staphylococcus epidermidis*, abscess, endocarditis, osteomyelitis) IgA nephropathy Lupus nephritis (WHO class III/IV)
Rapidly progressive GN	Presents as GN with AKI (oliguria, rising serum creatinine)	Antiglomerular basement membrane glomerulonephritis (kidney alone) or disease (kidney and lung involvement; also called Goodpasture syndrome) ANCA-associated vasculitis (microscopic polyangiitis, granulomatosis with polyangiitis, eosinophilic granulomatosis with polyangiitis) Immune complex–associated (IgA/IgA vasculitis, mixed cryoglobulinemia, SLE, PIGN)
Nephrotic syndrome	Proteinuria (>3.5 g/day), edema, high serum cholesterol, low serum albumin, urine lipids	Minimal change disease Focal segmental glomerulosclerosis MN MPGN Diabetic nephropathy Amyloid (myeloma, light-chain deposit disease, MGRS) Fibrillary GN
Asymptomatic proteinuria	Proteinuria <2 g/day/ ± CKD	IgA nephropathy, MN, MPGN, MGRS Hereditary glomerular disease (Alport syndrome) Tubulointerstitial disease (see Chapter 10)
Asymptomatic hematuria	Urinary RBCs >2/high-power field (spun sediment)	Low-grade glomerular disease (IgA nephropathy, thin basement membrane disease, Alport syndrome) Other (see Chapter 3)

GN, glomerulonephritis; IgA, immunoglobulin A; MN, membranous nephropathy; MGRS, monoclonal gammopathy of renal significance; MPGN, membranoproliferative glomerulonephritis; RBC, red blood cell; WHO, World Health Organization.

TABLE 7.2	General workup of patients suspected of having a glomerular disease

General recommendations

History: family history of kidney disease and hearing loss (Alport syndrome); a history of medications associated with nephrotic syndrome (NSAIDs, penicillamine, captopril, pamidronate, mercury); recent infection such as streptococcal (suggests PIGN) or viral infections (various GNs including granulomatosis with polyangiitis, anti-GBM, and immunoglobulin A nephropathy); history of cancer such as solid tumors (membranous nephropathy), Hodgkin (minimal change), or non-Hodgkin lymphoma (MPGN), history of systemic symptoms (sinusitis, melena/ hematochezia, cough, hemoptysis, rash, arthralgias).

Physical exam: look for features of nephrotic syndrome (pitting edema, xanthelasma); systemic features suggesting specific diagnoses, such as alopecia, arthritis, and facial rash (lupus); palpable purpura (cryoglobulinemia, endocarditis-associated GN, or lupus); hepatomegaly and clubbing of the nails (hepatitis B- or HCV-associated nephropathy); livedo reticularis (vasculitis).

Laboratory exam: routine electrolytes, glucose, liver function tests, albumin, cholesterol, 24-h urine protein and creatinine clearance (may be inaccurate in subjects with RPGN); serum and urinary protein electrophoresis, serum free light chains (in adults with proteinuria to rule out amyloidosis, light-chain deposition disease, or other forms of monoclonal gammopathies of renal significance.)

Radiologic studies: renal ultrasound to assess kidney size (normal 10–12 cm) to gauge if immunosuppression will be beneficial which is less likely in small kidneys.

Specific serologic tests for secondary causes

For nephrotic syndrome: human immunodeficiency virus antibody (focal segmental glomerulosclerosis); hepatitis B surface antigen (membranous); HCV antibody (membranous, MPGN, and cryoglobulinemia); rheumatoid factor and serum cryoglobulins (cryoglobulinemia secondary to HCV infection); antinuclear antibodies and anti-DNA antibody (lupus); serum and urine protein electrophoresis, serum free light chains (monoclonal gammopathy–related diseases); C3 and C4 (low levels suggest MPGN and/or cryoglobulinemia, or types V or III and IV + V lupus).

For acute GN or RPGN: streptozyme or antistreptolysin O titer; blood cultures (for PIGN); antinuclear antibodies and anti-DNA antibody (lupus); anti-GBM antibody (anti-GBM disease or syndrome); antineutrophil cytoplasmic antibody (microscopic polyangiitis, granulomatosis with polyangiitis, eosinophilic granulomatosis with polyangiitis); C3 and C4 (low C3 or C4 suggests PIGN, lupus nephritis, HCV-associated cryoglobulinemia, or MPGN).

Anti-GBM, anti-glomerular basement membrane; GN, glomerulonephritis; HCV, hepatitis C virus; MPGN, membranoproliferative glomerulonephritis; PIGN, postinfectious glomerulonephritis; RPGN, rapidly progressive glomerulonephritis.

Table 7.2 presents recommendations for the initial workup for those with either acute GN or nephrotic syndrome. Thorough history and physical examination may suggest a particular diagnosis, such as the history of a streptococcal skin or throat infection (postinfectious glomerulonephritis [PIGN]); systemic symptoms such as alopecia, facial rash, and arthritis (lupus nephritis); or the triad of weakness, arthralgias, and palpable purpura (hepatitis C virus [HCV]-associated cryoglobulinemia). Laboratory evaluation should include a careful examination of the urine sediment to look for signs suggestive of glomerular disease. Marked proteinuria with hyaline casts and a sediment with minimal numbers of red cells and leukocytes suggests nephrotic syndrome, whereas a sediment with red cells, +/− white cells, and red +/− white cell casts suggests an acute GN often secondary to lupus nephritis or PIGN. Red cells that are dysmorphic (showing irregular blebs) also suggest a glomerular cause of the hematuria. Renal function is assessed by the measurement of serum creatinine but estimated GFR tests are unreliable in the setting of rapidly changing renal function. Specific serologic tests recommended in the evaluation of these subjects are shown in Table 7.2. In addition, a renal ultrasound examination should be ordered to assess renal size; large kidneys are often seen with diabetic nephropathy, amyloid, nephritic syndrome, and human immunodeficiency virus (HIV) nephropathy, whereas small kidneys <9 cm in length suggest advanced or chronic disease and may limit the possibility for biopsy because of the increased risk of bleeding, and treatment because the disease may be too advanced at this stage.

Specific descriptions of the more common diseases presenting as acute GN or nephrotic syndrome are discussed below. Secondary causes of glomerular disease are discussed elsewhere, including glomerular diseases secondary to systemic lupus erythematosus (SLE) in Chapter 8, vasculitis in Chapter 9, and amyloid or monoclonal gammopathies in Chapter 11.

II. GLOMERULONEPHRITIS AND RAPIDLY PROGRESSIVE GLOMERULONEPHRITIS

A. Postinfectious Glomerulonephritis. This may be seen with streptococcal infection and is observed most commonly in children (ages 5 to 10 years), especially boys following an untreated acute streptococcal infection. Individuals commonly present 2 weeks (following throat infection) or 3 weeks (following skin infection) after the initial infection, with oliguria, weight gain, edema, and hypertension, and are noted to have a nephritic urinary sediment. Subclinical cases are common, especially in household contacts of the index case. The pathogenesis appears to be due to an immune reaction to certain streptococcal antigens. Throat cultures are usually negative when active GN is detected, but serologic tests including streptozyme and the antistreptolysin O titer are positive in most subjects, along with the presence of low serum C3 levels.

A kidney biopsy should be reserved for patients with an atypical presentation or in whom the disease does not improve spontaneously over a 2- to 3-week period. The biopsy usually shows glomerular hypercellularity due to both an infiltration of leukocytes and proliferation of endothelial and mesangial cells in the glomerulus. Immune complexes are demonstrated in the capillary wall by immunofluorescence (IF) microscopy, while electron microscopy reveals irregular subepithelial deposits or "humps" along the capillary loops.

Therapy is largely supportive with fluid and sodium restriction and administration of diuretics to control blood pressure and edema. Antihypertensive agents should be used to control blood pressure in those who fail to respond to more conservative measures. Immunosuppressive agents are generally not indicated. For those with prolonged kidney failure and a kidney biopsy that reveals glomerular crescents due to the proliferation of extraglomerular cells within Bowman's space, a trial of high-dose steroids may be considered but efficacy is unproven and carries serious potential risks.

Both the patient and family members should have throat cultures, and those with streptococcal infection require antibiotic treatment. Even with severe disease, children do well with supportive management; however, the presence of crescents on biopsy indicates a more guarded prognosis. Complete recovery is less common in adults, particularly in those with a creatinine clearance of <40 mL/min/1.73 m², persistent proteinuria of >2 g/day, or increased age. Recurrence of PIGN is rare.

Acute PIGN may also occur after or concurrent with other infections, especially in subjects with *Staphylococcus aureus* or *Staphylococcus epidermidis* GN, subacute or acute bacterial endocarditis, bacterial sepsis, visceral abscess, infected ventriculoatrial shunts, and osteomyelitis. There may be an IgA-dominant infection-related GN, usually with bacteremia with methicillin resistant of sensitive *S. aureus, Escherichia coli, S. epidermidis,* and *Klebsiella* in patients with comorbidities such as diabetes.

Treatment aimed at eradicating the primary infection is usually associated with recovery of GN in these patients.

B. **Immunoglobulin A Nephropathy.** IgA nephropathy patients have elevated levels of galactose-deficient O-glycan IgA1 which leads to immune complexes of antiglycan autoantibodies and galactose-deficient IgA1 and anti-O glycans. It is the most common form of GN in Asia and in industrialized nations, comprising 15% to 40% of all biopsy-proven GN. IgA nephropathy is distinctly uncommon in Africa and South America. Most cases occur in the second or third decade of life, with a male predominance. The most common clinical presentation is microscopic hematuria and nonnephrotic-range proteinuria in an asymptomatic individual; however, the classic presentation observed 10% to 15% of the time is an episode of gross or macroscopic hematuria, often occurring concurrently with an upper respiratory tract infection. Proteinuria is generally mild, but nephrotic syndrome is occasionally present. Renal function is usually normal or only mildly depressed, but the occasional patient may present as an RPGN or with AKI. No serologic tests have been found to be consistently helpful, and a kidney biopsy is required for diagnosis, although the absence of a depressed serum complement level suggests a noninfectious etiology for the GN.

Renal histology demonstrates a mild to moderate mesangial cell proliferation with extracellular matrix expansion. The diagnosis is confirmed by the demonstration of IgA deposits in the mesangium, often with coexistent IgG and C3 as demonstrated by IF microscopy. Electron microscopy demonstrates mesangial immune deposits. The biopsy is scored using the Oxford MEST-C classification (M—mesangial hypercellularity, E—endocapillary hypercellularity, S—segmental glomerulosclerosis, T—tubular atrophy/interstitial fibrosis, C—proportion of glomeruli with crescents [C0, C1 ≤ 25%, C2 ≥ 25%]).

IgA nephropathy is often slowly progressive; and within 20 years, 50% of the affected subjects will have developed either end-stage renal disease or demonstrate substantial loss of renal function. An increased risk for progression is associated with proteinuria >1 g/day, an elevated serum creatinine at presentation, hypertension, or significant glomerular or interstitial fibrosis on kidney biopsy. Treatment should be aimed at aggressive blood pressure control and reduction of proteinuria to <1 g/day with the administration of angiotensin-converting enzyme inhibitors (ACEIs) or angiotensin receptor blockers (ARBs). The efficacy of corticosteroids with >1 but <3.5 g/d of proteinuria despite ACEI or ARB treatment with an eGFR >50 mL/min/1.73 m², has not been proven in recent studies, although treatment can be considered. There should be extreme caution or avoidance of corticosteroids in those with eGFR < 30 mL/min/1.73 m², diabetes, obesity, active peptic ulceration, uncontrolled psychiatric illness, secondary disease, and latent infections. Those with nephrotic-range proteinuria, especially the minimal change variant of IgA nephropathy, are treated with corticosteroids.

Patients with IgA nephropathy who present with the syndrome of RPGN (>50% decline in eGFR in <3 months) and have crescentic nephritis on kidney biopsy may be treated aggressively with high-dose corticosteroids and cyclophosphamide (see below).

C. **Rapidly Progressive Glomerulonephritis.** RPGN presents clinically as AKI in the setting of a "nephritic" urinary sediment (red cell +/− white cell casts, proteinuria, microscopic hematuria). This is a medical emergency that requires immediate hospitalization and, usually, a kidney biopsy for specific diagnosis. Kidney biopsy in these subjects reveals a crescentic GN, in which there is proliferation of cells outside the glomerulus but within Bowman's space, often forming a "crescent" shape on histologic cross section. Categorization is further defined by the IF microscopic findings. The presence of IgG in a linear pattern along the glomerular basement membrane (GBM) defines anti-GBM GN when confined to the kidney or anti-GBM disease (Goodpasture syndrome) when there is lung involvement. The presence of Ig and complement in a "granular" pattern on the capillary wall suggests an immune complex–associated disease such as lupus nephritis, IgA nephropathy, or PIGN. The absence of immune deposits is observed with ANCA-associated vasculitis (microscopic polyangiitis, granulomatosis with polyangiitis, eosinophilic granulomatosis with polyangiitis) also known as pauci-immune GN. A description of each of the major categories of RPGN is shown in Table 7.3, and

TABLE 7.3	Rapidly progressive glomerulonephritis: major categories	
Immunofluorescence pattern of immunoglobulin	**Major etiologies**	**Serologic tests**
Linear staining	Anti-GBM disease (with pulmonary hemorrhage) or glomerulonephritis (restricted to the kidney)	Anti-GBM antibody positive
No staining	Vasculitis syndromes	
	Granulomatosis with polyangiitis	Usually PR3-ANCA positive
	Microscopic polyangiitis	Usually MPO-ANCA positive
	Eosinophilic granulomatosis with polyangiitis	
	Polyarteritis nodosa	ANCA negative
Granular staining	Immune complex diseases	
	Systemic lupus erythematosus	Antinuclear antibody positive, low C3, C4
	Immunoglobulin A nephropathy	Negative serologies
	Poststreptococcal glomerulonephritis	Streptozyme positive, low C3
	Membranoproliferative glomerulonephritis	Low C3 and/or C4

ANCA, antineutrophil cytoplasmic antibody; anti-GBM, antiglomerular basement membrane; MPO-ANCA, myeloperoxidase; PR3-ANCA, proteinase 3.

more details on lupus nephritis are provided in Chapter 8. Chapter 9 provides a description of the vasculitis syndromes.

Anti-GBM GN/syndrome typically presents in males in the second or third decade of life, with a second peak in subjects over 60 years of age. Some patients present with renal involvement only (termed anti-GBM GN or Goodpasture disease), whereas others present with pulmonary hemorrhage and nephritis (anti-GBM disease or Goodpasture syndrome); rarely, subjects may present with only pulmonary involvement. Classically, patients present with hemoptysis following an upper respiratory infection and have a nephritic urinary sediment. With pulmonary involvement, a history of smoking, or extensive hydrocarbon exposure is common. The chest x-ray shows pulmonary hemorrhage, and laboratory tests may demonstrate an iron-deficiency anemia from blood loss and varying levels of renal dysfunction. Circulating anti-GBM antibodies are present, and kidney biopsy reveals crescentic GN with linear staining of IgG and complement (C3) along the GBM. The antibody has been shown to be directed against the alpha-3 chain of type IV collagen, which is present in the glomerular and alveolar basement membranes.

Treatment of anti-GBM disease or syndrome includes high-dose intravenous steroids (e.g., methylprednisolone 500- to 1,000-mg daily × 3 days) followed by a course of oral prednisone for 6 months and cyclophosphamide for 3 months. Plasma exchange is also conducted daily until the anti-GBM antibody titer is no longer detectable. A conservative approach is considered for those without pulmonary hemorrhage who present with a serum creatinine >6.0 mg/dL, >85% crescents, or with severe fibrosis on kidney biopsy as renal function recovery is unlikely.

If kidney transplantation is necessary, the procedure should be delayed until anti-GBM antibody titers are low or undetectable to avoid rapid recurrence of the disease in the graft.

Treatment of pauci-immune (Chapter 9) GN and lupus nephritis (Chapter 8) are discussed elsewhere. For RPGN from crescentic IgA nephropathy induction therapy involves methylprednisolone (500 to 1,000 mg IV × 3 days) followed by oral steroids with oral or IV cyclophosphamide which is followed by azathioprine to reduce the potential toxicity that can occur with long-term cyclophosphamide administration, including infertility, bladder cancer, and leukemia.

III. NEPHROTIC SYNDROME. The nephrotic syndrome may occur because of both systemic and renal-limited disease processes. In the Western hemisphere, the most common cause of nephrotic syndrome is diabetic nephropathy (see Chapter 5). Another cause in the elderly is amyloidosis, which often occurs secondary to multiple myeloma (see Chapter 11). Other monoclonal gammopathy–related diseases can result in nephrotic syndrome, such as light-chain deposition disease (see Chapter 11). The overall management of nephrotic syndrome can be found in Chapter 3.

A. Minimal Change Disease. Minimal change disease (MCD), also called "nil disease" or "lipoid nephrosis," is the most common cause of idiopathic nephrotic syndrome in children between the age of 2 and 12 years but is also observed in 20% of adults with nephrotic syndrome. The onset is often acute and may be precipitated by a viral infection, allergy, bee sting, or immunization. Nephrotic syndrome has been reported in adults with Hodgkin lymphoma or other T-cell malignancies. Minimal change disease alone or with interstitial nephritis and AKI has also been reported with nonsteroidal anti-inflammatory drugs.

Clinical findings are a dramatic weight gain and pitting edema, usually in the presence of a normal blood pressure. The urinary sediment may show hyaline casts, and oval fat bodies, while red cells are usually absent. Renal function is usually near normal; however, AKI can be seen that may be due, at least in part, to volume contraction secondary to severe hypoalbuminemia. AKI can present in the elderly with vascular disease.

Children presenting with classic symptoms of MCD do not initially require biopsy and are treated empirically; however, the presence of hypertension or microscopic hematuria requires further evaluation.

Kidney biopsy reveals normal-appearing glomeruli by light microscopy in the absence of Ig by IF studies. Typically, the only abnormality is noted by electron microscopy, in which there is diffuse fusion or effacement of the foot processes of the glomerular visceral epithelial cells.

Treatment consists of oral corticosteroids (typically prednisone, 1 mg/kg/day). More than 90% of children with MCD will experience a complete remission within 4 to 8 weeks, but the majority (75%) require repeated courses of therapy due to relapse. Patients who relapse three or more times within a year, or who relapse prior to being tapered off steroids (steroid dependent), may require a 8 to 12 weeks of oral cyclophosphamide therapy. Children who fail to respond to corticosteroids require a kidney biopsy to establish the diagnosis and, quite possibly, to be considered for another therapy. Prednisone is also effective in inducing remission in adults with MCD, albeit at a lower rate of success than in children. In adults, a longer-daily or alternate-day administration of prednisone starting at 2 mg/kg every other day is required with 70% to 80% responding by 12 weeks of therapy. Frequent relapsing disease will often respond to cyclophosphamide, but the risk of using this agent in a benign disease must be considered carefully. Steroid sparing agents such as mycophenolate mofetil, calcineurin inhibitors and rituximab have been used in frequently relapsing disease with success.

B. Focal Segmental Glomerulosclerosis. Focal segmental glomerulosclerosis (FSGS) is currently the most common cause of nephrotic syndrome in young adults, accounting for 20% to 30% of all cases in many series. It is the most common primary glomerular disease which causes end-stage kidney disease in the United States. FSGS can be classified into primary, secondary, genetic, and unknown forms. Patients with primary FSGS typically present with the classic features of nephrotic syndrome and microscopic hematuria (50%). Primary FSGS may develop in a subject who has been treated repeatedly for MCD and who becomes progressively resistant to corticosteroids or be misdiagnosed as steroid-resistant MCD. Secondary FSGS results from reduced nephron mass or toxic effects from drugs or viral infections. Secondary causes of FSGS include heroin, interferon, pamidronate, vesicoureteral reflux, sickle cell disease, obesity, and HIV infection. Patients with secondary FSGS usually do not present with nephrotic syndrome as they usually have normal serum albumin levels and often no peripheral edema even with urine protein excretion >3.5 g/day, with or without renal impairment. Genetic forms of FSGS are due to mutations in podocytes and the slit diaphragm proteins. Patients with genetic FSGS are glucocorticoid resistant. Patients with childhood-onset genetic FSGS present with severe nephrotic syndrome. Patients with adult-onset genetic FSGS may present with either nonnephrotic- or nephrotic-range proteinuria and more slowly progressive CKD, or nephrotic syndrome. Unknown forms of FSGS may present clinically as secondary FSGS without a known cause or genetic mutation.

Kidney biopsy demonstrates a light microscopic pattern of segmental sclerosis of glomerular tufts, often with segmental increases in mesangial matrix and cellularity. There can be both normal-appearing and segmentally scarred glomeruli. Also, there is a predisposition for the involvement of juxtamedullary glomeruli. Both IgM and C3 deposits are often present in the sclerotic segments of the glomeruli, where they are thought to be trapped passively rather than having a pathogenetic role in the disease.

Treatment consists of prednisone at an average dose of 1 mg/kg body weight/day. Prolonged treatment of 5 to 8 months is often required, and even then, partial remission with a urine protein excretion <2 g/day or complete remission is observed in only 50% of patients. Favorable prognostic indicators include absence of tubulointerstitial disease on kidney biopsy, a normal or only modestly elevated serum creatinine, and nonnephrotic proteinuria. Failure to observe a decrease in urine protein excretion after 12 weeks of prednisone therapy in adults or after 8 weeks in children raises the likelihood of steroid resistance. Other steroid-sparing agents may be tried such as calcineurin inhibitors. As in all patients with nephrotic syndrome, the use of ACEIs or ARBs may help reduce proteinuria and control hypertension.

C. Membranous Nephropathy. MN is the most common cause of nephrotic syndrome in the middle-aged adults. Primary MN is caused by autoantibodies against the podocyte M-type phospholipase A2 receptor 1 (PLA2R) in approximately 80% of cases, and thrombospondin type 1 domain–containing 7A (THSD7A) in 5% to 10% of cases. MN usually presents as nephrotic syndrome, often with low-grade microhematuria and relatively well-preserved renal function. However, some patients have asymptomatic low-grade or nephrotic-range proteinuria that is discovered on routine urinalysis. The peak age of incidence is 40 to 60 years, and men predominate by a ratio of 2:1. Patients can lose 10 to 20 g protein/day and experience severe disability. While most cases are primary, secondary MN can be associated with the use of certain medications (penicillamine, captopril, or nonsteroidal agents), with certain viral infections (chronic hepatitis B and C viral infection), and with malignancies (lung, breast, gastrointestinal origin, and others). Occasionally, patients with SLE may develop MN (class V lupus glomerular disease, see Chapter 8). Rarely, MN may accompany other diseases (diabetes mellitus, autoimmune thyroiditis).

On kidney biopsy, the glomeruli typically appear normocellular with thickening of the GBM on light microscopy. Use of silver methenamine, which stains GBM, often reveals additional "spike-like" protrusions on the epithelial side of the GBM, which represent extensions of basement membrane-like material. IF microscopy demonstrates IgG and C3 along the capillary wall in a "granular" pattern, and electron microscopy reveals that the immune deposits are located on the outer side of the GBM under the epithelial foot processes ("subepithelial" region). PLA2R and THSD7A can be detected in biopsy tissue by these antibodies.

Management involves testing for anti-PLA2R and anti-THSD7A antibody levels along with tissue staining. If serum anti-PLA2R antibody is absent or low, and tissue staining for these antigens is negative, secondary causes of MN can be investigated by checking for hepatitis viruses, antinuclear antibodies, and thyroid antibodies, and age-appropriate malignancy screening (mammogram, chest x-ray, stool guaiac and colonoscopy, and prostate-specific antigen). Supportive therapy includes controlling the manifestations of nephrotic syndrome by reducing proteinuria with ACEIs or ARBs, treating hypercholesterolemia with statins, and reducing blood pressure to 125/75 mm Hg or less. In patients with markedly low serum albumin levels (<2.0 to 2.5 g/dL), there is a marked increase in risk for venous thrombosis, especially of the renal vein, and some clinicians recommend prophylactic warfarin therapy. More specific disease management is recommended for patients with MN who have features predictive of progression that include an elevated serum creatinine at presentation, proteinuria >8.0 g/day, high-titer PLA2R (>150 RU/mL) or the presence of hypertension. In these patients, some recommend use of the so-called "Ponticelli" regimen consisting of intravenous methylprednisolone for 3 days followed by oral prednisone on months 1, 3, and 5 and oral cyclophosphamide (2 to 2.5 mg/kg/day) on months 2, 4, and 6. One recent trial comparing rituximab to cyclosporine in primary MN resulted in fewer relapses with rituximab. For patients at low risk for ESRD (proteinuria <4 g/day, serum albumin >3, normal renal function) supportive therapy is advised. Patients with mild disease will likely not progress or may even spontaneously remit over a 5- to 10-year period. In contrast, subjects with marked proteinuria, elevated serum creatinine, and elevated anti-PLA2R titers (>150 RU/mL) frequently progress, and as many as 40% will eventually require dialysis or transplantation in the absence of therapy.

D. Membranoproliferative Glomerulonephritis. Patients with membranoproliferative glomerulonephritis (MPGN) may present with hematuria, variable proteinuria with some having the nephrotic syndrome along with normal or elevated serum creatinine. Classification may be based on mechanism of injury using IF microscopy. On kidney biopsy, glomeruli are hypercellular and lobular in appearance due to increased matrix with both mesangial and endothelial cell cellularity. Immune complexes or complements and parts of mesangial cells deposit between the GBM and endothelial cell cause thickening of the GBM on EM. Immune complex–mediated MPGN is caused by complement activation via the classical pathway. Patient may have normal/mildly decreased C3 and low C4 levels. IF shows positive Ig and complement staining. Immune complex MPGN is commonly from hepatitis C and patients may have features associated with circulating cryoglobulins (weakness, arthralgias, and palpable purpura) with vasculitis in some (livedo reticularis, leg ulcers, and pulmonary or cardiac involvement). Other infections such as endocarditis, infected shunts, abscesses, and parasitic infections can cause immune complex MPGN. Autoimmune diseases such as lupus will show "full-house" IF. MPGN due to monoclonal gammopathy may show either kappa or lambda light chains on IF or no staining. Complement-mediated MPGN shows predominantly complement staining without immune complexes on IF due to alternative complement pathway activation. Patients will usually have low serum C3 and normal C4 levels. C3 glomerulopathy encompasses C3 glomerulonephritis (C3GN) and C3 dense deposit disease (C3DDD). C3GN may be due to genetic mutations in complement inhibitory proteins, or monoclonal gammopathies. Monoclonal proteins may inhibit complement-regulating proteins causing C3GN. C3DDD affects children and young adults and are often due to C3 nephritic factors which are antibodies that make C3 convertase resistant to cleavage, resulting in alternative complement pathway activation. Thick ribbon-like deposits are seen along the basement membranes of glomeruli and tubules.

When patients with MPGN do not have immune complexes or complement on IF, damage may be via endothelial injury from thrombotic microangiopathies.

Treatment of MPGN consists of treating the underlying cause along with controlling hypertension and nephrotic syndrome with ACEIs/ARB, a low-salt diet, and diuretics. Patients with HCV-associated MPGN are treated with anti-viral therapy. Patients with autoimmune disease are treated according to the underlying autoimmune disease. Patients with MPGN and monoclonal deposits on biopsy may not have an identifiable clone found on serum and urine protein electrophoresis or serum free light chains, but therapy with proteasome inhibitors may be used (see Chapter 11). Patients with C3GN may be treated with immunosuppression such as mycophenolate mofetil and steroids while eculizumab has not shown consistent benefit.

The natural history of MPGN is complex; some patients have chronic and smoldering disease, whereas others manifest a progressive course. As many as 50% of patients may develop CKD after 15 to 20 years, and recurrence following transplantation is common.

E. **Fibrillary and Immunotactoid Glomerulonephritis.** Fibrillary GN causes nephrotic syndrome with or without microhematuria and a mild to moderately elevated serum creatinine in adults between 40 and 60 years of age. DnaJ homolog subfamily B member 9, has been identified in the individual fibrils. Malignancy, monoclonal gammopathy, autoimmune diseases, or infections have been associated with fibrillary GN in 30% to 50% of cases. The clinical presentation is often similar to MPGN, and by biopsy, the glomeruli may appear mildly hypercellular and contain IgG and C3 deposits. However, serum complement levels are normal, and electron microscopy reveals a characteristic finding of fibrillar deposits in the mesangium and subendothelial areas of the GBM. IF microscopy reveals Ig and C3 in the mesangium and capillary walls in a granular pattern. Amyloid is also characterized by fibrillary deposits, but in contrast to amyloidosis, the Congo Red stain is negative in fibrillary GN and the fibrillar deposits are larger in diameter (12 to 22 nm) and randomly organized. Another rare type of GN, immunotactoid GN, is also Congo Red negative, but fibrils are even larger in diameter (>30 nm), cylindrical, and arranged in parallel arrays. This disease is often associated with plasma cell dyscrasias, particularly chronic lymphocytic leukemia, B-cell lymphomas, and monoclonal gammopathies. No effective therapy has yet been described for fibrillary GN. Thus, the prognosis of fibrillary GN is guarded, and in one small series, 50% of affected patients progressed to end-stage renal disease. Patients with idiopathic fibrillary and immunotactoid GN who have low GFR and nephrotic-range proteinuria have been treated with rituximab.

IV. SUGGESTED READINGS

Floege J, Amann K. Primary glomerulonephritides. *Lancet.* 2016;387(10032):2036–2048.

Geetha D, Jefferson JA. ANCA-associated vasculitis: core curriculum 2020. *Am J Kidney Dis.* 2020; 75(1):124–137.

Herrera GA, Turbat-Herrera EA. Renal diseases with organized deposits: an algorithmic approach to classification and clinicopathologic diagnosis. *Arch Pathol Lab Med.* 2010;134(4):512–531.

Rodrigues JC, Haas M, Reich HN. IgA Nephropathy. *Clin J Am Soc Nephrol.* 2017;12(4):677–686.

Sethi S, Fervenza FC. Membranoproliferative glomerulonephritis—a new look at an old entity. *N Engl J Med.* 2012;366(12):1119–1131.

8 Renal Involvement in Systemic Lupus Erythematosus

Wai Lang Lau, Mark S. Segal

Systemic lupus erythematosus (SLE) is an autoimmune disease chiefly affecting the skin, kidneys, joints, serous membranes, and blood vessels. It is seen primarily in young women (age 18 to 40 years), especially African Americans, but can occur at any age. The 2019 EULAR/ACR criteria uses antinuclear antibodies (ANA) as an entry criteria; 22 criteria with individual weights (from 2 to 10) separated into seven clinical domains and three immunologic domains, with only the highest scoring item in each domain being scored; and 10 points are needed to diagnose SLE with a sensitivity of 96.1% and a specificity of 93.4%.

The hallmark of the disease is the presence of ANA in the serum. However, a positive ANA, especially at low titers (<1:40), is common in the normal population, particularly in older patients, and may also be observed in other collagen vascular diseases. In this regard, both the specific antigen and the pattern of staining may be helpful in distinguishing the various collagen vascular diseases. SLE is frequently associated with a diffuse (homogeneous) or speckled pattern of staining, whereas scleroderma is associated with a nucleolar or centromere pattern. Similarly, anti–double-stranded DNA and anti-Smith antibodies are highly specific for SLE, whereas anti-Scl70 suggests scleroderma, and anti-Ro and anti-La antibodies suggest Sjögren syndrome. Other antibodies often correlate with specific organ involvement, such as the presence of antiribosomal P antibodies (lupus cerebritis) and anti–Jo-1 antibodies (lung involvement). Antihistone antibodies suggest the presence of drug-induced lupus. However, it is critical to understand how the antibody titers are being determined. Anti–double-stranded DNA classically has been reported by the Crithidea immunofluorescence assay (reported as a titer), which is very specific for double-stranded DNA. More and more laboratories have been using an ELISA assay, reporting the results as ELISA units (EU), which may be positive if the serum contains antibodies for single-stranded DNA or histones. Finally, antiphospholipid antibodies suggest the potential for thrombotic complications.

Renal involvement is common in SLE and may occur in 30% to 50% of patients during the early course of their disease and in the majority (60% to 80%) if followed long term. There is a wide variety of clinical presentations (see below).

I. **CLINICAL PRESENTATION OF LUPUS NEPHRITIS**. Patients presenting with lupus nephritis often also have extrarenal manifestations. The most common extrarenal manifestations include low-grade fever, the classic malar or "butterfly" rash, Raynaud's phenomenon, hair loss, and arthralgias. Pleuritis, or pericarditis, or both, may be observed in up to 40% of patients. Other common findings include oral and skin ulcers, hepatosplenomegaly, normochromic anemia, mild leucopenia, and thrombocytopenia. While most cases are idiopathic, some cases of lupus are associated with certain drugs, including hydralazine, sulfonamides, procainamide, tumor necrosis factor alpha inhibitors, minocycline, quinidine, carbamazepine, and isoniazid. Renal involvement and anti–double-stranded DNA are rare in drug-associated lupus.

The renal manifestations of lupus are varied. Some patients have no evidence of renal involvement (class I lupus); in these patients, renal biopsy typically shows normal morphology, although some immune deposits may be present (Table 8.1). In contrast, others have minimal evidence of renal involvement, such as the presence of microscopic hematuria, low-grade (<2 g/day) proteinuria, and normal renal function. These patients typically have moderately elevated ANA titers and normal serum complement levels. Renal biopsy in these patients typically shows a mesangial pattern of disease (class II lupus nephritis) with immunoglobulin (Ig) G and C3 deposition in a mesangial pattern, and with mesangial hypercellularity with or without expansion of mesangial matrix. Both class I and class II variants of the disease are associated with a good renal prognosis, although, over the course of the illness, the renal disease could progress to a higher class with a worse prognosis.

The most serious presentation of lupus nephritis observed in 40% of patients includes severe hypertension, proteinuria, deteriorating renal function, and an active sediment. Some of these individuals are oliguric with daily increasing serum creatinine, thus manifesting as an acute renal failure. Extrarenal complications are also common, including cerebritis, pleuritis/carditis, and rash. In these patients, the ANA titer is often very elevated, and serum C3 and C4 levels are usually depressed. Antiphospholipid antibodies may be present and, if positive, can be associated with coexistent thromboses. Renal biopsy shows either class III or class IV lupus nephritis (Table 8.1). Class III is characterized by focal proliferative changes, whereas class IV manifests diffuse proliferative changes that involve both a proliferation of endogenous glomerular cells as well as an infiltration of leukocytes. Focal necrosis, crescents, or both may be present in severe cases. Immunofluorescence microscopy usually shows diffuse granular deposits of IgG and C3, often with IgA, IgM, and C4. Electron microscopy reveals subendothelial and mesangial immune deposits. Although class III and class IV lupus nephritis were regarded as separate entities in the past, it is evident that class III is most likely a milder form of class IV disease, and, hence, treatment for both classes is the same.

Another form of lupus nephritis presenting as nephrotic syndrome, often with only mildly reduced renal function, may also occur. These patients may not completely fulfill the criteria for SLE and often have low-titer ANA antibodies and normal serum complements. The renal biopsy in these patients shows a pattern consistent with membranous nephropathy with thickening of the basement membrane, the presence of IgG and C3 in a granular pattern on the capillary wall, and subepithelial immune deposits noted by electron microscopy (class V lupus; Table 8.1). Unlike idiopathic membranous nephropathy, there is usually evidence of mesangial immune deposits and tubuloreticular structures in the endothelial cells on electron microscopy, suggestive of a high interferon (IFN) state, which can be present in ~50% of lupus patients. Critically, the clinical signs and symptoms of each class of lupus are just a guide and an individual patient with any class of lupus can present with a more or less severe clinical phenotype. The histologic class of lupus nephritis can only be determined by a renal biopsy.

TABLE 8.1

Lupus nephritis according to ISN/RPS 2018 revision of the World Health Organization Classification System

	Normal (class I)	Mesangial (class II)	Focal segmental proliferative (class III)	Diffuse proliferative (class IV)	Membranous (class V)	Advanced sclerosing (class VI)	Lupus Podocytopathy
Light microscopy	Normal	Normal or diffuse mesangial hypercellularity	Focal <50% of glomeruli involved or diffuse >50% of glomeruli involved by mesangial and endocapillary hypercellularity +/− segmental necrosis +/− hyaline thrombi	Diffuse involvement of mesangial and endocapillary hypercellularity +/− segmental necrosis +/− hyaline thrombi	Diffuse thickening of the GBM and mesangial expansion	>90% of glomeruli be globally sclerotic with no evidence of ongoing activity	Normal glomeruli, FSGS +/− mesangial hypercellularity
Immunofluorescence microscopy	+/− Scant IgG and C3 in mesangium	Granular deposits of IgG and C3 in mesangium	Diffuse deposits of IgG, C3, and C4 in mesangium and capillary wall	Diffuse deposits of IgG, C3, and C4 in mesangium and capillary wall	Diffuse granular deposits of IgG and C3 in capillary wall +/− mesangium		Immune complex deposits absent or limited to mesangium
Immune deposits and other findings by electron microscopy	Negative	Mesangial	Subendothelial; mesangial	Subendothelial; mesangial	Subepithelial; diffuse foot process effacement		+/− Mesangial; diffuse foot process effacement
Notes	Absence of any structural abnormality	+/− mild abnormality on urine analysis	Hematuria and proteinuria on urinalysis, HTN, renal insufficiency (in class IV)	Hematuria and proteinuria on urinalysis, HTN, renal insufficiency (in class IV)	Nephrotic syndrome	There is no ongoing lupus activity	Nephrotic syndrome

GBM, glomerular basement membrane; IgG, Immunoglobulin G.

Patients may also present with elevation in creatinine, with proteinuria and hypertension, but without systemic signs of lupus. A renal biopsy at this time may show glomerulosclerosis without active lesions. When over 90% of the glomeruli are sclerosed and there is no indication of lupus activity, the lesion is classified as advanced sclerosing lupus nephritis (class VI lupus; Table 8.1).

Recently, there has been a distinct subgroup of lupus nephritis patients found: clinical SLE with predominant finding of nephrotic syndrome on presentation and by renal biopsy have lupus podocytopathy. Histologically, these patients exhibit either minimal change or focal segmental glomerulosclerosis by light microscopy, with associated class I/II lupus nephritis findings by immunofluorescence and electron microscopy. Serologically, patients have a positive ANA, a quarter may have a positive dsDNA, and hypocomplementemia is common. At present, the International Society of Nephrology/Renal Pathology Society classification does not include lupus podocytopathy as a class of lupus nephritis. However, given its distinct behavior, most clinicians believe this should be an independent type of lupus nephritis, not just a coexistent histologic lesion.

II. **MANAGEMENT AND PROGNOSIS.** Treatment of patients with lupus nephritis should be considered in two phases: induction and maintenance. Patients presenting with mild lupus nephritis (class I and class II) have no need for induction therapy and are managed conservatively, usually limiting corticosteroids to the minimal dose that controls the extrarenal manifestations of their disease. In addition, patients should be placed on hydroxychloroquine (Plaquenil) (200 to 400 mg/day) to limit extrarenal and renal flares. When using hydroxychloroquine, patients should receive a biannual complete fundoscopic exam by an ophthalmologist looking for signs of plaquenil toxicity. This toxicity is reversible with hydroxychloroquine discontinuation.

Patients presenting with acute lupus nephritis suggestive of class III or class IV disease are managed aggressively. If there is evidence of acute changes in renal function, the patient is hospitalized. Blood pressure is managed with sodium restriction, vasodilators, diuretics, and beta blockers. Angiotensin-converting enzyme inhibitors and angiotensin receptor blockers are usually avoided in the setting of acutely changing renal function because these agents may cause a temporary decrease in renal function. In severe cases, acute dialysis is indicated. After diagnostic renal biopsy, disease-specific treatment is initiated.

A. **Induction Therapy.** Induction therapy usually consists of high-dose (or pulse) methylprednisolone sodium succinate (Solu-Medrol, 500 to 1,000 mg intravenously daily × 3 days) followed by oral prednisone (1 mg/kg/day, max 60 mg that is gradually reduced beginning at 30 days). More recently the practice is to limit the daily dose of Solu-Medrol to 500 mg. The National Institutes of Health (NIH) protocol includes the use of pulse cyclophosphamide (Cytoxan) (0.5 to 1.0 g/m^2) monthly for 6 months, adjusting the dose based on the white blood count nadir at day 14 to 16. The Eurolupus protocol, which demonstrated equal efficacy, uses a lower-dose cyclophosphamide regimen (500 mg IV every 2 weeks for 6 doses). This lower-dose scheme greatly decreases traditional concerns about cyclophosphamide toxicity including infertility, infection, and oncogenicity.

An alternative induction agent utilizes mycophenolate mofetil (MMF; CellCept). This agent given at high doses (2 to 3 g/day) has been shown to be equally efficacious to the NIH cyclophosphamide regimen for lupus nephritis class III, IV, and V disease.

B. Maintenance Therapy. The most effective maintenance therapy is MMF (1,000 po BID) for up to 3 years following the end of induction therapy. While azathioprine is slightly less effective, it is a reasonable alternative in those who cannot tolerate MMF or its side effects. Some special considerations to help pick one over the other:

1. Cost—MMF tends to be more expensive.
2. Pregnancy—azathioprine can be given safely to women who desire to conceive.
3. Hyperuricemia/gout—MMF can be safely used with xanthine oxidase inhibitors.
4. Homozygosity for thiopurine methyltransferase mutation (<1% population)—these patients are at risk for severe myelosuppression with azathioprine and it should be avoided. Thiopurine methyltransferase activity should be tested prior to using azathioprine.

III. SPECIAL CASES. Patients with lupus podocytopathy are known to be very sensitive to glucocorticoid treatment alone. It is felt that this distinct entity is modulated more by a podocyte toxic "cytokine milieu" as opposed to an immune complex–mediated mechanism. However, just like with the idiopathic form, focal segmental glomerulosclerosis subtype of lupus podocytopathy is more difficult to treat, responding less often to glucocorticoids alone and necessitating more time to attain remission.

For patients with class V lupus nephritis, when to employ immunosuppression is debatable, though most nephrologists would treat when proteinuria approaches 3 g/day despite maximum use of ACE/ARB along with statins +/− mineralocorticoid receptor antagonists. For class V disease with heavy proteinuria, calcineurin inhibitors, cyclophosphamide, and MMF are all reasonable treatment options.

IV. SEVERE/REFRACTORY CASES AND FUTURE DIRECTIONS. There is an interest in multi-targeted therapy for challenging patients. A study of Chinese lupus nephritis patients with class IV disease or combined class IV/V disease, demonstrated the efficacy of prednisone, MMF (1,000 mg po BID), and tacrolimus (targeting a 12-hour trough of 5 to 7 ng/mL) over monthly cyclophosphamide for induction (6 months) and maintenance over 18 months.

Benlysta is the first new drug approved by the FDA for SLE in over a decade. Belimumab is a human monoclonal IgG1 antibody that binds to and inhibits soluble B-lymphocyte stimulator protein (also known as B-cell activating factor), a potent cytokine important for B-cell maturation. Its approval was based on its ability to improve disease course using the SLE responder index. This is a complicated scoring system that covers a host of organs affected by the disease, including the kidneys. More recently a phase 3 study specifically targeting patients with lupus nephritis (preliminary results) demonstrated that the addition of Benlysta to standard of care had better renal response as compared to placebo.

Rituximab (RTX) is a chimeric (mouse/human) monoclonal antibody directed against CD20, an antigen expressed on the surfaces of immature B cells. The investigators of the LUNAR (lupus nephritis assessment with RTX) study found that the addition of RTX (1,000 mg on days 1, 15, 168, and 182) to full induction with glucocorticoids and MMF was not superior to placebo in patients with class III/IV disease. Thus at this time, RTX is not considered a first-line induction agent for lupus nephritis. However, some observational studies suggest efficacy in patients who have failed induction therapy with other agents.

The lack of efficacy of RTX has been attributed to RTX not depleting B cell thoroughly enough. Obinutuzumab, a fully humanized monoclonal antibody directed against CD20, offers enhanced depletion of both peripheral and lymphoid tissue B cells and has demonstrated superior efficacy over RTX in lymphoma studies. In a phase 2 randomized controlled study, the addition of obinutuzumab in addition to standard of care offered an improved response over placebo in 125 patients (mostly Hispanics, 70% with class IV disease and 30% with class IV/V disease). The phase 3 study is underway—NCT 04221477.

Increased levels of IFN in patients with SLE were described 40 years ago and were later identified as type I IFN. Observational studies found that patients treated for malignancy with IFN-alpha could develop a lupus-like disease. Anifrolumab, a monoclonal antibody against the IFN-alpha receptor 1, blocks the effects of IFN-alpha. Anifrolumab is currently being tested in a phase 2 study versus placebo as an addition to standard of care in patients with proliferative lupus nephritis.

In the past 2 decades, the knowledge of the intracellular pathway downstream of cytokine receptors has increased tremendously. Inhibition of the receptor-associated kinases provides a novel approach in suppressing multiple cytokines simultaneously. Small and orally active molecules that inhibit the intracellular Janus kinases (JAKs) are now available and are being tested in SLE treatment.

Finally, there is voclosporin, a more potent derivative of cyclosporine; a new calcineurin inhibitor with a better metabolic profile, fewer adverse effects, and no need for therapeutic drug monitoring. Preliminary results of a phase 3 study adding voclosporin to standard of care, offered a greater renal response compared to placebo. This will likely be an addition to our toolbox of lupus nephritis treatments very soon.

This is indeed a very exciting time in research and pharmaceutical development for lupus nephritis treatment. Considering the age demographic of most lupus patients and the known high renal morbidity that is associated with this form of nephritis, the need for the continued quest for safer and more effective treatment options is paramount.

V. SUGGESTED READINGS

Appel G, Contreras G, Dooley MA, et al. Mycophenolate vs cyclophosphamide for induction treatment of lupus nephritis. *J Am Soc Nephrol*. 2009;20(5):1103–1112.

Contreras G, Pardo V, Leclercq O, et al. Sequential therapies for proliferative lupus nephritis. *N Engl J Med*. 2004;350(10):971–980.

Houssiau F, Vasconcelos C, D' Cruz D, et al. Immunosuppressive therapy in lupus nephritis: the Euro-lupus Nephritis trial, a randomized trial of low-dose versus high-dose intravenous cyclophosphamide. *Arthritis Rheum*. 2002;46(8):2121–2131.

Liu Z, Zhang H, Liu Z, et al. Multitarget therapy for induction treatment of lupus nephritis: a randomized trial. *Ann Intern Med*. 2015;162(1):18–26.

Rovin B, Furie R, Latinis K, et al. Efficacy and safety of rituximab in patients with active proliferative lupus nephritis: the lupus nephritis assessment with rituximab study. *Arthritis Rheum*. 2012;64(4):1215–1226.

9 Renal Vasculitis

Negiin Pourafshar, Michael Choi

Vasculitis is characterized by inflammation and necrosis of blood vessels, with subsequent tissue ischemia. Virtually any size or type of blood vessel, in any organ, can be affected. There is considerable overlap within the spectrum of the vasculitides, but certain patterns are recognized based on the size of vessels and organs affected. This chapter will review antineutrophil cytoplasmic antibody (ANCA)-associated vasculitis (AAV) and the immune complex IgA vasculitis and the medium-vessel vasculitis polyarteritis nodosa (PAN).

I. **ANCA-ASSOCIATED VASCULITIS.** AAV can be divided into 3 clinical diseases described below but may also be classified by ANCA serology (proteinase or PR3-ANCA vs. myeloperoxidase or MPO-ANCA) as clinical outcomes (higher mortality with (MPO-ANCA) and relapse rates (higher with PR3-ANCA) are more closely associated with ANCA specificity (Table 9.1). It is felt that infection or inflammation prime neutrophils resulting in movement of MPO and PR3 from intracellular neutrophil granules to the cell surface. ANCAs bind to MPO or PR3 and activate neutrophils which release reactive oxygen species, proteases, and with neutrophil cell death, neutrophil extracellular traps (NETs). These NETs contain MPO, PR3, and complement components which cause endothelial injury (see Fig. 9.1).

A. **Granulomatosis with Polyangiitis.** Granulomatosis with polyangiitis (GPA) is a primary systemic vasculitis, predominantly affecting small- and medium-sized arteries of the respiratory tract and kidneys.

1. **Clinical picture.** GPA is most common in Caucasians 50 to 70 years of age. Disease hallmarks are necrotizing granulomata of the upper and lower respiratory tract and necrotizing glomerulonephritis. Patients commonly present with epistaxis, hemoptysis, or sinusitis, and radiographic pulmonary nodules that change or cavitate. Constitutional symptoms, rash, arthritis, serositis, and neuritis also occur. PR3-ANCA is found in 70% to 75% of patients, MPO in 20%, and no ANCA in 5% of patients. Serial titers of PR3-ANCA are sometimes useful in monitoring disease activity.

2. **Renal involvement.** Clinical renal disease may be preceded by extrarenal manifestations, although evidence for involvement of the kidneys can be found in most patients, with urinalysis showing hematuria, red cell casts, and proteinuria. Renal function may be impaired in only a small proportion of patients initially but characteristically function deteriorates in most. Kidney biopsy usually shows focal or diffuse necrotizing pauci-immune glomerulonephritis. Rapidly progressive glomerulonephritis (RPGN) is associated with crescents ("crescentic" glomerulonephritis) and fulminant renal failure. The term pauci-immune describes the scarcity of immune deposits

| TABLE 9.1 | ANCA-associated vasculitis | | |

	Granulomatosis with polyangiitis (GPA)	**Microscopic polyangiitis (MPA)**	**Eosinophilic granulomatosis with polyangiitis (EGPA)**
Autoantibodies directed against antigen	PR3 (C-ANCA): 70–75% MPO (p-ANCA): 20% ANCA negative: 5%	MPO (P-ANCA): 60% PR3 (C-ANCA): 30% ANCA negative: 10%	MPO (P-ANCA): 50% PR3 (C-ANCA): 10%
Age/Race	Caucasians; fifth to seventh decade	Southern Europeans or Asian descent; sixth to eighth decade	
Respiratory tract/Lungs	Necrotizing granulomata of the upper and lower respiratory tract. Respiratory involvement is more common than MPA. May present with epistaxis, hemoptysis, or sinusitis	Necrotizing vasculitis without granulomatous inflammation	Necrotizing granulomatous inflammation of the respiratory tract; asthma and eosinophilia
Renal involvement	Focal or diffuse necrotizing pauci-immune glomerulonephritis; RPGN is associated with crescentic glomerulonephritis and fulminant renal failure	Involves small and medium arteries and commonly presents as RPGN but the kidney disease course may be more indolent than GPA	Less common renal involvement
Neurologic involvement	Peripheral neuropathy and mononeuritis multiplex	Peripheral neuropathy; less common mononeuritis multiplex	
Relapse	Higher risk of relapse	Lower relapse risk than GPA	

seen on immunofluorescence and electron microscopy. Small amounts of Immunoglobulin (Ig) G and C3 may be seen on biopsy. For GPA, pathognomonic granulomas are common in the respiratory tract, but are typically absent in the kidney.

B. Microscopic Polyangiitis. Microscopic polyangiitis (MPA) involves small and medium arteries and commonly presents as RPGN.

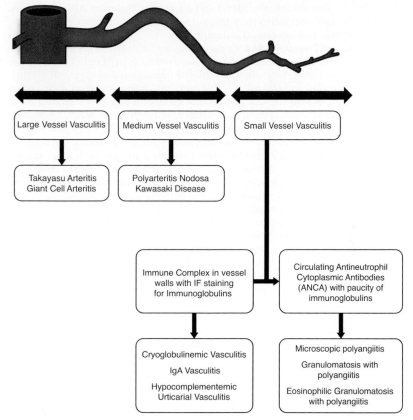

FIGURE 9.1: Renal vasculitis. Predominant distribution of renal vascular involvement by a variety of vasculitides. The heights of the trapezoids represent the relative frequency of involvement of different portions of the renal vasculature by the three major categories of vasculitis. *EGPA,* Eosinophilic granulomatous polyangiitis; *GPA,* granulomatous polyangiitis; *HSP,* Henoch–Schönlein purpura. (*Comprehensive Clinical Nephrology*, ISBN: 978-1-4557-5838-8 Copyright © 2015, 2010, 2007, 2003, 2000 by Saunders, an imprint of Elsevier Inc.)

1. **Clinical picture and renal involvement.** Patients with MPA present at 60 to 80 years of age and patients are often of Southern Europeans or Asian descent. Patients with MPA may demonstrate multisystem involvement with glomerulonephritis being common. The kidney disease course may be more indolent than GPA. Urinalysis and renal biopsy findings are similar to GPA. Patients with MPA may be MPO positive (60%), PR3 positive (30%), or ANCA negative (10%). The presence of anti-myeloperoxidase antibodies is suggestive, but not diagnostic, of this entity.

C. **Eosinophilic Granulomatosis with Polyangiitis.** Eosinophilic granulomatosis with polyangiitis (EGPA) is similar to GPA with necrotizing granulomatous inflammation of the respiratory tract and small to medium vessels, but different in that asthma and eosinophilia are associated with this disease. ANCA is positive in only 50% of patients (usually MPO) and affects the kidney in 20% of patients. The ANCA-positive patients may develop necrotizing crescentic GN. There may be eosinophilic rich interstitial inflammation.

D. Management and Prognosis of AAV. Early, aggressive treatment is indicated if there is evidence of major organ disease and should not be delayed until kidney biopsy results are available. Treatment is initiated (induction therapy) with methylprednisolone (500 to 1,000 mg intravenously on 3 successive days, followed by oral prednisone(1 mg/kg/day, 60 to 80 mg maximum for 2 to 4 weeks followed by tapered dose) which is combined with either intravenous or oral cyclophosphamide or rituximab. Pulse cyclophosphamide (15 mg/kg every 2 to 3 weeks for 3 to 6 months intravenously) is associated with lower toxicity, but a higher relapse rate, than oral administration (initially 2 mg/kg/day). Rituximab is effective for induction therapy with patients who have a serum creatinine <4.0 mg/dL not on mechanical ventilation in the RAVE trial. This may be the preferred option for relapsing disease and in those with PR3 disease. Induction treatment that combines either regimen with plasma exchange has been used for severe acute kidney injury, those with pulmonary hemorrhage, and those with concurrent anti-GBM disease. The PEXIVAS trial did not show improved outcomes with plasma exchange for the first two conditions.

Maintenance immunosuppressive therapy is generally started after 3 to 6 months from the start of induction therapy. After induction therapy with corticosteroids and cyclophosphamide, a trial showed that patients switched to azathioprine after 3 to 6 months had equivalent relapse rates to those who continued on oral cyclophosphamide at 2 years. After corticosteroid and cyclophosphamide induction therapy, a trial showed that fixed rituximab doses every 6 months were found to be superior to azathioprine. It is suggested that after induction therapy with rituximab, maintenance therapy with either azathioprine or rituximab therapy be continued. The optimal rituximab schedule for maintenance therapy is unknown. The optimal duration of maintenance therapy is unknown, but therapy is generally continued for at least 24 months after induction therapy with trials suggesting this should be longer. Adjunctive or alternative therapies include trimethoprim-sulfamethoxazole, azathioprine, methotrexate, and mycophenolate mofetil (MMF). Remission can be achieved in more than 90% of patients, although almost one-half relapse at some time. End-stage renal disease (ESRD) develops in about 20% to 25% of patients. Treatment-related toxicity is a significant problem and antimicrobial and osteoporosis prophylaxis should be used. Recurrence of vasculitis after transplantation occurs in about 0.01 to 0.02 episodes per patient per year.

II. IMMUNOGLOBULIN A VASCULITIS. Immunoglobulin A vasculitis (IgAV), formerly called Henoch–Schonlein purpura, affects small vessels and capillaries.

Immune complexes containing IgA are deposited in the skin and kidneys. The extrarenal manifestations help differentiate this disease from IgA nephropathy.

A. Clinical Picture. IgAV is relatively common in children who typically present with abdominal pain, bloody diarrhea, edema, and polyarthralgia. In adults, the disease tends to act similarly to other small-vessel vasculitides, and IgA deposition is needed to make the diagnosis. Skin involvement that is seen in all patients ranges from urticaria to palpable purpura, classically distributed over the buttocks and dependent extensor surfaces of the extremities. Skin biopsy reveals leukocytoclastic vasculitis, with IgA deposits seen in the newest lesions. Older adults with no identifiable etiology for the development of IgAV should have age-appropriate malignancy screening.

B. **Renal Involvement.** Evidence of renal involvement is not universal, but ranges from all degrees of hematuria to acute nephritis with acute kidney injury and hypertension. Kidney disease follows onset of systemic symptoms from a few days to a month later. Children generally have mild involvement, but adults are more likely to develop moderate to severe disease. Proteinuria, sometimes in the nephrotic range, is common. Histologically, changes identical to IgA nephropathy are seen, with IgA deposits in the glomerular mesangium. IgG and C3 deposition may also be detected, but serum complement levels are usually normal. A mild focal segmental glomerulonephritis is characteristic of the disease, although necrosis and crescents can occur in severe cases. The severity of glomerulonephritis does not correlate with the extent of extrarenal disease. Renal outcomes are significantly worse in adults compared to children.

C. **Management and Prognosis.** IgAV is usually self-limiting over weeks to months. Relapses, usually milder than the initial episode, may occur. Supportive therapy with fluid and sodium restriction and appropriate treatment of hypertension is usually sufficient in those with proteinuria <1 g/day. The glomerulonephritis usually resolves, albeit with residual hematuria that does not necessarily have implications for future deterioration of renal function. Although there is no evidence that corticosteroids alter the course of the disease, adult patients have been treated with >1 g/day of proteinuria, elevated serum creatinine, or crescentic glomerulonephritis on biopsy. Intravenous and oral corticosteroids, cyclophosphamide, rituximab, and MMF have been suggested for treatment of patients with severe crescentic glomerulonephritis (>20% to 25%), but there have been no controlled trials to support these measures. The extent of renal disease generally determines the long-term prognosis. Nephrotic syndrome, acute kidney injury, and crescents on biopsy are poor prognostic features. Recurrence after transplantation occurs, notably in living related donor allografts.

III. **POLYARTERITIS NODOSA.** (PAN is a primary vasculitis of primarily medium and occasionally small-sized arteries that involves many organs, notably the kidneys, nervous system, and heart. Aneurysms ("nodosa") form subsequent to healing and fibrosis. The condition is rare.

A. **Clinical Picture.** The incidence of PAN increases between the ages of 40 and 60 years and usually presents as fever, weight loss, and muscle and joint pain. Inflammation of vessels with intimal proliferation reduces organ perfusion and causes ischemia and thrombosis. Renin-dependent hypertension due to glomerular ischemia is very common. Approximately 70% of patients develop cardiac disease, including ischemia and pericarditis, and half experience abdominal pain and bloody diarrhea. Mononeuritis multiplex and polyneuropathy occur frequently. Central nervous system involvement tends to occur late and may cause seizures and stroke. PAN is associated with hepatitis B antigenemia, intravenous drug abuse, and hairy cell leukemia. Biopsy of a clinically affected organ or celiac or renal arteriography may be used in diagnosis; arteriography shows characteristic aneurysms and irregular constrictions.

B. **Renal Involvement.** Nearly all patients have some evidence of renal disease, ranging from minimal findings on urinalysis to gross hypertension, hematuria, flank pain, and acute kidney injury. The arcuate and interlobular arteries are primarily affected. Glomerular ischemia leads to fibrinoid necrosis, sclerosis, and patchy cortical infarction but little cell proliferation. The fall in the glomerular filtration rate generally results from reduced glomerular perfusion. Although up to one-third of patients may also have glomerulonephritis, crescentic glomerulonephritis is rare in PAN and some authorities consider the presence of glomerulonephritis, signifying capillary involvement, indicative of small-vessel vasculitis not PAN. Healing of the vessel wall leaves changes similar to hypertensive nephrosclerosis, but in PAN the elastic lamina is destroyed rather than reduplicated. Renal disease is the major cause of death.

C. **Management and Prognosis.** Early treatment is essential and succeeds in 10-year survival rates of 80%. Relapse is rare. Cyclophosphamide and corticosteroids are given for non–hepatitis B-associated PAN. Plasmapheresis and antiviral therapy may be effective in the presence of hepatitis B positivity. Younger patients with limited disease may be managed with steroids alone.

IV. SUGGESTED READINGS

Audemard-Verger A, Terrier B, Dechartres A, et al. Characteristics and management of IgA vasculitis (Henoch-Schönlein) in adults: data from 260 patients included in a French Multicenter Retrospective Survey. *Arthritis Rheumatol.* 2017;69(9):1862.

Geetha D, Jefferson JA. ANCA-associated vasculitis: core curriculum 2020. *Am J Kidney Dis.* 2020; 75(1):124–137.

Jennette JC, Falk RJ. Renal and systemic vasculitis. In: Johnson RJ, Feehally J, eds. *Comprehensive Clinical Nephrology.* 3rd ed. Mosby, 2007:275–290.

Jennette JC, Nachman PH. ANCA glomerulonephritis and vasculitis. *Clin J Am Soc Nephrol.* 2017; 12(10):1680–1691.

Mukhtyar C, Flossmann O, Hellmich B, et al. Outcomes from studies of antineutrophil cytoplasm antibody associated vasculitis: a systematic review by the EULAR systemic vasculitis task force. *Ann Rheum Dis.* 2008;67(7):1004–1010.

Rovin BH, Caster DJ, Cattran DC, et al. Management and treatment of glomerular diseases (part 2): conclusions from a kidney disease: improving Global Outcomes (KDIGO) Controversies Conference. *Kidney Int.* 2019;95(2):281–295.

Walsh M, Merkel PA, Peh C-A, et al. Plasma exchange and glucocorticoids in severe ANCA-associated vasculitis. *N Engl J Med.* 2020;383:622–631.

10 Renal Involvement in Thrombotic Microangiopathy and Scleroderma

Mohammed A. Alshehri, Michael Choi

I. **THROMBOTIC MICROANGIOPATHY.** Thrombotic microangiopathy (TMA) encompasses a group of acquired and inherited syndromes and diseases that have identical pathologic features. They can be classified as thrombotic thrombocytopenic purpura (TTP), Shiga-toxin–associated hemolytic uremic syndrome (HUS) or typical HUS, atypical HUS (aHUS), and TMA secondary to drugs or systemic diseases. A successful outcome relies on the early identification and treatment or removal of the culprit agent.

TMAs are associated with pregnancy, malignant hypertension, infections, systemic diseases such as antiphospholipid syndrome, scleroderma, and systemic lupus erythematosus, transplantation and medications (vascular endothelial growth factor [VEGF] inhibitors, tacrolimus, mitomycin C, interferon [IFN]-beta, ticlopidine, and quinine). The most common initial event is endothelial injury resulting in platelet microthrombi, platelet consumption, hemolytic anemia, and variable renal and neurologic manifestations. TTP is caused by ADAMTS-13 (a disintegrin and metalloproteinase with thrombospondin type 1 motif, member 13) activity <10% from antibodies or deficiency. This results in accumulation of unusually large multimers of von Willebrand factor to trigger platelet aggregation and microthrombi in vessels. Approximately half of the patients with aHUS have an underlying inherited or acquired alternative pathway complement abnormality which leads to unchecked activation of terminal complement in endothelial cells. TMAs may rarely be associated with metabolic abnormalities (e.g., Cobalamin deficiency).

A. **Clinical Picture.** The presentation correlates with the specific distribution of microangiopathic lesions which vary in these entities. Both renal and neurologic manifestations can occur which can overlap. Typical HUS predominantly affects the kidneys of young children after an acute diarrheal illness. Shiga-toxin–producing bacteria, usually *Escherichia coli* O157:H7 can be identified on stool culture. Stool PCR testing to detect Shiga toxin is becoming widely available. Other infectious causes include human immunodeficiency virus, *Shigella dysenteriae,* and *Streptococcus pneumoniae.* The incidence of TTP peaks in the third to fourth decade and is more common in women. Cerebral vessel microthrombi cause fluctuating neurologic symptoms including confusion, seizures, and paresis. More than 90% of patients with TTP and HUS have purpura at presentation. Epistaxis, hematuria, gastrointestinal hemorrhage, and

Coombs negative hemolytic anemia with elevated LDH and low haptoglobin are common. The peripheral blood smear shows schistocytes, burr cells, and helmet cells. Thrombocytopenia is common; however, there may be renal involvement without thrombocytopenia. Low C3 levels are present in only 30% to 50% of patients with aHUS.

Other findings may include fever, myalgias, and arthralgias. A diagnosis of aHUS is presumed if ADAMTS-13 activity is >10%, test for Shiga-toxin–producing organisms are negative, and there are no obvious secondary causes of TMA. The Kidney Disease: Improving Global Outcomes (KDIGO) conference on aHUS and C3GN recommended testing for genes that may cause complement dysregulation in every patient with suspected aHUS.

B. **Renal Involvement.** Proteinuria and microscopic or gross hematuria are common. More than one-half will have acute kidney injury of varying severity at some time, but renal involvement tends to be more common and more severe in HUS and other TMAs compared to TTP. Prolonged anuria, the need for early dialysis, and proteinuria that persists after recovery are risk factors for developing chronic kidney disease.

Kidney biopsy reveals glomerular endothelial cell hypertrophy and expansion of the subendothelial space. Platelet and fibrin thrombi deposition occlude glomerular capillaries and afferent arterioles and cause ischemia and necrosis. Immunofluorescence microscopy is usually negative.

C. **Management and Prognosis.** Typical HUS is usually self-limiting. Supportive therapy includes dialysis and bowel rest. In *E. coli* O157:H7 infection, antibiotics are usually held unless there is bacteremia, as they may increase Shiga-toxin release by dying bacteria.

Untreated TTP is almost invariably fatal within 3 months. Plasma exchange (PE) with fresh frozen plasma replacement to provide ADAMTS13 and remove possible antibodies has increased survival to 90%. In adult patients, PE should start as early as possible when TTP is suspected. Glucocorticoids and rituximab have been used with PE for TTP.

In aHUS, progression to ESRD and mortality has decreased after the introduction of anticomplement therapy in 2011. Eculizumab is a humanized monoclonal antibody that binds to C5 and prevents formation of the membrane attack complex, and it is indicated in patients with aHUS. Meningococcal vaccination and prophylactic antibiotics should be administrated as the risk of infection with encapsulated organisms increases with the complement blockade. Data regarding the optimal duration of treatment is limited. Patients require close monitoring, particularly in the first year, when the recurrence rate is higher. Some genetic mutations are associated with a higher recurrence rate of aHUS than others. Detailed genetic testing can help in guiding whether long-term treatment should be continued. Complement mutations may play a role in secondary forms of TMAs such as pregnancy if the presentation is not suggestive of hemolysis, elevated liver enzyme, and low platelets (HELLP) syndrome.

Improvement in platelet count and serum lactic acid dehydrogenase correlates with the treatment response. Platelet infusions may be detrimental and should only be given in the face of life-threatening hemorrhage. Historically, splenectomy and nephrectomy have been reported as rescue therapies in refractory TTP and HUS, respectively. With refractory TTP, caplacizumab (blocks VWF–platelet interaction), high-dose glucocorticoids, and rituximab have been used. Overall, renal and neurologic sequelae are more likely in aHUS and adult forms of HUS and in TTP. Relapses occur but are less common and milder in typical HUS. Recurrence after transplantation is more common in aHUS.

II. PROGRESSIVE SYSTEMIC SCLEROSIS (SCLERODERMA). Systemic sclerosis is a disease of uncontrolled proliferation of collagen associated with obliterative vascular lesions which mainly affects the skin, lungs, gastrointestinal tract, and kidneys.

A. Clinical Picture. Progressive systemic sclerosis (PSS) is a relatively rare disease, most common in middleaged women. Arterial walls become thickened, leading to the narrowing and eventual obliteration of the lumen. Skin involvement is seen in 90% of patients: Ischemic ulcers, subcutaneous calcinosis, Raynaud's phenomenon, telangiectasia, and sclerodactyly may occur. Extradermatologic manifestations may predominate in some patients who experience an acute diffuse onset and include esophageal dysmotility, pulmonary interstitial fibrosis, cardiomyopathy, polymyositis, and arthralgias. Most patients demonstrate positive antinuclear antibodies, but their absence cannot exclude the diagnosis. Anti–DNA-topoisomerase (Scl-70) antibodies are highly specific for PSS, and their presence is associated with more extensive disease and a higher risk of interstitial lung disease. Anticentromere antibodies are usually associated with limited cutaneous systemic sclerosis. Positive RNA polymerase III antibody is associated with an increased risk of scleroderma renal crisis (SRC).

B. Renal Involvement. Approximately one-half of all patients with PSS have clinical evidence of renal involvement. Acute kidney injury accounts for more than one-third of all deaths. Obliterative arterial lesions, mainly preglomerular, are seen on kidney biopsy. There is a concentric proliferation of smooth muscle cells in the media that migrate into the intima, producing an "onion skin" appearance. Basement membrane thickening and fibrinoid necrosis may be seen in the glomeruli and tubulointerstitium, along with immunoglobulin M and C3 deposition, tubular atrophy, and edema. Urinalysis is usually unremarkable, although ischemic glomerulosclerosis may cause hematuria. Renal disease is complicated by the SRC in approximately 20% of patients. This occurs more commonly in winter and is characterized by the abrupt onset of hyperreninemic hypertension and the potential to progress to kidney failure within weeks. It is likely initiated by renal vasoconstriction due to cold-induced vasospasm, hypovolemia, or heart failure. The use of high-dose steroids and cyclosporine has been associated with SRC. Although hypertension is a typical finding of SRC, normotensive SRC has been reported, although patients may have higher blood pressures than their usual baseline. Rarely, SRC can occur without sclerodermatous skin changes, and the diagnosis can be challenging.

C. Management and Prognosis. Management and prognosis are dependent on the pattern of organ involvement. Overall mortality from renal, cardiac, or respiratory failure approaches 65% at 7 years after diagnosis. About one-third of patients with SRC progress to end-stage renal disease (ESRD).

Control of blood pressure is paramount and is usually achieved with ACE inhibition. Early use of these agents can stabilize and improve renal function. Other therapy includes prostacyclin analogs, phosphodiesterase type 5 inhibitors, and endothelin-1 antagonists for pulmonary vascular disease, immunomodulatory drugs for interstitial lung disease, calcium channel blockers for Raynaud's phenomenon, and proton pump inhibitors for esophageal reflux. Cold avoidance, good nutrition, and skin care are also important. Poor vascular access may cause problems in maintenance hemodialysis. Continuous ambulatory peritoneal dialysis is often more successful, although compromised peritoneal vasculature may reduce dialysis efficiency. PSS is associated with poor graft survival after transplantation.

III. SUGGESTED PRACTICAL APPROACH. Adult patients with TMA:

- TTP should be presumed and PE should be started after tests for ADAMTS13 activity. Workup for Shiga toxin should be performed regardless of the GI symptoms.
- If ADAMTS13 activity is >10% and there is no evidence of Shiga toxin, TTP and typical HUS are excluded, there should be strong consideration for starting Eculizumab.
- Continue the workup for secondary causes of TMA. Genetic testing should be individualized.

IV. SUGGESTED READINGS

Batal I, Domsic RT, Medsger TA, et al. Scleroderma renal crisis: a pathology perspective. *Int J Rheumatol.* 2010;2010:543704e.

Brocklebank V, Wood KM, Kavanagh D. Thrombotic microangiopathy and the kidney. *Clin J Amer Soc Nephrol.* 2018;13(2):300–317.

Goodship THJ, Cook HT, Fakhouri F, et al. Atypical hemolytic uremic syndrome and C3 glomerulopathy: conclusions from a "Kidney Disease: Improving Global Outcomes" (KDIGO) controversies conference." *Kidney Int.* 2017;91(3):539–551.

Kavanagh D, Sheerin N. Thrombotic microangiopathies. In: Yu A, ed. *Brenner and Rector's The Kidney.* 11th ed. Elsevier; 2020.

Mouthon L, Bussone G, Berezné A, et al. Scleroderma renal crisis. *The J Rheumatol.* 2014;41(6):1040–1048.

Thurman JM, Frazer-Abel A. Thrombotic microangiopathies. In: Lerma EV, Rosner MH, Perazella MA. eds. *CURRENT Diagnosis & Treatment: Nephrology & Hypertension.* 2nd ed. McGraw-Hill; 2020. https://accessmedicine.mhmedical.com/content.aspx?

11 Monoclonal Gammopathy–Related Kidney Diseases

Michael Choi

I. **INTRODUCTION.** Multiple myeloma (MM) and other monoclonal gammopathies commonly cause kidney disease via intact or components of the immunoglobulin. Almost 50% of patients with MM develop kidney disease sometime during course of their illness with 20% to 50% of patients with newly diagnosed MM having acute kidney injury (AKI) or chronic kidney disease (CKD) at the time of diagnosis. MM is characterized by the presence of 10% clonal plasma cells in bone marrow or serum monoclonal intact immunoglobulin spike (M-spike) of >3 g/dL and at least one myeloma-defining event such as hyperCalcemia, Renal impairment from cast nephropathy, Anemia, and/or Bone lesions (CRAB). The serum free light-chain (FLC) ratio of kappa to lambda is normally 0.26 to 1.65. The normal ratio increases to 0.37 to 3.17 with renal impairment. A serum FLC ratio of >100 of involved to uninvolved light chain with the level of the uninvolved chain >10 mg/dL, >60% plasma cells, and >1 bone lesion by MRI strongly predict progression to symptomatic myeloma. Patients who do not exhibit any of the myeloma-defining events of CRAB, but meet the requirement for M-spike or clonal plasma cells are classified as having smoldering MM. Patients without myeloma-defining events but have M-spike of <3 g/dL or clonal plasma cells of <10% are classified as having monoclonal gammopathy of undermined significance (MGUS). Approximately 1% per year of MGUS patients progress to MM. There is a newer classification that describes monoclonal gammopathy–related kidney damage but without overt malignancy known as monoclonal gammopathy of renal significance (MGRS). Such hematologic malignant and premalignant conditions lead to monoclonal immunoglobulin or immunoglobulin fragments to cause kidney damage via direct or indirect toxicity. This chapter will discuss pathogenesis, clinical presentation, evaluation, and treatment of various kidney diseases that occur due to monoclonal gammopathies.

II. **LIGHT-CHAIN CAST NEPHROPATHY.** Light-chain cast nephropathy results in kidney disease due to overproduction of immunoglobulin free light chains which cause tubular injury, obstructive casts, and inflammation. It is the most common cause of kidney disease in MM patients. Light-chain cast nephropathy usually occurs with high levels of serum FLCs >100 mg/dL.

In MM, excretion of light chain can range from 100 mg to >20 mg/day which is far more than the normal excretion of <30 mg/day. Upon filtration, these light chains bind uromodulin (also known as Tamm–Horsfall mucoprotein), creating dense intratubular casts leading to obstruction with giant-cell reaction and interstitial inflammation. Once kidney injury occurs, it often progresses rapidly within days to weeks. Factors associated with aggravating monoclonal gammopathies include volume depletion from hypercalcemia, infections, and nephrotoxic agents such as NSAIDs.

Serum FLC, serum protein electrophoresis (SPEP), and immunofixation (IFE) are the main tests toward establishing the diagnosis of light-chain nephropathy. Serum FLC is very sensitive with 100% of patients having >50 mg/dL compared with SPEP (85%) and IFE (95%). On urine protein electrophoresis (UPEP), Bence Jones proteinuria (monoclonal FLC) is the predominant urine protein excreted with <10% as albumin. Although a kidney biopsy is not required, it is the gold standard for diagnosing cast nephropathy. Light microscopy (LM) often reveals sparing of the glomeruli with giant cells and intense interstitial infiltrates surrounding casts in distal tubules that may be fractured in appearance. Immunofluorescence (IF) shows casts staining for a single light chain, while electron microscopy (EM) may show crystalline features.

The overall goal of treatment is to reverse kidney injury as soon as possible due to the strong association between cast nephropathy and early mortality in patients with MM. Treatment consists of antimyeloma therapy (e.g., cyclophosphamide, bortezomib, and dexamethasone), and fluid management. The treatment goal is to decrease serum FLC by at least 60% within 3 weeks of therapy to help with renal recovery. In patients without heart failure or oliguric AKI, intravenous fluids are given to reach a urine output of 3 L/day in order to decrease light-chain concentration in tubules and correct volume depletion, hypercalcemia, and hyperuricemia. The role of extracorporeal removal of light chains is not clear. There are conflicting results in the MYRE and EuLITE trials on the benefits of high cutoff dialysis membranes which use a larger pore size than conventional high-flux dialysis filters to remove FLCs. In the MYRE trial, there was more hemodialysis independence at 6 months compared to that in standard therapy (57% vs. 34%), but no mortality difference at 12 months. Similarly, plasmapheresis can also be useful in removing FLCs, but trials have not shown a consistent benefit.

III. AMYLOIDOSIS. Amyloidosis is a systemic disease caused by protein misfolding leading to self-aggregation and formation of fibrils which commonly cause glomerular disease. There are over 30 types of amyloid. Immunoglobulin-related amyloidosis due to plasma-cell dyscrasia or B-cell lymphoproliferative diseases include immunoglobulin light-chain (AL) amyloid representing 95% of cases followed by heavy- and light-chain (AHL) amyloidosis, with heavy-chain (AH) amyloidosis being the least common. All three subtypes of immunoglobulin-related amyloidosis have similar clinical presentations with proteinuria present in nearly 75% of patients. Proteinuria is predominantly albumin (nearly 70%) on UPEP, with median levels of 5.8 g/day. Half of these patients also have elevated serum Cr, with 20% having levels >2.0 mg/dL. One study revealed that 41.6% of patients with renal manifestations required renal replacement therapy. Due to the systemic nature of the disease, patients may present with heart failure, peripheral neuropathy, orthostatic hypotension, easy bruisability, or solely kidney involvement. High suspicion for amyloidosis should prompt immediate workup.

Immunoglobulin-mediated amyloidosis is considered a low tumor burden disease. Less than 10% of patients with immunoglobulin-related amyloidosis meet the criteria for MM, and these patients are classified as MGRS. Initial evaluation should include SPEP, UPEP, IFE, and serum FLC. In immunoglobulin-related amyloidosis, the combination of SPEP and serum IFE detects monoclonal protein in 66% to 88%, whereas the combination of UPEP and urine immunofixation electrophoresis (UIFE) has a detection rate of 67% to 80%. Serum FLC assay detects abnormalities in 78% to 88% of patients. Together these tests can detect immunoglobulin protein in the majority of patients, but a tissue biopsy is required for diagnosis.

In the kidney, amyloid deposits are found in vessel walls, glomeruli, and the tubular interstitium. Under LM, amyloid deposits are eosinophilic. Congo Red stains are positive for amyloid, and this appears apple green under polarized light. IF reveals light-chain restriction for AL, both light and heavy-chain restriction for AHL, with heavy-chain restriction for AH. EM shows 7- to 12-nm amyloid fibrils which are randomly arranged within the mesangium, interstitium, and vessel walls.

The goal of treatment is to reduce production of amyloid, limit further organ damage, and allow for tissue amyloid regression. Over the past decade, median survival has increased from 18 months to 5 years. Treatment currently depends on whether patients are eligible for autologous hematopoietic cell transplantation (HCT). If eligible for HCT, it is recommended patients receive induction therapy with an anti–plasma-cell proteasome inhibitor-based regimen (either CyBorD or bortezomib-melphalan-dexamethasone known as BMD) followed by HCT with melphalan. If not eligible for HCT, then patients should be treated with CyBorD or BMD therapy. Addition of the anti–CD 38 antibody daratumumab to CyBorD appears promising for increasing complete hematologic response and increasing renal response. Assessing response to treatment should be based on SPEP and serum FLC assays. Ultimately, kidney transplantation can also be an option in conjunction with bortezomib-based chemotherapy and HCT, especially in patients without significant cardiac involvement or MM.

IV. MONOCLONAL IMMUNOGLOBULIN DEPOSITION DISEASE. In contrast to amyloidosis, light- or heavy-chain fragments in monoclonal immunoglobulin deposition disease (MIDD) do not form fibrils, do not stain with Congo Red, and usually only involve the kidney, although there may be cardiac or hepatic involvement (35%). There are three types of MIDD based on composition of deposits which include light-chain (LCDD), heavy-chain (HCDD), or light- and heavy-chain deposition disease (LHCDD). LCDD is the most common and accounts for 80% of biopsy-proven MIDD cases.

Patients with LCDD typically present with proteinuria or nephrotic syndrome with or without renal insufficiency. Patients with renal impairment often progress to ESKD requiring dialysis. Approximately 60% to 80% of patients with LCDD are classified as MGRS, with an underlying lymphoproliferative disorder. MM is present in 20% of patients with LCDD. Workup for LCDD is similar to AL amyloidosis with serum FLC assay revealing abnormality in almost all patients in contrast to serum and urine IFE (64% and 68%, respectively). LM often reveals nodular mesangial sclerosis which is periodic acid-Schiff (PAS) stain positive with thickening of the tubular basement membrane. IF shows linear staining of light chain in tubular basement membranes and glomeruli with 80% being kappa and 20% lambda. EM shows tubular and subendothelial deposits with a powdery appearance. Treatment for LCDD uses anti–plasma-cell proteasome inhibitor therapy with bortezomib-based regimens along with HCT.

HCDD is a rare MIDD with similar clinical characteristics to LCDD but involves deposition of only heavy chains. The heavy chains are truncated due to a deletion of constant domain 1 (CH1) which makes them unable to link to the light chain. Most commonly involved heavy chain is IgG. Diagnostic workup and treatment are similar to LCDD, along with the kidney biopsy findings. LM shows similar features to LCDD with mesangial nodular glomerulosclerosis with Congo Red stain negative, PAS positive, and thickening of tubular basement membrane. EM shows fine granular electron-dense deposits within the inner aspect of the glomerular basement membrane.

LHCDD is the least common type of MIDD which consists of both heavy- and light-chain deposition. The pathogenic features are not well understood, as deletion of the constant domain that leads to pathogenicity in HCDD has not been demonstrated in LHCDD. LHCDD has similar clinical characteristics, diagnostic workup, and treatment as the other MIDDs. Microscopic findings are also similar with the exception that IF reveals staining for both heavy and light chains.

V. MEMBRANOPROLIFERATIVE GLOMERULONEPHRITIS/C3 GLOMERULOPATHY/ PROLIFERATIVE GLOMERULOENEPHRITIS WITH MONOCLONAL IgG DEPOSITS.

Membranoproliferative glomerulonephritis (MPGN) represents a histologic pattern of glomerular injury from infections, autoimmune diseases, and complement dysregulation. A retrospective study after reviewing kidney biopsies of 64 patients with MPGN, not infected with hepatitis B or C, revealed that 41% had monoclonal gammopathy. Clinically, patients with MPGN from monoclonal gammopathies present similarly to other glomerulonephritis. Urine studies often show hematuria with dysmorphic red cells, occasional red cell casts, and variable amount of proteinuria. Renal function can be normal to severely impaired. Diagnostic tests to determine if MPGN is due to monoclonal gammopathy are similar to the ones discussed with other monoclonal-related kidney diseases including SPEP, UPEP, immunofixation, and serum FLC. C3 glomerulopathy (C3G) has an MPGN pattern and proliferative glomerulonephritis with monoclonal IgG deposits (PGNMID) usually does as well, although the latter may have an endocapillary proliferative or membranous GN pattern.

Patients with PGNMID most commonly present with nephrotic syndrome, kidney dysfunction, and hematuria, similar to other glomerulonephritis. PGNMID mimics immune complex glomerulonephritis. On IF, 50% of biopsies stain for IgG3 kappa deposition at the glomeruli followed by IgG3 lambda in 15%. EM reveals granular nonorganized electron-dense deposits limited to glomeruli. The treatment for patients with PGNMID depends on the presence of detectable B- or plasma-cell clone or serum/urine monoclonal protein. Up to 70% to 80% do not have detectable monoclonal gammopathy on SPEP, UPEP, IFE, serum FLC, or bone marrow aspirate. Examining IF using special techniques has revealed polyclonal Ig deposition on biopsy. If there is a detectable clone from plasma cells, VCD (bortezomib, cyclophosphamide, dexamethasone) may be used while RCD (rituximab, cyclophosphamide, dexamethasone) may be used for clones from B cells. If no clones are detected by bone marrow, empiric therapy based on the postulated origin of the clone (B cells vs. plasma cells) could be initiated. One study using this strategy for 16 patients demonstrated an 88% renal response and 38% complete renal response (urine protein

<0.5 g/day). If patients progress to ESRD, then the goal is no longer to preserve kidney function but to treat extrarenal involvement. Treatment should be continued in those awaiting kidney transplant as recurrence rate is extremely high with 90% showing recurrence within 6 months post-transplant.

C3G has an MPGN pattern and is composed of C3 glomerulonephritis (C3GN) and dense deposit disease due to overactivation of the alternative complement pathway. Although the exact mechanism is not known, it is postulated that the monoclonal gammopathy plays a central role in activation of the alternative complement pathway. The clinical presentation is similar to other MPGN as described above. Some cases of C3G were originally misdiagnosed as postinfectious GN as the glomerular disease followed an upper respiratory infection including streptococcus species. LM does not reveal any unique features and can appear as classic MPGN. IF does help in distinguishing as it shows C3 deposits along glomerular, tubular, and Bowman's capsule basement membrane with minimal to no immunoglobulin which rules out immune–complex mediated diseases. EM may show subendothelial, mesangial, and less frequent subepithelial deposits which are less intense than other deposition diseases. In addition to kidney biopsy, there are special serum tests that are now available to help diagnose C3G. In addition to serum C3 and C4, antibody testing against various C3 nephritic factors are available which are sensitive but not specific. Some of these nephritic factors include C3NeF, C3bBb, and C5NeF (most common). The treatment is based on low-quality evidence, but approach is similar to PGNMID using clone-based chemotherapy if detected versus other conventional immunosuppressive agents.

VI. OTHER GLOMERULAR DISEASES ASSOCIATED WITH MONOCLONAL GAMMOPATHY. Cryoglobulins are immunoglobulins that precipitate at cold temperatures, and dissolve at higher temperatures often caused by infections, especially hepatitis C, autoimmune disorders, and lymphoproliferative disorders. Type I cryoglobulinemia is caused and diagnosed by monoclonal immunoglobulins in serum while type II cryoglobulinemia has both monoclonal and polyclonal immunoglobulins. Patients with cryoglobulinemia due to lymphoproliferative disorders commonly present with skin, joints, and nervous system involvement. In type I cryoglobulinemia, 20% to 30% of patients have glomerulonephritis which may cause hematuria (41%), nephrotic syndrome (22%), CKD (13%), and AKI (9%). Type II cryoglobulinemic glomerulonephritis from dysproteinemia is rare.

Type I cryoglobulinemia is often associated with MGUS and MM especially with the IgG subtype while type II is most commonly associated with B-cell lymphoproliferative disorders. On LM, features are similar to typical MPGN with mesangioproliferative, endocapillary, membranoproliferative, and crescentic glomerulonephritis. Eosinophilic intracapillary deposits known as "cryoplugs" may be present. IF shows granular staining of monoclonal immunoglobulin in capillary walls and mesangium. EM also has similar MPGN findings of mesangial, subendothelial, and subepithelial electron-dense deposits. The data for treatment is limited to case reports and case series with chemotherapy and immunosuppressive therapy to treat the underlying monoclonal disease process. Plasmapheresis has also been used in severe cases with unclear efficacy.

Fibrillary glomerulonephritis (FGN) and immunotactoid glomerulopathy are rare disorders with prevalence of <1.4% in kidney biopsy series. The major distinguishing factor between the two diseases is the presence of a heat shock protein known as DNAJB9 within glomeruli of patients with FGN. The role of DNAJB9 in the pathogenesis of FGN is unclear but it is postulated to be involved in creating antigen–antibody aggregation. The clinical presentation is similar to typical GN with hematuria, proteinuria, and variable kidney impairment. LM shows typical MPGN features. Immunohistochemistry shows staining for the unique protein DNAJB9 within glomerular capillary walls and mesangium of patients with FGN as well as IgG, C3, Kappa, and lambda. EM shows random fibrillar deposits in mesangium and glomerular capillary walls that are larger (13 to 20 nm) than the ones present in amyloidosis.

Immunotactoid glomerulopathy differs from FGN by the absence of DNAJB9, and presence of microtubules that are organized in parallel arrays and are larger (mean 31 nm) than fibrils in FGN. FGN and immunotactoid glomerulopathy are difficult to treat due to lack of randomized controlled trials with a limited number of cases. No therapies have clearly shown to be beneficial, and more than half the patients progress to renal failure. Treatment targets the underlying disease if identified (malignancy such as CLL with immunotactoid glomerulopathy, monoclonal gammopathy, autoimmune disease) with chemotherapy or immunosuppressive therapy.

VII. CRYSTALLINE PODOCYTOPATHY AND PROXIMAL TUBULOPATHY. Crystalline podocytopathy is an extremely rare disease characterized by deposition of light chains that crystallize within podocytes resulting in nephrotic syndrome. Histologically, LM shows FSGS features, immunohistochemistry stains for light chains while EM shows the distinguishing feature of crystalline structures on podocytes. Due to limited data, treatment approach ranges from being conservative to involving chemo therapy or immunosuppressive agents.

Light-chain proximal tubulopathy (LCPT) is very rare and caused by crystallization of light chains within proximal tubules. Pathogenesis is thought to be due to pathologic light chains that cannot be degraded and lead to accumulation within proximal tubules upon reabsorption from filtrate. The initial clinical presentation of LCPT is unique in comparison to other monoclonal gammopathy–related kidney diseases since it rarely affects GFR but does impair tubular function. Patients will present with signs of Fanconi syndrome with aminoaciduria, normoglycemic glycosuria, proximal renal tubular acidosis (RTA), hypophosphatemia, and hypouricemia. Light chains depositing within the distal tubules due to decreased reabsorption of light chain can cause a type 1 RTA. Light-chain kappa is present in 95% of patients, specifically V-kappa 1, which blocks lysosomal degradation. Noncrystalline LCPT is rare and reveals patchy tubular injury. IF stains for kappa light chain within crystals. EM is diagnostic showing polygonal, rectangular, rod-shaped, or needle-like crystalline inclusions within proximal tubular cells. Treatment of the underlying hematologic disease with antiproteosome therapy while conservatively managing electrolyte abnormalities. Overall, LCPT may lead to a slow progression of chronic kidney disease over several years with low-grade proteinuria. As with the other rare monoclonal-related kidney diseases, more cases and treatment trials are needed to build a more robust approach to therapy.

VIII. SUMMARY

Diagnosis	Clinical presentation	Pathophysiology	Kidney biopsy
Light-chain cast nephropathy	AKI proteinuria which is predominantly light chain	Light chain binds uromodulin-creating intratubular casts resulting in obstruction and inflammation	**LM:** Giant cells in distal tubules with intense infiltrates, spares glomeruli. **IF:** Single light-chain casts. **EM:** Crystalline features.
Monoclonal Immunoglobulin amyloidosis	Monoclonal light-chain (AL) amyloidosis Monoclonal heavy-chain (AH) amyloidosis Monoclonal light- and heavy-chain (AHL) amyloidosis	Proteinuria (mostly albumin), kidney impairment	Monoclonal proteins self-aggregate to form fibrils which deposit within glomeruli	**LM:** Amyloid stains for Congo Red and appears apple green under polarized light, spikes along GBM. **IF:** Light-chain restriction for AL and AHL, heavy-chain restriction for AH and AHL. **EM:** Amyloid fibrils as solid and randomly arranged 8–12-nm deposits within mesangium, interstitium, and vessel walls, spikes along GBM.

(*continued*)

Diagnosis		Clinical presentation	Pathophysiology	Kidney biopsy
Monoclonal immunoglobulin deposition disease (MIDD)	Light-chain deposition disease (LCDD)	Nephrotic syndrome with or without renal insufficiency	Deposition of pathologic light chain	**LM:** Nodular glomerulosclerosis with Congo Red stain negative, PAS positive, and thickening of tubular basement membrane. **IF:** Linear light chain in tubular basement membranes and glomeruli with 80% being kappa and 20% lambda. **EM:** Fine granular electron-dense deposits within the inner aspect of the glomerular basement membrane and outer aspect of the tubular basement membrane.
	Heavy-chain deposition disease (HCDD)		Deposition of heavy chains that is truncated due to a deletion of constant domain 1 (CH1) which makes them unable to link to the light chain	**LM, IF, and EM:** Similar to LCDD.
	Light- and heavy-chain deposition disease (LHCDD)		Deposition of both heavy- and light-chain but pathogenesis is unclear	**LM, IF,** and **EM:** Similar to LCDD and HCDD.

Membranoproliferative glomerulonephritis	Proliferative GN with monoclonal deposits (PGNMID)	Hematuria, variable proteinuria, and kidney impairment typical of MPGN	Deposition of monoclonal immunoglobulin with glomerular inflammation	**LM:** Endocapillary proliferative glomerulonephritis with membranous features, classic MPGN features. **IF:** 50% stain for IgG3 kappa deposition at the glomeruli followed by IgG3 lambda in 15%. **EM:** Granular nonorganized electron-dense deposits.
	C3 glomerulopathy	Typical MPGN, may follow upper respiratory infection	Activation of alternative complement pathway	**LM:** Classic MPGN features. **IF:** C3 deposits along glomerular, tubular, and Bowman's capsule basement membrane. **EM:** Subendothelial, mesangial, and less frequently subepithelial deposits which are less intense than other deposition diseases.
Rare monoclonal gammopathies	Type I cryoglobulinemic GN	Most commonly present with extrarenal symptoms involving skin, joints, and nervous system. 20% present with typical GN: hematuria, nephrotic syndrome, CKD, and AKI	Deposition of monoclonal immunoglobulin	**LM:** Typical MPGN: mesangioproliferative, endocapillary, membranoproliferative and crescentic glomerulonephritis. See intracapillary deposits ("cryoplugs"). **IF:** Granular staining of monoclonal immunoglobulin in capillary walls and mesangium. **EM:** MPGN findings of mesangial, subendothelial, and subepithelial electron-dense deposits.

(*continued*)

Diagnosis		Clinical presentation	Pathophysiology	Kidney biopsy
	Fibrillary glomerulonephritis (FGN)	Typical GN: hematuria, proteinuria, and variable kidney impairment	DNAJB9 plays a central role in pathogenesis of FGN through unclear mechanism, possibly through antigen–antibody aggregation	**LM:** Typical MPGN features. **IF:** DNAJB9 protein within glomerular capillary walls and mesangium. **EM:** Random fibrillar deposits (20 nm) in mesangium and glomerular capillary walls that are larger than the ones present in amyloidosis.
	Immunotactoid glomerulopathy		Formation of microtubules that are larger than fibrils in FGN	**LM, IF:** Similar to FGN but does not stain for DNAJB9. **EM:** Microtubules organized in parallel arrays (~30 nm).
Crystalline monoclonal gammopathy	Crystalline podocytopathy	Nephrotic syndrome	Deposition of light chains that crystallize within podocytes	**LM:** Typical FSGS features: Focal and segmental glomerulosclerosis and mesangial sclerosis. **IF:** Stains for light chains. **EM:** Crystalline structures in podocytes.
	Light-chain proximal tubulopathy (LCPT)	Rarely affects GFR, signs of Fanconi syndrome: aminoaciduria, normoglycemic glycosuria, proximal renal tubular acidosis (RTA), hypophosphatemia, and hypouricemia	Crystallization of pathologic light chains (V-kappa 1) that cannot be degraded and lead to accumulation within proximal tubules	**LM:** Varying degree of tubular atrophy and interstitial fibrosis. **IF:** Kappa light chain within crystals. **EM:** Polygonal, rectangular, rod shaped, or needle-like crystalline inclusions within proximal tubular cells.

IX. SUGGESTED READINGS

Bridoux F, Leung N, Hutchison CA, et al. Diagnosis of monoclonal gammopathy of renal significance. *Kidney Int.* 2015;87(4):698–711. doi: 10.1038/ki.2014.408

Fernández de Larrea C, Verga L, Morbini P, et al. A practical approach to the diagnosis of systemic amyloidoses. *Blood.* 2015;125(14):2239–2244. doi: 10.1182/blood-2014-11-609883

Hogan JJ, Alexander PA, Leung N. Dysproteinemia and the kidney: core curriculum 2019. *Am J Kidney Dis.* 2019;74:822–836. doi 10.153/j/ajkd.2019.04.029

Hutchison CA, Bradwell AR, Cook M, et al. Treatment of acute renal failure secondary to multiple myeloma with chemotherapy and extended high cut-off hemodialysis. *Clin J Am Soc Nephrol.* 2009;4(4):745–754. doi: 10.2215/CJN.04590908

Leung N, Bridoux F, Nasr SH. Monoclonal gammopathy of renal significance. *N Engl J Med.* 2021;384(20):1931–1941. doi:10.1056/MEJMra181097

Rosenstock JL, Markowitz GS, Valeri AM, et al. Fibrillary and immunotactoid glomerulonephritis: distinct entities with different clinical and pathologic features. *Kidney Int.* 2003;63(4):1450–1461. doi: 10.1046/j.1523-1755.2003.00853.x

Stokes MB, Valeri AM, Herlitz L, et al. Light chain proximal tubulopathy: clinical and pathologic characteristics in the modern treatment era. *J Am Soc Nephrol.* 2016;27(5):1555–1565. doi: 10.1681/ASN.2015020185

12 Tubulointerstitial Nephritis

Wen Shen

I. **DEFINITION AND DESCRIPTION.** *Tubulointerstitial nephritis* (TIN) refers to the inflammation, cellular infiltration, and fibrosis of the renal tubules and interstitium, with relative sparing of the glomeruli early in the disease. A variety of infectious, allergic, and infiltrative diseases can cause TIN. Although tubulointerstitial inflammation can be seen with many glomerular diseases, the glomerular abnormalities are the predominant or primary features of these conditions. The clinical spectrum of TIN ranges from acute interstitial nephritis (AIN), with a sudden onset of acute renal failure requiring renal replacement therapy, to chronic interstitial nephritis, with a smoldering course culminating in end-stage renal disease (ESRD). Table 12.1 lists the causes of acute and chronic TIN.

II. **PATHOGENESIS.** TIN is an immunologic response to diverse etiologic agents. Drugs are among the most common cause of TIN. Drug-induced TIN usually results from cell-mediated hypersensitivity reactions and is termed allergic interstitial nephritis. The interstitial inflammation and edema as well as damage to tubular cells result in tubular obstruction and acute kidney injury. Generally, this inflammation is reversible once the offending agent is withdrawn, but prolonged exposure leads to irreversible and progressive renal insufficiency.

Chronic interstitial nephritis has an insidious onset. It is characterized by tubular cell atrophy, tubular dilatation, and interstitial fibrosis. It is commonly associated with tubular dysfunction, Fanconi syndrome, type IV renal tubular acidosis with hyperkalemia, and low–molecular-weight proteinuria.

The fibroblast is the primary cell type responsible for chronic fibrosis. The tubular epithelial cells constitute the major source of fibroblasts by a process called epithelial–mesenchymal transdifferentiation (EMT). These EMT cells secrete extracellular matrix. Fibrogenesis is enhanced by proteinuria and hypoxia. Proteinuria promotes tubular epithelial cell secretion of cytokines, whereas hypoxia activates fibroblasts and triggers EMT. Transforming growth factor-beta 1 (TGF-β1) acts as a chemoattractant for fibroblasts, induces proliferation of fibroblastic cells, and increases the transcription of genes encoding proteins of the extracellular matrix. TGF-β1 also inhibits the production of metalloproteinases that degrade the matrix and increases the production of tissue inhibitors of metalloproteinases, which are their natural inhibitors. These reactions result in expansion of tissue matrix, interstitial fibrosis, and tubular atrophy. Activation of nuclear factor kB by oxidative stress or TGF-β1 causes transcription and release of other proinflammatory cytokines. Activation of the renin–angiotensin system contributes to maintaining this cycle of inflammation and fibrosis.

TABLE 12.1 Causes of tubulointerstitial nephritis	
Acute tubulointerstitial nephritis	**Chronic tubulointerstitial nephritis**
Hypersensitivity reactions (penicillin, sulfonamides, nonsteroidal anti-inflammatory drugs)	Drugs (analgesics, lithium, cyclosporine, tacrolimus)
Immunologic disease (SLE, Goodpasture syndrome)	Proton pump inhibitor, antibiotics (beta lactams, cephalosporins, sulfonamides, rifampin, vancomycin, ethambutol, erythromycin), diuretics, allopurinol
Acute transplant rejection	
Infections	Heavy metals (lead, cadmium, mercury)
Bacterial (associated with chronic obstruction or reflux)	Obstructive uropathy, nephrolithiasis, reflux disease
Viral (BK polyoma virus, cytomegalovirus, hantavirus, human immunodeficiency virus, hepatitis B)	Immunologic diseases (SLE, Sjogren syndrome, primary glomerulopathies, sarcoidosis)
Fungal < histoplasmosis	Vasculitis (antineutrophil, cytoplasmic antibody-associated, Wegener granulomatosis)
	Chronic allograft nephropathy
Parasitic (leishmania, toxoplasmosis)	Atherosclerotic kidney disease (ischemic nephropathy, cholesterol, microemboli)
	Metabolic diseases (hypercalcemia, cystitis, hyperoxaluria)
	Genetic diseases (Alport syndrome, medullary cystic kidney)
	Miscellaneous (Balkan endemic nephropathy, Chinese herb, *Aristolochia* nephropathy)

SLE, systemic lupus erythematosus.

III. CLINICAL PRESENTATION AND DIAGNOSIS. AIN is encountered in 2% to 3% of renal biopsies. Chronic interstitial nephritis accounts for 5% of cases of ESRD in the United States. Drug exposure accounts for the majority of cases of AIN. Other causes include sarcoidosis, Legionella, leptospirosis, streptococcal, and viral infections. Renal biopsy generally does not show any immune deposits, but the interstitial infiltrates are rich in T cells. The major histologic changes are interstitial edema and marked interstitial infiltrates that can include eosinophils, plasma cells, and neutrophils. Granuloma formation is characteristic of sarcoidosis but is not commonly seen on biopsy and can occur in any form of AIN.

Common clinical features are listed in Table 12.2. Fever, rash, white cells and/or white cell casts in urinalysis, eosinophilia, and eosinophiluria are typically absent in nonsteroidal anti-inflammatory drug (NSAID)-associated AIN. Eosinophiluria (eosinophils >1% of urinary white cells by Hansel stain) has a sensitivity and specificity of 67% and 83%, respectively, for the diagnosis of AIN after exclusion of those due to NSAIDs. Therefore, the absence of eosinophiluria does not exclude the diagnosis of AIN. Pyuria is also variable, being present in >90% of methicillin-induced AIN, but in <50% of cases induced by NSAIDs, and

TABLE 12.2 Clinical features of acute and chronic tubulointerstitial nephritis

Acute tubulointerstitial nephritis	Chronic tubulointerstitial nephritis
Begins abruptly with acute renal failure	Insidious onset
Occurs within days of exposure to offending drug or several months to NSAIDs	Often diagnosed incidentally on routine screening or evaluation of hypertension
Rash, fever eosinophilia, eosinophiluria, and elevated immunoglobulin E	Patients are usually asymptomatic
Tubular function abnormalities ± Fanconi syndrome	Hypertension is common
	Elevation in serum creatinine, tubular dysfunction (renal tubular acidosis), or Fanconi syndrome
Proteinuria is usually absent or mild ± microscopic hematuria ± sterile pyuria	Proteinuria is usually mild (<1 g/day) and of low molecular weight
Renal biopsy may be required to make a definitive diagnosis	Renal biopsy shows interstitial fibrosis, tubular atrophy, arteriolar sclerosis, and mononuclear cell infiltrate
NSAID-induced tubulointerstitial nephritis may present with nephritic-range proteinuria from minimal change disease	Papillary necrosis with analgesic nephropathy causes gross hematuria, flank pain ± obstruction

NSAID, nonsteroidal anti-inflammatory drug.

at 50% in other drug-induced causes. If it is drug related, TIN occurs between 1 and 3 weeks after exposure to the medication with an average of 10 days. Renal sonogram reveals increased cortical echogenicity and enlarged or normal-sized kidneys. Peripheral eosinophilia, eosinophiluria, and hypocomplementemia are frequent findings in atheroembolic renal disease seen after intravascular procedures, trauma, and thrombolytic therapy in patients with extensive atherosclerosis. A renal biopsy is generally not needed to establish the diagnosis except in patients who present with advanced renal failure, or when the history and laboratory findings do not lead to a clear diagnosis, and in cases where renal function does not improve after the offending agent is discontinued.

IV. TREATMENT OF ACUTE TUBULOINTERSTITIAL NEPHRITIS. In most cases, cessation of the offending agent results in quick recovery and complete resolution, although some patients progress to chronic kidney disease. If no sign of improvement is observed within a few days of discontinuation, renal biopsy or empiric therapy with corticosteroids may be considered. Although controlled trials are lacking, many authors suggest using prednisone at 1 mg/kg for 2 to 6 weeks, with rapid tapering of the dose. Retrospective studies have shown that corticosteroid therapy improves recovery time of TIN, and reduced the risk of incomplete renal recovery, especially when started early. However, in some studies, renal function did not differ after corticosteroid treatment and supportive care groups in the retrospective studies.

V. TREATMENT OF CHRONIC TUBULOINTERSTITIAL NEPHRITIS. Treatment depends on the cause but includes adequate blood pressure control and management of anemia. There is no role for corticosteroid therapy in chronic TIN. Some experimental therapies with the inhibitors of EMT, bone morphogenic protein-7, hepatocyte growth factor, TGF-β, and fibroblast signal transduction are under investigation to arrest tubulointerstitial fibrosis.

A. **Nonsteroidal Anti-Inflammatory Drug-Induced Acute Interstitial Nephritis with Nephrotic Syndrome.** All nonselective NSAIDs and COX-2 inhibitors can cause this syndrome of acute kidney injury, interstitial infiltrates composed of T lymphocytes, and minimal change glomerulonephritis. Affected patients present with hematuria, ±pyuria, ±white cell casts, proteinuria, and an acute rise in plasma creatinine concentration. The manifestations of an allergic reaction (fever, rash, eosinophilia, and eosinophiluria) are typically absent. Spontaneous resolution generally occurs within weeks to months after therapy is discontinued. There is no clear evidence that corticosteroid therapy is beneficial in this setting. However, a course of prednisone may be warranted in patients whose acute kidney injury persists more than 1 to 2 weeks after discontinuation of the offending agent.

B. **Aristolochic Acid Nephropathy.** This syndrome of chronic TIN was first reported in Belgium, where 14 cases of advanced renal failure were reported in women using Chinese herbs at a weight loss clinic. The histologic findings include severe tubular atrophy and interstitial fibrosis without inflammatory infiltrates or glomerular damage. The pathogenesis is not clearly understood, but the nephrotoxicity of aristolochic acid (AA) was confirmed in animal models. There is no specific therapy for this disease, which follows a progressive course to ESRD. Due to the high incidence of cellular atypia and carcinogenesis, regular surveillance with urinary cytology is recommended. Renal transplantation can be successful in these patients.

C. **BK Polyoma Viral Nephritis.** This syndrome of acute kidney injury and interstitial nephritis is seen in up to 5% of renal allograft recipients after about 1 year of transplantation. Its incidence has increased sharply since the introduction of more potent immunosuppressive agents. The clinical manifestations resemble those of acute rejection and include renal dysfunction, resulting in either an acute or slowly progressive rise in serum creatinine. The urinalysis is consistent with interstitial nephritis. A renal biopsy is needed to establish the diagnosis and to rule out concomitant acute cellular rejection. Specific findings include the characteristic intranuclear viral inclusions, which can be confirmed by a positive immunohistologic or in situ hybridization for the BK virus. Therapy requires reducing the degree of immunosuppression while closely monitoring for acute cellular rejection. Antiviral therapy with cidofovir or leflunomide has been shown to have efficacy in some studies, but the results are not consistent. These agents have not shown a superior effect to reducing immunosuppressant dose alone. Therefore, they should not be routinely used to treat BK viral nephritis. Serial urinary and blood PCR for BK polyoma virus should be performed to monitor the response to therapy and to detect a relapse.

D. **Tubulointerstitial Nephritis and Uveitis Syndrome.** Tubulointerstitial nephritis and uveitis syndrome (TINU) is a rare disorder predominantly affects young women and has no identifiable risk factors. Diagnosis requires both TIN and uveitis but remains a diagnosis of exclusion. Patients with uveitis present with red painful eyes bilaterally associated with photophobia and decreased vision. Constitutional symptoms include fever, weight loss, fatigue, malaise, anorexia, asthenia, abdominal and flank pain, arthralgias, myalgias, headache, polyuria, and/or nocturia. Laboratory findings may include eosinophilia, anemia, abnormal liver function tests, and an elevated erythrocyte sedimentation rate. The renal disease is self-limited and requires no specific treatment, except in patients with progressive renal dysfunction. The role of immunosuppressive therapies in treating TINU is not well established. But uveitis should be treated with topical or systemic corticosteroids and should be managed by an ophthalmologist. Refractory cases of uveitis can be treated with azathioprine, methotrexate, cyclosporine, or mycophenolate mofetil. Human leukocyte antigen (HLA) DR and DQ alleles have been reported to be associated with TINU and might be the risk alleles.

E. **TIN Associated with Inflammatory Bowel Disease**. TIN has been associated with inflammatory bowel disease (IBD). The occurrence of TIN in IBD may be secondary to systemic inflammation, susceptibility to autoimmunity, exposure to medications, genetic predisposition, malnutrition, and infection. Inflammation and disease activity in IBD have been shown to correlate with low–molecular-weight proteinuria. Mesalamine, a frequently used agent to treat IBD, is a well-known medication associated with TIN.

F. **IgG4-Associated Immune Complex Multiorgan Autoimmune Disease**. Multiorgan autoimmune disease (MAD) has been linked to TIN. The patients present with C3 and C4 hypocomplementemia and TIN along with other organ involvement such as autoimmune pancreatitis, lymphadenopathy, sialadenitis, and retroperitoneal fibrosis. Interstitial IgG4-positive plasma-cell infiltration and C3 deposition are frequently observed in addition to elevated serum IgG and IgE levels. IgG4-associated TIN usually responds well to corticosteroids.

VI. SUGGESTED READINGS

Gonzalez E, Gutierrez E, Galeano C, et al. Early steroid treatment improves the recovery of renal function in patients with drug-induced acute interstitial nephritis. *Kidney Int*. 2008;73(8): 940–946.

Iwano M, Neilson EG. Mechanisms of tubulointerstitial fibrosis. *Curr Opin Nephrol Hypertens*. 2004;13(3):279–284.

Joyce E, Glasner P, Ranganathan S, et al. Tubulointerstitial nephritis: diagnosis, treatment, and monitoring. *Pediatr Nephrol*. 2017;32(4):577–587.

Rodriguez-Iturbe B, Johnson RJ, Herrera-Acosta J. Tubulointerstitial damage and progression of renal failure. *Kidney Int*. 2005;68(Suppl 99):S82–S86.

Rossert J. Drug-induced acute interstitial nephritis. *Kidney Int*. 2001;60(2):804–817.

Schwarz A, Krause PH, Kunzendorf U, et al. The outcome of acute interstitial nephritis: risk factors for the transition from acute to chronic interstitial nephritis. *Clin Nephrol*. 2000;54(3):179–190.

13

Renal Involvement in Viral Diseases and HIV

Saraswathi Gopal

Viruses cause a diverse array of diseases in the kidney and the genitourinary tract. Pathologic mechanisms include cytopathic injury through direct invasion of the cells, immune complex–mediated damage, or as part of sepsis-related multi-organ failure (systemic inflammatory response syndrome). This chapter reviews the spectrum of renal involvement associated with various viral infections.

I. **HUMAN IMMUNODEFICIENCY VIRUS INFECTION.** Patients infected with the human immunodeficiency virus (HIV) may develop numerous renal complications. They are at risk for acute kidney injury (AKI) and chronic kidney disease (CKD) (Fig. 13.1). Any condition that presents as AKI can lead to CKD if not promptly addressed. In addition, fluid and electrolyte abnormalities are common. In particular, hyponatremia is frequently observed and, in most cases, is due to volume depletion with water retention from the appropriate stimulation of antidiuretic hormone. Patients with HIV infection may also be at risk for developing the syndrome of inappropriate secretion of antidiuretic hormone in association with infection or drug use. Some patients manifest hyponatremia (often with hyperkalemia) as an indication of adrenal insufficiency secondary to HIV infection. Disorders of potassium, calcium, and magnesium balance may also be seen. Management of these disorders is discussed in Chapters 17 to 20.

A. **Acute Kidney Injury in the HIV-Infected Patient.** AKI is a frequent complication in patients with HIV infection, especially those with the clinical picture of acquired immune deficiency syndrome (AIDS). Diagnosis is essentially the same as in any patient who manifests a rising level of blood urea nitrogen or serum creatinine (see Chapter 35). Ruling out prerenal causes is critical because many patients may develop volume depletion secondary to diarrhea and poor oral intake. The usual causes of AKI such as sepsis and the use of radiocontrast agents are also common. Postrenal causes may also occur secondary to obstruction from stones or tumors or autonomic dysfunction of the bladder.

There are also specific etiologies of AKI that one should consider in the HIV-infected patient. A major category relates to the nephrotoxicity of various drugs commonly used to treat HIV-infected patients, including aminoglycosides, amphotericin B, foscarnet, and pentamidine. Acyclovir and valacyclovir, when used at high doses, and particularly in patients with pre-existing renal insufficiency, may lead to high urinary concentrations of these drugs, resulting in crystal formation and acute tubular obstruction (appearing as needle-like crystals on urinary sediment examination). Certain protease inhibitors, notably indinavir and atazanavir, have been found to cause acute nephrotoxicity by forming intratubular crystals and nephrolithiasis leading to microscopic

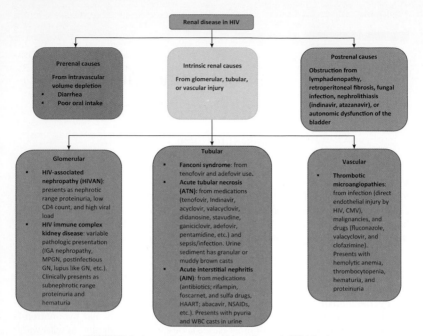

FIGURE 13.1: Approach to evaluate kidney disease in HIV infection.

and, occasionally, gross hematuria and renal failure. Nucleoside reverse transcriptase inhibitors such as abacavir can cause acute interstitial nephritis, leading to AKI. The use of the nucleotide reverse transcriptase inhibitor, tenofovir fumarate, has been associated with development of the Fanconi syndrome, AKI due to injury to the proximal tubule, and nephrogenic diabetes insipidus. The use of high-dose sulfadiazines to treat toxoplasmosis may be associated with crystalluria (appearing as "haystacks") in AKI. Acute interstitial nephritis may also develop secondary to the use of rifampin, foscarnet, or the sulfa class of antibiotics.

In addition to drug toxicities, HIV infection can be associated with an acute thrombotic microangiopathy (TMA) believed to be due to endothelial cell injury and clinically similar to thrombotic thrombocytopenic purpura or hemolytic uremic syndrome. Finally, HIV may be associated with a variety of glomerular diseases, some of which may present with a relatively acute deterioration in renal function (see below).

There is little doubt that AKI contributes to mortality and morbidity in HIV-infected patients, although sepsis remains the leading cause of death. Apart from management of AKI, treatment should also be directed at the underlying cause of AKI. The decision to initiate renal replacement therapy for AKI in HIV-infected patients should be made using the same clinical criteria as in non–HIV-infected patients.

B. **Chronic Kidney Disease in HIV-Infected Patient.** HIV-associated nephropathy (HIVAN) presents as nephrotic range proteinuria and renal failure in patients with high viral load and low CD4 counts. The disease usually presents in patients with acquired immunodeficiency syndrome (AIDS) who have a CD4 cell count $<200 \times 10^3$ cells/mL, but it may occur at any stage, including the acute presentation of HIV infection. The pathologic lesion associated with HIVAN is collapsing form of focal segmental glomerulosclerosis (FSGS). Other findings include microcystic renal tubular dilatation, interstitial inflammation, fibrosis, and tubuloreticular inclusion bodies. Since the introduction of HAART, the prevalence of HIVAN has decreased significantly due to adequate viral suppression. HIVAN is disproportionately more common in people of African descent. This has been associated with the high prevalence of specific APOL1 (apolipoprotein 1) gene risk variants (G1 and G2) in this population. These specific risk variants of APOL1 gene are hypothesized to have evolved to provide innate resistance against infection from *Trypanosoma brucei* subspecies. Interaction between environmental factors and APOL1 gene risk variants (G1 and G2) determine the strength of association between these genetic variants and HIVAN. The use of highly active antiretroviral therapy is central to the effective treatment of HIV-associated nephropathy. In addition, the use of angiotensin-converting enzyme inhibitors or angiotensin receptor blockers will help with proteinuria control and can eventually slow the progression of the disease. Untreated HIVAN can rapidly progress to end-stage renal disease (ESRD).

HIV infection leads to aberrant regulation of the immune system resulting in polyclonal gammopathy and immune complex formation. These immune complexes deposit in the kidney resulting in HIV immune–mediated kidney disease. Histologically, it manifests as varying degrees of endocapillary proliferation and inflammation presenting either as IgA nephropathy, postinfectious glomerulonephritis, lupus-like glomerulonephritis, membranoproliferative glomerulonephritis, mesangial proliferative glomerulonephritis, or membranous nephropathy. In the absence of clear evidence regarding the most effective therapy for HIV immune–mediated kidney disease, HAART is used in patients with this condition. The role of immunosuppressive therapy is controversial.

A small number of HIV-infected patients have developed TMA. This manifests as hemolytic anemia, thrombocytopenia, hematuria, proteinuria with or without neurologic deficits, and fever. HIV has direct cytotoxic effect on the endothelial cells and can precipitate TMA. Other coexisting conditions like malignancies, opportunistic infections, and medication use (fluconazole, valacyclovir, and clofazimine) can also play a role in the pathogenesis of TMA in patients with HIV infection.

In the early days of treatment of end-stage renal failure due to HIV, hemodialysis provided little long-term survival, as most patients died from the infectious complications of their HIV. After the introduction of HAART, many HIV-infected patients do well on hemodialysis. There is no difference in survival benefit between hemodialysis and peritoneal dialysis in patients with HIV infection. During hemodialysis, standard universal protocol is used, no isolation is required. Effluent from peritoneal dialysis should be treated as contaminated fluid since HIV can survive in the effluent fluid tubing for a variable amount of time. Some centers perform kidney transplantation in selected HIV-infected patients who have maintained normal levels of CD4 cells and have undetectable viral loads. Renal allograft survival has been reported to compare favorably with that of uninfected patients receiving renal transplantation.

II. OTHER VIRUS INFECTION
A. Hepatitis B Virus. Kidney disease in chronic hepatitis B infection presents as immune complex–mediated glomerulonephritis. Common manifestations

are membranous nephropathy (MN), membranoproliferative glomerulone-phritis (MPGN) and immune complex–related vasculitis, that is, polyarteritis nodosa (PAN). Other associations include mesangioproliferative glomerulo-nephritis and IgA nephropathy. The prevalence of HBV-associated kidney dis-ease depends on the geographic prevalence of HBV infection. Membranous nephropathy is more common in children whereas MPGN is the common manifestation in adults with chronic HBV infection. HBV-associated renal disease is treated with antiviral therapy. Kidney Disease Improving Global Outcomes (KDIGO) recommends the use of interferon or oral antiviral agents that consist of either one of the nucleotides (adefovir dipivoxil, tenofovir diso-proxil fumarate, tenofovir alafenamide) or nucleoside (lamivudine, entecavir, and telbivudine) analogs. Entecavir or tenofovir is usually preferred based on efficacy profile. If tenofovir is used, tenofovir alafenamide is preferred since it is associated with a low risk of nephrotoxicity compared to tenofovir diso-proxil fumarate. Corticosteroids may be given for a short period (<6 months) in patients who present with rapidly progressive glomerulonephritis (crescen-tic glomerulonephritis). Hepatitis B patients undergoing dialysis are placed in isolation in addition to standard universal protocol since HBV is highly viable on environmental surfaces.

B. **Hepatitis C Virus.** Kidney disease is one of the more common extrahepatic mani-festations present in patients with chronic HCV. The most common HCV-related nephropathy is MPGN, usually in the context of mixed cryoglobulinemia. Other manifestations include membranous nephropathy and PAN. HCV-infected patients should be evaluated for proteinuria, hematuria, hypertension, and a reduced glomerular filtration rate. Patients who are found to have renal abnor-malities should undergo testing for cryoglobulins, hypocomplementemia, and a positive rheumatoid factor. A kidney biopsy should be considered in patients with renal impairment. Treatment involves antiviral therapy; the development of potent direct-acting antiviral agents (DAAs) against HCV has enabled suc-cessful eradication of HCV with minimal side effects. They also cause resolu-tion of cryoglobulinemia, and glomerular lesions. Glecaprevir-pibrentasvir and sofosbuvir containing combinations are the commonly used DAAs. In addition to antiviral therapy, patients with severe cryoglobulinemia or PAN are treated with immunosuppressive therapy.

C. **Cytomegalovirus (CMV).** CMV infection occurs most commonly in immunocompro-mised individuals including those who have HIV, cancer and those who are organ transplant recipients. Infection with CMV can cause a viral syndrome (with fever, fatigue, myalgias, and leucopenia) or tissue invasive disease (like gastritis, duo-denitis, pneumonitis, etc.). The incidence of CMV infection in organ transplant recipients depends on the donor and recipient CMV serology profiles. Patients present with AKI in the setting of findings of systemic infection. CMV infec-tion is associated with a risk of acute rejection in renal transplant recipients. Diagnostic modalities include serology, qualitative and quantitative polymerase chain reaction (PCR), pp65 antigenemia, culture, and histopathology. Pathologic findings on renal biopsy include tubulointerstitial nephritis with lymphocytes and plasma cells along with cytomegaly (in tubular and endothelial cells) and viral inclusion bodies (characteristic intranuclear basophilic inclusion bodies with surrounding halo called "owl's eye-type nuclear inclusions"). Diagnosis is confirmed by immunohistochemical staining for CMV. The drugs of choice for CMV syndrome and tissue-invasive CMV disease are valganciclovir or intrave-nous ganciclovir. The treatment is usually continued for a minimum of 2 weeks or until the clinical symptoms have resolved and the virus is undetectable on quantitative analysis.

D. Polyoma Virus (BK). Polyoma virus–associated nephropathy (PVAN) is an important infection in renal allograft recipients mostly occurring within the first year after renal transplantation. Infection with polyoma virus is ubiquitous, with a seroprevalence rate of 70% to 90% in adults. This virus exhibits tropism for the renal tubular cells and immunosuppression leads to reactivation of the latent infection causing graft dysfunction. Characteristic histologic findings on renal biopsy include epithelial cell enlargement, karyomegaly, intranuclear viral inclusion bodies along with varying degrees of interstitial inflammation. Diagnosis is confirmed by immunohistochemistry (using an antibody to SV40 large T antigen) or electron microscopy showing virions of 40-nm diameter. Monitoring using nucleic acid testing of BKV in blood and urine is recommended for early detection of infection. Decoy cells seen on urine cytology originate from infected renal tubular cells with nuclei altered by viral inclusions. The presence of decoy cells is a sensitive (~99%) measure but has a low positive predictive value (29%). The mainstay of therapy is reduction of the immunosuppressive therapy. Secondary medications like cidofovir, leflunomide, and fluoroquinolones have been used to treat PVAN with variable results.

E. Parvovirus (B19). Parvovirus has been associated with collapsing FSGS, endocapillary and mesangioproliferative glomerulonephritis. Proliferative glomerulonephritis presents as nephrotic syndrome with hypocomplementemia after a prodrome of fever, rash, and arthritis. Apart from glomerular disease, parvovirus infection can also cause pure red cell aplasia in renal transplant recipients and a transient aplastic crisis in ESRD patients. Serology is of limited value in diagnosis, PCR is used to confirm infection. There is no specific therapy for parvovirus infection. Spontaneous recovery is the norm in immunocompetent individuals. In immunosuppressed individuals, reduction of immunosuppression, and/or intravenous immunoglobulin (IVIG) can help recovery.

F. Other Viruses. Hantavirus infection is caused by inhalation of aerosolized viral particles from infected rodents' urinary or fecal secretions. Hantaviruses affect lungs and kidneys. It is responsible for "hemorrhagic fever with renal syndrome (HFRS)." Clinically, patients with HFRS present with sudden onset of flu-like syndrome with fever, myalgia, and headache followed by gastrointestinal symptoms and AKI. Pathogenic mechanisms leading to renal dysfunction include direct damage to vascular endothelium, complement activation, and cytokine-mediated damage to the tubulointerstitial space. Acute tubulointerstitial nephritis with mononuclear cells and CD8+cell infiltration is the most prominent finding in renal histopathology. Therapy is restricted to supportive care. There is no specific treatment for hantavirus.

Dengue viral infection is caused through the bite of the infected female Aedes aegypti. AKI occurs in 10% to 30% of patients infected with dengue and mostly occurs in patients with dengue hemorrhagic fever or dengue shock syndrome. AKI occurs as a result of hypovolemia, capillary leak, or rhabdomyolysis. Glomerulonephritis has also been reported in dengue infections and could be due to immune-complex deposition or direct viral damage to the kidneys. Treatment includes supportive measures.

Patients with moderate to severe SARS-CoV2 infection can have AKI. Renal impairment has been attributed to intravascular volume depletion, tubulointerstitial nephritis, rhabdomyolysis, and multiorgan failure. Infection with SARS-CoV2 has been associated with glomerular lesions as well (minimal change disease, collapsing glomerulopathy, and immune-mediated glomerular disease). Our understanding of renal involvement in SARS-CoV2 infection continues to evolve.

III. SUGGESTED READINGS

Cohen SD, Kopp JB, Kimmel PL. Kidney diseases associated with human immunodeficiency virus infection. *N Engl J Med.* 2017;377(24):2363–2374.

D'Agati V, Appel GB. HIV infection and the kidney. *J Am Soc Nephrol.* 1997;8(1):139–152.

Daugas E, Rougier P, Hill G. HAART-related nephropathies in HIV-infected patients. *Kidney Int.* 2005;67(2):393–403.

Gupta SK, Eustace JA, Winston JA, et al. Guidelines for the management of chronic kidney disease in HIV-infected patients: recommendations of the HIV Medicine Association of the Infectious Disease Society of America. *Clin Infect Dis.* 2005;40(11):1559–1585.

Lai AS, Lai KN. Viral nephropathy. *Nat Clin Pract Nephrol.* 2006;2(5):254–262.

Szczech LA, Gupta SK, Habash R, et al. The clinical epidemiology and course of the spectrum of renal disease associated with HIV infection. *Kidney Int.* 2004;66(3):1145–1152.

Hereditary Diseases

14 Renal Cystic and Other Hereditary Diseases

Wen Shen

Renal cysts are fluid-filled cavities with epithelial linings. Simple renal cysts increase in frequency with age but are of little clinical importance. Ultrasound examination of simple renal cysts reveals a homogeneous pattern without internal echoes or calcium. Computed tomography (CT) scanning shows an attenuation value close to that of water, no enhancement with intravenous contrast, no thickening or irregularity of the cyst wall, and a smooth interface with the renal parenchyma. Cysts that lack these criteria are termed *complex* and require further evaluation as some may be malignant neoplasms.

Three adult cystic diseases cause significant complications: autosomal dominant polycystic kidney disease (adult-type ADPKD), medullary sponge kidney, and medullary cystic disease (Table 14.1). An autosomal recessive polycystic kidney disease is encountered predominantly in children. It presents with abdominal mass, liver involvement that can include portal hypertension, and renal failure. Acquired cystic disease is encountered in patients who have received dialysis treatment for several years.

Renal cysts develop from tubules, predominantly in the distal nephron, with which they retain continuity initially. As the cysts accumulate glomerular filtrate, they enlarge and eventually become isolated from the glomerulus. Thereafter, cyst expansion depends on the transepithelial transport of solutes (predominantly chloride) and fluid. Cyst formation involves proliferation of epithelial cells with production of excessive basement membrane, loss of polarity of the tubular cells, and cellular production of cytokines with ongoing tubule (cyst wall) solute secretion, followed by osmotic flow of water. Recent studies in animal models of ADPKD have demonstrated that agonist-activated cyclic adenosine monophosphate (cAMP) mediates solute transport, and leads to cyst proliferation and fluid secretion. While tubular epithelial cAMP is stimulated by many agonists, a special role for arginine vasopressin (AVP) is shown by a remarkable reduction in cyst growth in animal models of PKD treated with vasopressin type 2 (V_2) receptor antagonists, or in those with a congenital abnormality that prevents AVP action (the Brattleboro rat).

I. AUTOSOMAL DOMINANT POLYCYSTIC KIDNEY DISEASE

A. **Clinical Presentation and Diagnosis.** ADPKD is caused by mutations in the polycystin-1 or polycystin-2 genes that encode large proteins expressed in the kidneys and blood vessels. Polycystin is expressed at the base of the cilia that are found in many cells, including the renal tubular epithelium, where they dictate cell polarity and cell calcium influx during shear stress that activates cAMP and other pathways. ADPKD affects 1 in 400 to 1,000 Americans. It accounts for

TABLE 14.1 Clinical features of major renal cystic diseases

Feature	Simple renal cysts	Polycystic kidney disease	Acquired cystic disease	Medullary sponge kidney	Medullary cystic kidney disease
Incidence	1:10	1:600	Common in dialysis patients	1:5,000	Rare
Typical age at presentation	Older age	20–40 y	Variable	40–60 y	Variable
Inheritance	None	Autosomal dominant	None	Autosomal dominant	Mainly autosomal dominant
Cyst location	Variable	Mainly distal tubules	Variable	Collecting duct	Corticomedullary
Flank pain or hematuria	Rare	Frequent	Rare	With stones or infection	None
Major complications	Rare	Hypertension UTIs Renal stones Aneurysm	Renal cell carcinoma	UTIs Renal stones	Salt wasting Polyuria
Renal failure	Absent	Likely over time	Associated with pre-existing renal failure	Rare	Variable

15% of the cases of end-stage renal disease (ESRD). Approximately 85% of the cases are caused by a dominant gene located on the short arm of chromosome 16 (the PKD-1 gene) while 5% to 10% of cases result from an abnormal gene located on the long arm of chromosome 4 (the PKD-2 gene), which causes a milder phenotype of the disorder. ADPKD is associated with congenital hepatic fibrosis, hepatic cysts (in 50% of patients; the frequency increases with age), Budd–Chiari syndrome, pancreatic cysts, and colonic diverticula. Cholangio-carcinoma and cysts in the gonads, epididymis, and central nervous system occur rarely. Cardiac valvular abnormalities are present in 25% of patients and renal tubular dysfunctions manifest as impaired acidification and concentrating ability and diminished citrate excretion, predisposing to renal stones occur in some. Renal adenomas are present in 20% of patients but are rarely malignant. Cystic calcification is common. Proteinuria is usually mild (<1 g/day). Endothelial dysfunction of blood vessels contributes to hypertension, that is exacerbated by the activation of the renin–angiotensin and sympathetic nervous systems. Anemia is less common than anticipated from the degree of renal failure because of persistent erythropoietin production.

B. **Screening.** The screening test of choice for ADPKD is renal ultrasound. The diagnosis requires a family history and at least two cysts in the kidneys before age 30; at least two cysts in each kidney aged 30 to 59 and four cysts in each kidney aged more than 60. CT and magnetic resonance imaging (MRI) are more sensitive and require more cysts for diagnosis. An imaging study is not sufficient to diagnose ADPKD when the family history is negative. Genetic testing should be considered when a definite diagnosis is required, such as a young family member being evaluated for kidney donation. Fewer than 25% of ADPKD-1 gene carriers have detectable renal cysts before the age of 30 years. Screening of a presymptomatic, normotensive subject born from an affected parent is not recommended currently given that an effective treatment is still not available.

C. **Classification of Disease Progression.** Predicting the risk of ADPKD progression is important to identify the patients who may benefit from specific treatment and to project their prognosis. The Mayo classification system uses a measurement of single total kidney volume (TKV) at any age to categorize patients into five prognostic classes: class 1A, 1B, 1C, 1D, and 1E. Classes 1C to 1E are the high-risk groups to develop ESRD. The TKV can be calculated by TKV calculator: https://www.mayo.edu/research/documents/pkd-center-adpkd-classification/doc-20094754. CT or MRI without contrast that measures coronal and sagittal length is required for the calculation. The Mayo classification provides the assessment of disease progression risk in patients with typical ADPKD.

D. **Treatment.** Suppression of vasopressin signaling by the vasopressin V_2 receptor antagonist tolvaptan has been shown to slow the growth of renal cysts and reduce the increase of TKV. Both of the phase 3 trials Tolvaptan in Patients with Autosomal Dominant Polycystic Kidney Disease (TEMPO) and Tolvaptan in Later Stage Autosomal Dominant Polycystic Kidney Disease (REPRISE) trials demonstrated that tolvaptan slowed estimated glomerular filtration rate (eGFR) decline in patients with ADPKD. Adverse effects associated with tolvaptan include thirst, polyuria, nocturia, and polydipsia. Liver injury with elevated liver enzymes and potential liver failure has been reported and must be closely monitored during the therapy. Since there was no significant difference in eGFR decline between tolvaptan and placebo in patients with low risk of disease progression, tolvaptan is recommended for use in patients with high risk of progression as assessed by Mayo imaging classification (TKV >750 mL), or a history of decline in eGFR greater than 5 mL/min/1.73 m^2 in 1 year or at least 2.5 mL/min/1.73 m^2 per year for 5 years.

E. Complications and Management. Hypertension occurs early and is frequent. It may be caused by renin release due to cyst expansion causing focal renal ischemia. Inhibition of renin–angiotensin–aldosterone system with angiotensin-converting enzyme inhibitor (ACEI) or an angiotensin receptor blocker (ARB) is the first choice of treatment. Hypertension usually responds but occasionally acute renal failure can occur because angiotensin II is required to maintain an adequate ultrafiltration pressure in glomeruli located downstream of a cyst causing vascular obstruction. Aggressive treatment of hypertension is warranted, especially because the patient may have an undetected cerebral aneurysm. Based on the data from the large Halt Progression of Polycystic Kidney Disease Trial (HALT-PKD) study, aiming for blood pressure <110/75 mm Hg in patients younger than 50 years with preserved renal function and GFR >60 mL/min/1.73 m^2 could provide cardiac benefits and reduce the rate of cyst growth.

Pain in the flank can indicate cyst hemorrhage, cyst infection, or nephrolithiasis. Cyst hemorrhage usually resolves with bed rest and analgesia. Some patients develop calcium oxalate or uric acid stones (see Chapter 21). Renal cell carcinoma (RCC) can occur in ADPKD although it is not common. Nephrectomy is not recommended unless patients suffer from intractable pain from large cysts, recurrent and severe infection, suspicion of RCC, uncontrolled cyst hemorrhage that failed to respond to intra-arterial embolization, ventral hernia due to large kidney size, or limited space for kidney transplant.

Renal insufficiency progresses to ESRD by age 60 in approximately one-half of patients. Women have a less aggressive course than men. ESRD develops earlier in African Americans. Hemodialysis is often preferable to peritoneal dialysis because of the limited peritoneal space as a result of enlarged kidneys. Living-related kidney donors must be screened carefully with genetic tests since gene carriers may not show cysts even when they are 30 years old.

Headache of sudden onset in ADPKD could suggest subarachnoid hemorrhage from rupture of an intracerebral aneurysm. The initial test is a noncontrast CT scan of the head followed by a lumbar puncture if the scan is negative and subarachnoid hemorrhage remains a possibility. Conventional angiography is used to localize a bleeding intracerebral aneurysm. Early intervention by surgical clipping or coil embolization reduces recurrent bleeding.

Intracerebral aneurysm affects 5% to 10% of patients with ADPKD but routine screening is not generally recommended. Screening with MRI angiography is reserved for patients with either a previous or family history of bleeding from a ruptured aneurysm, or for those with high-risk occupations. Aneurysms >5 mm require neurosurgical evaluation.

F. Prognosis. Patients with PKD2 gene have a better prognosis since cysts occur later and the declining of GFR is slower. Other risk factors associated with ADPKD progression are hypertension, proteinuria, early onset of symptoms, and male gender. The Mayo classification system can be used to predict the prognosis.

II. ACQUIRED CYSTIC DISEASE. Simple renal cysts are common and increase with age. Usually, these are single, unilateral, and benign.

Acquired cystic disease in patients with ESRD can be benign, but malignant cysts develop occasionally. Ultrasound screening is recommended for patients on dialysis >7 years.

III. MEDULLARY SPONGE KIDNEY. Although medullary sponge kidney is a congenital anomaly, it does not usually present until age 40 to 60 years. There is marked enlargement of the medullary and inner papillary portions of the collecting ducts. Approximately one-fourth of patients have hemihypertrophy of the body.

Medullary sponge kidney is associated with recurrent hematuria and urinary tract infections, nephrolithiasis, polyuria from an inability to concentrate the urine, and distal renal tubular acidosis. Diagnosis is made by intravenous pyelography or contrast computed tomography which show striations in the papillae or cystic collections of contrast medium in ectatic collecting ducts. Patients with renal tubular acidosis require treatment with alkali. Those with renal calculi should drink enough fluids to maintain at least 2 L of urine output per day. Those with hypercalciuria should receive a thiazide diuretic.

IV. MEDULLARY CYSTIC DISEASE. This takes several forms, each of which is uncommon. Juvenile nephronophthisis is autosomal recessive. Medullary cystic disease is an autosomal dominant disease. Renal–retinal dysplasia refers to medullary cystic disease associated with retinal degeneration, familial retinitis pigmentosa, and pigmentary optic atrophy. The kidneys have small, thin-walled cysts at the corticomedullary junction. The childhood form presents with polydipsia, polyuria, anemia, lethargy, and growth retardation. It usually progresses to ESRD before the age of 20. The adult form presents with salt-wasting nephropathy that may require large amounts of salt and fluids to combat orthostasis.

V. VON HIPPEL-LINDAU DISEASE. Von Hippel–Lindau disease is an uncommon autosomal dominant disorder of retinal angiomas, central nervous system hemangioblastomas, pancreatic cysts, renal cysts, and bilateral or multicentric RCCs. Therefore, the diagnosis mandates regular surveillance for renal neoplasms and early referral to surgery. Pheochromocytomas occur in one-third of patients.

VI. TUBEROUS SCLEROSIS. Tuberous sclerosis is an uncommon autosomal dominant disorder characterized by epilepsy, mental retardation, adenoma sebaceum, ash-leaf skin pigmentation, angiomyolipoma of the kidneys, renal cysts, and, occasionally, pheochromocytomas.

VII. SICKLE CELL NEPHROPATHY. Patients with sickle cell nephropathy can present with microscopic or gross hematuria from medullary congestion caused by sickling of erythrocytes at the low partial pressure of oxygen in the medulla. This can lead to papillary necrosis. Conservative treatment for a crisis entails infusion of hypotonic fluid and diuretics. Patients may have tubular defects manifest as a concentrating defect, acidosis, hyperphosphatemia, hyperuricemia, or hyperkalemia. The development of focal segmental glomerulosclerosis with interstitial fibrosis is heralded by proteinuria and progresses to renal failure. Renal transplant can be successful, but nephropathy can reoccur.

VIII. Alport syndrome, familial thin membrane disease, and nail-patella syndrome are discussed in Chapter 15.

IX. SUGGESTED READINGS

Bergmann C, Guay-Woodford LM, Harris PC, et al. Polycystic kidney disease. *Nat Rev Dis Primers.* 2018;4(1):50.

Nobakht N, Hanna RM, Al-Baghdadi M, et al. Advances in autosomal dominant polycystic kidney disease: a clinical review. *Kidney Med.* 2020;2(2):196–208.

Schrier RW, Abebe KZ, Perrone RD, et al. HALT-PKD trial investigators. *N Engl J Med.* 2014; 371(24):2255.

Torres VE, Chapman AB, Devuyst O, et al. Tolvaptan in later-stage autosomal dominant polycystic kidney disease. *New Eng J Med.* 2017;377(20):1930–1942.

15 Genetic Glomerular and Tubular Disorders

Michael Lipkowitz, Limeng Chen

There has been an explosion of knowledge about genetic causes of glomerular and tubular diseases in the last decade. This review will touch on only a few of the most prominent disorders.

I. GLOMERULAR DISEASES

A. Disorders of the Podocyte and Slit Diaphragm (Table 15.1).

The integrity of the podocyte foot processes and slit diaphragms are maintained by interactions of many proteins that comprise or regulate the slit diaphragm itself or foot process, or interact with the intracellular actin cytoskeleton. Mutations can result in inherited nephrotic syndrome (Table 15.1).

Clinical presentation. These disorders most commonly present as steroid-resistant nephrotic syndrome (SRNS) in childhood, although with more available genetic testing, many have been found also to present in adolescence or adulthood. The autosomal recessive (AR) form of the gene causing congenital nephrotic syndrome of the Finnish type (NPHS) presents with severe early-onset disease with diffuse mesangial sclerosis and rapid progression to renal failure.

Diagnosis. This requires kidney biopsy and genetic testing. These should be performed for SRNS in children, where 25% have a genetic cause. Some 55% of mutations detected in adults with FSGS have been in the gene for collagen IV usually associated with Alport syndrome. There are important benefits to making a genetic diagnosis. First, this may predict prognosis; second, most of these disorders do not respond to immunosuppression so that the complications of this therapy can be avoided, and for some genes there are emerging therapies; third, this helps predict the risk of posttransplant recurrence, that is generally low; fourth, some mutations have associated sequelae such as nephroblastoma in Wilms tumor 1 mutations that require screening and are mutation dependent; finally, family screening and counseling can be planned.

Treatment. At present, treatment remains supportive. For early-onset disease such as congenital nephrotic syndrome of the Finnish type, albumin and nutrient infusion have been required for supportive care, control of edema, and infection protection. In very severe neonatal cases unilateral nephrectomy with RAS inhibition and indomethacin, or total nephrectomy followed by dialysis and transplantation have been employed. RAS inhibition has been recommended based on its relatively low toxicity and general benefits for proteinuria, but data are minimal. There is no good support for immunosuppression. There are a few mutations for which specific therapies have been suggested.

TABLE 15.1 Podocyte **slit** diaphragm–related genes causing steroid-resistant nephrotic syndrome

Disorder	Gene	Inheritance	Protein	Pathophysiology	Clinical features	Tests	Treatment
Congenital nephrotic syndrome of the Finnish type	NPHS1	AR	Nephrin	Forms slit diaphragm, anchors to actin cytoskeleton	FSGS or DMS, early-onset childhood, rare adult	Genetic, renal biopsy	Albumin infusion, nutritional support, nephrectomy and transplant, RAS inhibition
Congenital nephrotic syndrome type 2	NPHS2	AR	Podocin	Anchors nephrin in plasma membrane	FSGS or DMS; early, adolescent, or adult	Genetic, renal biopsy	RAS inhibition, nutritional support, edema control
Familial nephrotic syndrome type 3	PLCE1	AR	Phospholipase Cε1	Cell signaling, regulation of podocyte structure	Early-onset, isolated DMS or FSGS	Genetic, renal biopsy	RAS inhibition, nutritional support, edema control
CD2AP mutations	CD2AP	AD	CD2AP	Adapter protein connecting slit diaphragm to actin cytoskeleton	Childhood-onset FSGS	Genetic, renal biopsy	RAS inhibition, nutritional support, edema control
Actinin-4 mutations	ACTN4	AD	α-Actinin-4	Actin filament crosslinking protein	Adult-onset FSGS		RAS inhibition
Denys–Drash syndrome	WT1	AD	Wilms tumor 1	Tumor suppressor, kidney development	Childhood-onset DMS, male pseudohermaphroditism, risk for nephroblastoma	Genetic, renal biopsy	Screen for nephroblastoma
TRPC6 mutations	TRPC6	AD	TRPC6	Receptor-activated calcium channel regulates actin cytoskeleton–slit diaphragm complex	Childhood- or adult-onset FSGS	Genetic, renal biopsy	RAS inhibition

AR, autosomal recessive; AD, autosomal dominant, FSGS, focal segmental glomerulosclerosis, DMS, diffuse mesangial sclerosis; RAS, renin–angiotensin system.

B. Disorders of the Glomerular Basement Membrane (Table 15.2). There are a number of genes that affect the structure and function of the glomerular basement membrane (GBM).

   1. Alport syndrome. This was originally described as an X-chromosome–linked disorder with resulting male predominance and lesser severity in women with one normal and one affected X chromosome. Subsequent identification of mutations in the type IV collagen α3, 4, and 5 chains, that normally form a trimer, has led to the recognition that there are also autosomal dominant (AD) and AR forms of Alport's and digenic forms where genes for different chains are affected (Table 15.2). Some families have high-frequency hearing loss, anterior lenticonus, posterior polymorphous corneal dystrophy, or rarely retinal flecks. Leiomyomatosis of the female genitalia or esophagus occurs in some families. Kidney biopsy reveals a thickened and laminated GBM containing granules of varying density and sizes with the splitting of the basement membrane. There is tubule dropout and interstitial fibrosis. Immunofluorescence for the collagen IV α chain may be absent or interrupted in the GBM and skin for X-linked and α5 AR variants, and can be seen in women carriers with α5 mutations. Benign familial hematuria (thin basement membrane disease) is a variant of AD Alport syndrome. Anti-GBM disease occurs in 3% of transplant recipients.

   The initial presenting feature is microscopic or more rarely gross hematuria, followed eventually by proteinuria and progressive CKD in the more severe forms. Early disease is often missed if there is no family history since early in the course biopsy can be negative or show only thin basement membranes. Almost all X-linked and AR patients eventually develop ESKD but there is more variable incidence and severity in patients with AD.

   Genetic testing is recommended for diagnosis and is useful in FSGS also, since a number of childhood and early adult patients with FSGS have Alport's.

   There is no FDA-approved treatment for Alport's. Several large observational studies have shown significant benefit from RAS inhibition. Current recommendations are to treat with RAS inhibition for overt proteinuria in all patients and to treat for hematuria or microalbuminuria in those whose mutations suggest severe disease. Female carriers for X-linked disease should be monitored closely and treated similarly if evidence of renal disease develops.

   2. Nail-patella syndrome. This is an AD condition with variable penetrance caused by mutations in LIM homeobox transcription factor 1β (LMX1β) that regulates podocyte production of α3 and 4 collagens. This results in lucencies in the GBM and in podocyte effacement. Some children have nephrotic syndrome and nail dysplasias.

II. DISORDERS OF TUBULES (Table 15.3)

   1. Bartter syndrome. This is defined as metabolic alkalosis and hypokalemia with polyuria, polydipsia, normal to increased urine calcium, normal BP or hypotension, and usually growth and mental retardation. Onset occurs usually antenatally or in childhood. The causes are mutations that either inhibit luminal Na-K-2CL uptake in the thick ascending limb, prevent recycling of K into the lumen via ROMK channels, or prevent Cl efflux through the basolateral cell membrane Cl channels. Mutations have been found in the specific channels or in proteins that regulate expression of these channels (Barrtin, calcium-sensing receptor, CaSr). Na loss activates the RAAS

TABLE
15.2 Glomerular basement membrane disorders

Disorder	Gene	Inheritance	Protein	Pathophysiology	Clinical features	Tests	Treatment
Alport's X-linked (60–70% of Alport's)	COL4A5	X-linked	Type IV collagen $\alpha5$ chain	Dysregulated $\alpha345$ trimer formation in GBM	Hematuria, proteinuria, renal failure in 100% of men and 30% of women. Sensorineural hearing loss, lenticonus	Genetic, kidney biopsy, skin biopsy for $\alpha5$ mutations	RAS inhibition for overt proteinuria, for hematuria or microalbuminuria or for severe mutations
Alport's autosomal dominant (includes thin basement membranes; 25–30% of Alport's)	COL4A3, COL4A4	AD	Type IV collagen $\alpha3$ or $\alpha4$	Dysregulated $\alpha345$ trimer formation in GBM	Variable penetrance and findings including hematuria, FSGS, fibrosis, CKD	Genetic, biopsy	RAS inhibition for proteinuria, CKD care
Alport's autosomal recessive (10–15% of Alport's)	COL4A3 and/ or COL4A4	AR	Type IV collagen $\alpha3$ or $\alpha4$	Mutations on both chromosomes (in trans); Dysregulated $\alpha345$ trimer formation in GM	Nearly 100% risk of ESRD. Findings similar to X-linked except risk equal for males and females. Specific mutations strongly predict outcomes	Genetic, biopsy	RAS inhibition; CKD care
Nail-patella syndrome	LMX1B	AD	LIM homeobox transcription factor 1β (LMX1β)	Regulates podocyte production of $\alpha3$ and $\alpha4$ collagen	Nephrotic syndrome in 40%, dysplastic nails, hypoplastic patella	Genetic, biopsy	RAS inhibition; CKD care

AR, autosomal recessive; AD, autosomal dominant; RAS, renin-angiotensin system; GBM, glomerular basement membrane.

TABLE

15.3

Renal tubule–related genes

Disorder	Gene	Inheritance	Protein	Pathophysiology	Clinical features	Tests	Onset
Bartter syndrome, types I–IV	SLC12A1; KCNJ1; CLCNKB; BSND (IVa) CLCNKA and CLCNKB (IVb)	AR; AR or autosomal digenic; digenic	NKCC2; ROMK; CLC-Kb; Barttin (β-subunit of CLC-Ka and CLC-Kb, IVa) CLC-Ka and CLC-Kb (IVb)	Inhibition of TAL sodium reabsorption due to loss of luminal Na-K-2Cl uptake, luminal K recycling, or basolateral Cl efflux	Maternal hydramnios, polyuria, dehydration Growth retardation, low normal BP, hypokalemia, metabolic alkalosis, renin–angiotensin system activation	Serum and urine electrolytes, renin and aldo levels, genetic testing	Neonatal period, infancy, childhood
Bartter syndrome, type V	MAGED2	X-linked	melanoma-associated antigen D2	Mutations prevent chaperone function as for Na-K-2Cl in the luminal membrane	Very early onset of polyhydramnios, prematurity, massive and persistent salt wasting and polyuria, with high mortality	Serum and urine electrolytes, renin and aldo levels, genetic testing	Neonatal period
Autosomal dominant hypocalcemia with Bartter syndrome	CASR	AD	Calcium-sensing receptor	Activating mutation of TAL calcium-sensing receptor causes decrease in ROMK potassium efflux and Na-K-2Cl uptake	Familial hypocalciuric hypercalcemia with Bartter	Serum and urine electrolytes, renin and aldo levels, genetic testing	Infancy

(continued)

TABLE 15.3 Renal tubule–related genes (Continued)

Disorder	Gene	Inheritance	Protein	Pathophysiology	Clinical features	Tests	Onset
Gitelman syndrome	*SLC12A3; CLCNKB*	AR	Thiazide-sensitive sodium chloride cotransporter; chloride channel CLCNKB	Decreased Na uptake in the DCT due to loss of NaCl cotransport in the lumen or Cl exit basolaterally	Low normal BP, hypokalemia, metabolic alkalosis, RAS activation, low serum magnesium, hypocalciuria	Serum and urine electrolytes, renin and aldo levels, genetic testing	Children, juvenile
Dent disease, type 1; type 2	*CLCN5 OCRL*	X-linked, AR	ClC-5 chloride channel OCRL 5-phosphatase	Regulates early endosomes and proximal tubule protein reabsorption	Low-molecular-weight proteinuria, hypercalciuria, nephrolithiasis, nephrocalcinosis, rickets, and renal failure	Serum and urine electrolytes, renal imaging, genetic testing	Infancy, children
Lowe oculocerebrorenal syndrome (congenital cataracts and mental retardation)	*OCRL*	X-linked, AR	OCRL protein	5-phosphatase, regulates early endosomes	Glaucoma, mental retardation, hypotonia, Fanconi syndrome, growth failure, developmental delay		Neonatal period, Infancy

AR, autosomal recessive; AD, autosomal dominant, RAS, renin-angiotensin system; DCT, distal convoluted tubule; ROMK, renal outer medullary potassium channel; TAL, thick ascending limb.

system resulting in compensatory K and H secretion. Diagnosis is made by measuring serum and urine electrolytes, renin, aldosterone and genetic testing.

Treatment consists of electrolyte replacement. If hypokalemia is severe, treatment with inhibitors of distal K^+ secretion such as amiloride, spironolactone, or indomethacin can be used. RAS inhibition has also been used successfully, but can cause hypotension. Kidney transplantation has been performed occasionally in refractory cases.

2. **Gitelman syndrome.** This is defined as metabolic alkalosis and hypokalemia with normotension, hypocalciuria, and hypomagnesemia. The cause is inactivating mutations in the thiazide-sensitive NaCl cotransporter of the distal convoluted tubule. The hypokalemia can cause polyuria and nocturia, and with hypomagnesemia can cause muscle cramps.

Diagnosis and treatment are similar to Bartter syndrome. The main differentiating features are later-onset, hypocalciuria and hyomagnesemia, although there can be significant overlap that requires genetic testing to resolve.

3. **Dent disease.** This is a syndrome of low–molecular-weight proteinuria, hypercalciuria, nephrolithiasis, nephrocalcinosis, rickets, and renal failure. It is caused by mutations of the CLCN5 or ORCL genes that regulate lysosome acidification and protein reabsorption. Treatment is to decrease urinary calcium by Na restriction and the use of thiazide diuretics. Patients with renal failure can be transplanted successfully without disease recurrence.

III. DISORDERS CAUSING CKD

A. **Sickle Cell Nephropathy.** This can present with microscopic or gross hematuria from medullary congestion caused by sickling of erythrocytes at the low partial pressure of oxygen in the medulla and can lead to papillary necrosis. Sickle cell disease or sickle trait can interact with the apolipoprotein L1 (APOL1) risk genotype to accelerate disease progression. Conservative treatment for a crisis entails infusion of hypotonic fluid and use of diuretics. Patients may have tubular defects manifest as a concentrating defect, renal tubular acidosis, hyperphosphatemia, hyperuricemia, or hyperkalemia. The development of focal segmental glomerulosclerosis with interstitial fibrosis is heralded by proteinuria and progresses to renal failure. Renal transplant can be successful, but nephropathy can reoccur.

B. **Fabry Disease.** This is an X-linked lysosomal storage disease from inactivation of the gene for α-galactosidase that leads to the accumulation of globotriaosylceramide (GB3), renal failure, and eventually to death from cardiovascular or cerebral dysfunction. Early symptoms are pain (acroparesthesias), angiokeratomas/telangiectasias, and GI problems. There are characteristic corneal opacifications. Diagnosis is often unsuspected. Renal disease onset is usually in the fourth decade and includes proteinuria, isosthenuria, Fanconi syndrome, and progressive CKD. Renal occurs less frequently in women. Diagnosis is by biopsy which shows characteristic "zebra bodies" on electron microscopy, that are lysosomes filled with GB3 in an onion skin pattern. Light microscopy shows podocyte and endothelial cell vacuolation. Treatment is replacement of α-galactosidase by regular infusion that is offered to all men with classic X-linked disease, and women who have signs and symptoms of disease. Treatment slows progression of renal disease especially if started early and reduces pain, but does not prevent cardiovascular or neurologic disease.

C. APOL1-Related Kidney Disease. The gene for APOL1 is expressed in humans and primates and confers resistance to trypanosomes that cause sleeping sickness. Recently 2 mutations that enhance trypanolytic function have been detected in high frequencies in Africans from trypanosome endemic areas. African Americans (AA) with 2 copies of the mutant gene are at higher risk to develop kidney disease. This was first shown for FSGS, that has a 17-fold increased risk while risk for developing HIVAN is 29- to 89-fold, hypertensive ESKD is 7- to 11-fold, nondiabetic, CKD is 3- to 4-fold, and lupus nephritis is 2.5- to 3-fold. Interestingly, the progression but not the incidence of diabetic nephropathy is increased. There is increased risk of loss of transplanted kidneys with the risk genotype, but no effect of kidney loss based on recipient genotype. These APOL1 mutations are responsible for about half the excess risk of kidney disease in AA compared to Caucasians and may double the lifetime risk of ESKD from 8% to 15%. The mutant genes are present in about 50% of AA patients with hypertension-attributed ESKD, and in about 75% of AA patients with FSGS.

The mechanism of APOL1 kidney disease has not yet been defined. APOL1, expression is increased by interferon that may explain its relationship to FSGS in HIVAN and now in COVID-19–related kidney disease. There is no specific therapy for APOL1-related kidney disease. RAS inhibition and SGLT2 inhibitors remain the recommended therapies. There are no concrete recommendations for genetic testing.

IV. SUGGESTED READINGS

Devuyst O, Knoers NV, Remuzzi G. Rare inherited kidney diseases: challenges, opportunities, and perspectives. *Lancet.* 2014;383(9931):1844–1859.

Downie ML, Lopez Garcia SC, Kleta R, et al. Inherited tubulopathies of the kidney: insights from genetics. *Clin J Am Soc Nephrol.* 2021;16(4):620–630. doi: 10.2215/CJN.14481119

Kashtan CE, Ding J, Garosi G. Alport syndrome: a unified classification of genetic disorders of collagen IV α345: a position paper of the Alport syndrome classification working group. *Kidney Int.* 2018;93(5):1045–1051.

Mrad FCC, Soares SBM, de Menezes Silva LAW, et al. Bartter's syndrome: clinical findings, genetic causes and therapeutic approach. *World J Pediatr.* 2021;17(1):31–39. doi: 10.1007/s12519-020-00370-4

16

Genetic Forms of Hypertension

Gajapathiraju Chamarthi, Rajesh Mohandas, Limeng Chen

Blood pressure is a polygenic trait that is influenced by lifestyle and environmental factors. Thus, most patients with hypertension do not have a genetic basis for the increased blood pressures. However, rare single-gene mutations have been identified that can cause hypertension. A few important syndromes relevant to nephrology practice are discussed in this chapter.

I. **GLUCOCORTICOID REMEDIABLE HYPERTENSION.** Glucocorticoid remediable hypertension (GRA) or familial hyperaldosteronism type 1 is an autosomal dominant disorder caused by a chimeric gene resulting from an unequal crossover of CYP11β1 and CYP11β2 genes, driving excessive aldosterone synthesis under the influence of adrenocorticotropic hormone (ACTH).

A. **Pathogenesis.** In a normal physiologic state, aldosterone synthesis is increased by angiotensinogen II or hyperkalemia and requires the CYP11β2 (aldosterone synthase) enzyme that is expressed only in the zona glomerulosa of the adrenal gland. Similarly, cortisol synthesis is regulated by ACTH and requires the CYP11β1 (11β-hydroxylase) enzyme that is expressed only in the zona fasciculata of the adrenal gland. In GRA, unequal crossing over of the genes results in a chimeric gene consisting of the regulatory region of the 11β-hydroxylase gene and the coding sequence of CYP11β2, resulting in the synthesis of aldosterone synthase in the zona fasciculata under the regulation of ACTH. Excessive production of aldosterone causes hypertension in these patients.

B. **Clinical Features, Diagnosis, and Treatment.** Early-onset of severe hypertension, a strong family history of hypertension, and hemorrhagic strokes secondary to ruptured cerebral aneurysms are clues to diagnose this disorder. Aldosterone levels are increased, and renin is suppressed. Hypokalemia may be present but is often less common than in patients with primary hyperaldosteronism. Persistent suppression of aldosterone during the dexamethasone suppression test or increased urinary excretion of the metabolites 18-hydroxycortisol and 18-oxocortisol, that are produced due to the abnormal presence of aldosterone synthase in the zona fasciculata, are suggestive of the diagnosis. Genetic analysis can establish the diagnosis and is the preferred method for diagnosis of this disease. Low-dose glucocorticoid given to suppress ACTH release is the treatment of choice and can improve blood pressure control. Mineralocorticoid receptor (MR) blockers such as spironolactone can be added for further control of hypertension.

II. **PSEUDOHYPOALDOSTERONISM TYPE II (GORDON SYNDROME).** Gordon syndrome is an autosomal dominant disorder caused by abnormalities of the with-no-lysine

(WNK) family of kinases, resulting in increased activation of thiazide-sensitive Na-Cl cotransporter (NCC) leading to hypertension, hyperkalemia, and hyperchloremic metabolic acidosis.

A. **Pathogenesis.** WNK family consists of WNK1, WNK2, WNK3, and WNK4 kinases that regulate phosphorylation of SPAK (Sterile 20-related proline-alanine-rich kinase), which in turn phosphorylates and activates the NCC. Mutations in WNK1 and WNK4 kinases result in increased activity of NCC, leading to increased sodium and chloride reabsorption, volume expansion, and hypertension. Increased uptake of sodium in the distal convoluted tubule results in decreased sodium delivery to the collecting duct. Decreased ENaC activity and subsequent decrease in luminal negativity result supress the activity of ROMK and H-K ATPase, resulting in hyperkalemia and acidosis. The WNK kinases also regulate ROMK channels. Mutations of WNK kinases can directly reduce the expression of potassium channels, thereby limiting the transport of potassium from cells into the tubular lumen and contributing to hyperkalemia. Also, mutations in Cullin 3 and Kelch 3, that are two proteins that regulate WNK1 and WNK4, have been identified as cause of Gordon syndrome.

B. **Clinical Features, Diagnosis, and Treatment.** Hyperkalemia with normal renal function is typically the initial presenting feature and often precedes hypertension, which manifests in the second decade of life. In addition to hyperkalemia, patients often have hyperchloremic metabolic acidosis, low fractional excretion of sodium, and suppressed plasma renin levels. Aldosterone levels are variable and usually are not suppressed despite volume overload due to stimulation from hyperkalemia. In severe forms of Gordon syndrome, patients can present with intellectual impairment, failure to thrive, and short stature. Thiazide diuretics that block the NCC and low-salt diet are effective in controlling hypertension and correcting the biochemical abnormalities.

III. **LIDDLE SYNDROME.** Liddle syndrome is a rare autosomal dominant disorder characterized by constitutively increased activity of the epithelial sodium channel (ENaC), resulting in increased sodium reabsorption independent activation of the mineralocorticosteroid (MR).

A. **Pathogenesis.** ENaC is composed of alpha, beta, and gamma chains. Nedd4 binds to the beta or gamma subunits of ENaC, facilitating endosomal degradation and recycling of the ENaC. In Liddle syndrome, mutations in genes coding for beta or gamma subunits of ENaC (SCNN1B or SCNN1G) result in deletions of proline-rich regions that facilitate binding of Nedd4. The inability to retrieve the ENaC channel from the apical membrane results in constitutive expression of the ENaC channel on the apical surface of principal cells, that increases sodium reabsorption and causes volume expansion. The excessive reabsorption of sodium by ENaC accentuates the lumen-negative electrical gradient, promoting the secretion of potassium and hydrogen ions into the lumen, causing hypokalemia and metabolic alkalosis.

B. **Clinical Features, Diagnosis, and Treatment.** Patients present with severe hypertension in teenage years accompanied by hypokalemia and metabolic alkalosis. There is usually a history of other family members with severe hypertension at a young age. Laboratory tests reveal suppressed plasma renin and aldosterone levels secondary to volume expansion. Urinary aldosterone excretion rates are low. A definitive diagnosis requires genetic testing for mutations of the ENaC channel. ENaC blockade with potassium-sparing diuretics such as amiloride or triamterene and low-salt diet will lower the blood pressure and normalize potassium levels. Spironolactone is not effective in Liddle syndrome, as the increased activity of the ENaC channel is independent of aldosterone mediated activation of the MR.

IV. SYNDROME OF APPARENT MINERALOCORTICOID EXCESS. The syndrome of apparent mineralocorticoid excess (AME) is an autosomal recessive disorder caused by inactivating mutations of the 11β-hydroxysteroid dehydrogenase type 2 (11β-HSD2) enzyme, resulting in activation of the MR by cortisol.

A. Pathogenesis. Aldosterone, as well as cortisol, can bind to and activate the MR. In the normal physiologic state, the cortisol concentration is severalfold higher than the aldosterone levels. The specificity of the distal nephron to respond to aldosterone is achieved by the 11β-HSD2 enzyme, that metabolizes cortisol to cortisone thereby, rendering it unable to bind or activate the MR. Deficiency of 11β-HSD2 due to genetic mutations or acquired inhibitors such as glycyrrhizin acid found in licorice can cause activation of the MR by cortisol, resulting in hypertension and hypokalemia.

B. Clinical Features, Diagnosis, and Treatment. Early onset of severe hypertension in childhood, hypokalemia, metabolic alkalosis, along with suppressed renin and aldosterone levels, should suggest a possible diagnosis of AME. Other clinical features, such as low birth weight, failure to thrive, hypercalciuria, and polyuria, can be present. Increased ratio of cortisol metabolites (tetrahydrocortisol [THF] and allotetrahydrocortisol [alloTHF]) compared to cortisone metabolites (tetrahydrocortisone [THE]) or an increased free cortisol/free cortisone ratio in 24-hour urine collection is suggestive of AME. It is important to rule out licorice ingestion, which has a similar presentation as AME. Genetic testing is available for confirmation. MR blockers such as spironolactone and eplerenone are the first-line medications to control hypertension. Further blockade of ENaC with amiloride or triamterene may be required to control hypertension, and potassium supplementation may be necessary to correct hypokalemia.

V. CONGENITAL ADRENAL HYPERPLASIA. These are a group of autosomal recessive disorders caused by inherited abnormalities of enzymes regulating adrenal steroid biosynthesis. Defects in 11β-hydroxylase or 17α-hydroxylase enzymes result in increased deoxycortisol and deoxycorticosterone metabolites. These have mineralocorticoid activity, thereby causing hypertension.

A. Pathogenesis. Normally, 11β-hydroxylase converts deoxycorticosterone and deoxycortisol to corticosterone and cortisol, respectively. 17α-hydroxylase converts progesterone and pregnenolone to 17–OH–progesterone and 17-OH pregnenolone, respectively, which are precursors for cortisol and adrenal androgen synthesis. Deficiencies of either of these enzymes result in decreased cortisol production, leading to increased ACTH secretion. ACTH increases the production of adrenal hormones resulting in the accumulation of steroid precursors such as deoxycortisol and deoxycorticosterone that have potent mineralocorticoid activity, thereby causing hypertension.

B. Clinical Features, Diagnosis, and Treatment. Early-onset of hypertension, hypokalemia, metabolic alkalosis with suppressed renin and aldosterone levels are common features to both these disorders. The presence or absence of hyperandrogenism can help in distinguishing between these two enzyme deficiencies. In congenital adrenal hyperplasia (CAH type IV 11β-hydroxylase deficiency), the enzyme defects result in excessive adrenal androgens production leading to precocious puberty in males and virilization in females. In CAH type V

TABLE
16.1 Overview of the causes, clinical features, and treatment of monogenic forms of hypertension

Disorder	Inheritance	Pathophysiology	Clinical features	Renin	Aldo	Tests	Treatment
GRA	AD	Chimeric gene CYP11β1/CYP11β2 leading to excessive aldosterone under the regulation of ACTH	Early-onset of HTN, strong family history of early onset of HTN and hemorrhagic strokes	↓	↑	Genetic test	Low-dose glucocorticoids, spironolactone, amiloride, or triamterene
Gordon syndrome	AD	Mutations in WNK 1/4, CUL3, and KLHL3, causing overactivation of NCC	Hyperkalemia with normal renal function, metabolic acidosis, and HTN	↓	Variable	Genetic test	Low-sodium and potassium diet, thiazide diuretics
Liddle syndrome	AD	Constitutively overactive ENaC	Early-onset of HTN, hypokalemia, and metabolic alkalosis	↓	↓	Genetic test	Low-salt diet, amiloride or triamterene
AME	AR	Inactivating mutation of 11β-HSD2 allowing cortisol to act on MR	Early-onset of HTN, low birth weight, hypokalemia, metabolic alkalosis, polyuria, and growth retardation	↓	↓	Increased (THF+ aTHF)/(THE). Free cortisol / cortisone. Genetic test	Low-salt diet, spironolactone, amiloride, or triamterene

CAH	AR	Adrenal enzyme defect: 11β-hydroxylase, 17α-hydroxylase resulting in accumulation of precursors that have mineralocorticoid action	HTN, hypokalemia, metabolic alkalosis. *11β-hydroxylase defects*: virilization in females and precocious puberty in males. *17α-hydroxylase defects*: primary amenorrhea in females and ambiguous genitalia in males	$\downarrow$ $\downarrow$	Steroid profile after ACTH stimulation test. Genetic test	Glucocorticoids, spironolactone
Geller syndrome	AD	Mutations in the MR allowing it to be activated by progesterone	Severe hypertension during pregnancy	$\downarrow$ $\downarrow$	Genetic test	Low-salt diet, delivery of the fetus

AME, apparent mineralocorticoid excess; CAH, congenital adrenal hyperplasia; GRA, glucocorticoid remediable aldosteronism; AD, autosomal dominant; AR, autosomal recessive; ENaC, epithelial sodium channel; ACTH, adrenocorticotropic hormone; MR, mineralocorticoid receptor; NCC, sodium chloride cotransporter; HTN, hypertension; Aldo, Aldosterone; WNK, with no lysin kinases; 11β-HSD2, 11β-hydroxysteroid dehydrogenase 2; ↑, increased; ↓, decreased; THF, tetrahydrocortisol; aTHF, allotetrahydrocortisol; THE, tetrahydrocortisone.

(17α-hydroxylase deficiency), the inability to synthesize adrenal sex hormones results in males presenting with ambiguous genitalia and females presenting with amenorrhea and delayed sexual development. Evaluation of steroid profile after ACTH stimulation can lead to appropriate diagnosis, and genetic testing can be done for confirmation. Corticosteroids in doses just sufficient to block the ACTH secretion is the cornerstone of therapy for these disorders. Hypertension can be controlled with MR antagonists, such as spironolactone.

VI. GELLER SYNDROME. Geller syndrome is an extremely rare autosomal dominant disorder caused by mutations of the MR that usually presents with dramatic hypertension complicating pregnancy.

A. Pathogenesis. In a healthy state, hormones that lack 21-hydroxyl groups such as progesterone and cortisone are incapable of activating the MR, whereas in Geller syndrome, mutations in MR result in reconfiguration of the hormone-binding site, enabling it to be activated by progesterone, in addition to aldosterone.

B. Clinical Features, Diagnosis, and Treatment. The onset of hypertension usually occurs in the second or third decade. Patients present with severe exacerbation of hypertension during pregnancy, when the progesterone levels are elevated 100-fold. Suppressed renin and aldosterone levels are usually evidenced by laboratory evaluation. Patients typically do not have proteinuria or edema, differentiating it from preeclampsia. Genetic testing can confirm the diagnosis. Delivery of the fetus results in decreased progesterone levels and is the mainstay of treatment for hypertension. Treatment in nonpregnant females and males has not been established. Spironolactone is often ineffective in blocking the mutated MR.

VII. CONCLUSION. Monogenic forms of hypertension should be suspected in younger patients with severe hypertension, characteristic biochemical abnormalities, or a family history of hypertension at a young age. The clinical and biochemical features are summarized in Table 16.1. Genetic tests can confirm the diagnosis. Knowledge of the underlying genetic defect is essential to choose specific therapeutic agents to control hypertension in these patients effectively.

VIII. SUGGESTED READINGS
Ehret G. Genetic factors in the pathogenesis of hypertension. In: Post TW, ed. *UpToDate*. UpToDate Inc; 2020. Accessed July 15. https://www.uptodate.com/contents/genetic-factors-in-the-pathogenesis-of-hypertension
Freehally J, Floege J, Tonelli M, et al. *Comprehensive Clinical Nephrology*. 6th ed. Elsevier; 2019.
Garovic VD, Hilliard AA, Turner ST. Monogenic forms of low-renin hypertension. *Nat Clin Pract Nephrol*. 2006;2(11):624–630.
Levanovich PE, Diaczok A, Rossi NF. Clinical and molecular perspectives of monogenic hypertension. *Curr Hypertens Rev*. 2020;16(2):91–107.
Raina R, Krishnappa V, Das A, et al. Overview of monogenic or mendelian forms of hypertension. *Front Pediatr*. 2019;7:263.

Disorders of Water, Electrolytes, and Acid-Base Regulation

17 Dysnatremia and Disorders of Water Balance

Charles S. Wingo, Mark S. Segal

Under physiologic conditions, the osmolality of all body fluids is tightly regulated and maintained within a narrow range (285 to 295 mOsm/kg H_2O) by alterations in water intake and excretion. Water homeostasis is dependent on: (1) access to water and an intact thirst mechanism; (2) appropriate renal regulation of solutes and water; (3) the magnitude of extrarenal solute and water losses; (4) intact antidiuretic hormone (ADH) biosynthesis, release, and action to changes in serum osmolality and intravascular plasma volume. Derangements of water balance are reflected as changes in serum osmolality (S_{osm}), which largely result from changes in serum sodium concentration (S_{Na}).

I. **NORMAL WATER BALANCE**. Total body water (TBW) constitutes ~60% of lean body mass (LBM) in men and ~50% in women. TBW is distributed between the intracellular compartment (two-thirds) and the extracellular compartment (one-third). Three-fourths of the extracellular fluid (ECF) volume is interstitial lymph fluid and one-fourth is intravascular. Osmotic equilibrium is maintained between the intracellular and extracellular compartments by fluid shifts across cell membranes that are freely permeable to water.

Potassium salts are the predominant intracellular osmoles and sodium salts are the major extracellular osmoles. Because most cell membranes are freely permeable to water, S_{osm} is the same as ECF osmolality and intracellular fluid (ICF) osmolality. Because S_{Na} is usually a major constituent of ECF osmolality, S_{Na} directly correlates with S_{osm}. Derangements in blood urea nitrogen (BUN) or glucose concentrations can also alter S_{osm} and are included in the calculation of S_{osm}:

$$S_{osm} \text{ (mOsm/kg } H_2O) = 2S_{Na} \text{ (mEq/L)} + (\text{glucose [mg/dL]}/18) + (\text{BUN [mg/dL]}/2.8)$$

This calculation should correlate to within 10 mOsm/kg H_2O of the measured S_{osm}. A greater disparity (an "osmolar gap") could be due to an error of measurement, pseudohyponatremia, or the presence of another osmotically active solute such as mannitol or ethylene glycol. Thus, confirming serious disturbances in S_{Na} by measurement of S_{osm} is important and provides additional diagnostic information. "Ineffective osmoles" such as urea and ethanol can alter S_{osm} but do not affect water distribution between the intracellular and extracellular compartments because they are membrane permeable. "Effective osmoles" such as sodium, mannitol, and glucose (in the absence of insulin) are distributed mainly extracellularly and can cause fluid shifts across the cell membrane.

Relatively small increases in S_{osm} are sensed by the hypothalamus and stimulate thirst and ADH secretion. Hypotension and hypovolemia (>10% reduction of circulating plasma volume) can also stimulate thirst and ADH secretion through nonosmotic mechanisms. Thirst is the principal defense against hyperosmolality, whereas renal water excretion is the ultimate defense against hypoosmolality. ADH binds to the arginine vasopressin (AVP) receptor 2 (V_2 receptors) in the collecting duct to affect an increase in water permeability promoting net water reabsorption into the interstitium. Maximal ADH action reduces urine volume to ~500 mL/day and increases urine osmolality (U_{osm}) to 800 to 1,400 mOsm/kg H_2O. Complete absence of ADH results in a large diuresis of up to 15 to 20 L/day with a U_{osm} of 40 to 80 mOSm/kg H_2O depending on the fluid intake. Any factor that impairs ADH release, tubular responsiveness to ADH, or medullary hypertonicity will also limit urinary concentrating ability.

S_{Na} is a measurement that reflects the balance of body sodium and water. Changes in total body sodium alter effective circulating volume, whereas changes in S_{Na} usually reflect changes in water balance. Therefore, S_{Na} does not necessarily correlate with either effective circulating volume or with renal sodium excretion.

II. HYPONATREMIA (S_{Na} <135 mEq/L). This is the most frequent electrolyte abnormality in hospitalized patients, with an incidence of 1% to 2%.

A. Pathophysiology. Hyponatremia occurs by (a) excess water intake (water intoxication) with normal renal function, which rarely occurs, or (b) a continued (solute-free)[1] water intake with decreased renal diluting capacity. Appropriate excretion of a water load requires the following:

1) Adequate glomerular filtration without excessive proximal reabsorption to deliver tubular fluid to the diluting segments of the nephron (ascending limb of Henle and early distal convoluted tubule); thus azotemia of any cause (prerenal, renal, or obstruction) reduces water excretion;

2) Normal function of diluting segments of the nephron; thus loop and thiazide diuretics can disrupt this function;

3) Suppression of ADH to prevent reabsorption of water in the collecting ducts; thus inappropriate production or administration of ADH can lead to hyponatremia.

B. Classification. A diagnostic decision tree is presented in Figure 17.1. Initial evaluation of hyponatremia includes simultaneous measurement of S_{osm} and S_{Na} and an assessment of the effective circulating volume (as an index of total body sodium). Accurate serial recordings of body weight and intake–output records may be valuable. Signs of *hypovolemia* include poor skin turgor, dry mucous membranes, dry axillae, flat neck veins, tachycardia, and postural changes in vital signs (hypotension or relative tachycardia). Common laboratory manifestations of hypovolemia include hemoconcentration (increased hematocrit and serum protein), an increased BUN-to-creatinine ratio, an increased uric

---

[1]The term "free-water" is frequently used by nephrologists and dates from concepts formulated during the time when clearance experiments were the primary means to deduce renal function. This term is an abbreviation for, "solute-free water," which is equivalent to simply "water" the term largely used in this chapter.

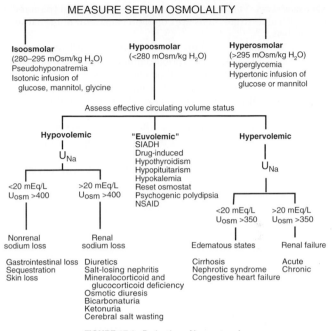

FIGURE 17.1: Evaluation of hyponatremia.

acid, and a U_{Na} of <20 mEq/L. *Hypervolemia* is usually manifested by an elevated jugular venous pressure and peripheral or presacral edema. Hemodilution (decreased hematocrit and serum protein) and a decreased BUN-to-creatinine ratio are often observed, whereas the U_{Na} is less helpful since it may be low ($U_{Na} < 20$) in individuals with congested heart failure or cirrhosis or high ($U_{Na} > 20$) in these same states when the patient is on a diuretic.

III. ISOOSMOLAR HYPONATREMIA. Pseudohyponatremia (artifactual depression of the S_{Na}) can occur when the fraction of plasma that is water (normally 92% to 94%) is decreased by excessive amounts of lipids or proteins. This may occur with severe hyperlipidemias (usually triglyceridemia >1,500 mg/dL) or hyperproteinemias such as Waldenström macroglobulinemia or multiple myeloma (serum protein >10 g/dL). In these instances, the measured S_{osm} will be normal, but the serum osmolar gap will be increased. Pseudohyponatremia must be distinguished from the true, potentially serious hyponatremia with normal S_{osm}, also with an increased serum osmolar gap, that can occur with infusions of isosmotic, sodium-free solutions such as glycine in certain urologic procedures.

IV. HYPOOSMOLAR HYPONATREMIA

A. Hypovolemic Hyponatremia. In this condition, a total body sodium deficit is present that is in excess of water losses. Either renal or nonrenal sodium losses result in contracted effective circulating volume that enhances isosmotic reabsorption of fluid in the proximal tubule. This limits fluid delivery to the distal diluting segments and with significant hypovolemia, nonosmotic stimulation of thirst and nonosmolar stimulation of ADH release also compound the hyponatremia.

B. Nonrenal Sodium Loss. Vomiting, diarrhea, and sequestration (pancreatitis, peritonitis) of gastrointestinal fluids are common causes for nonrenal sodium loss.

C. Renal Sodium Loss

1. **Diuretic administration.** All diuretics that inhibit NaCl reabsorption in the diluting segment can lead to hyponatremia by this mechanism. This is most frequently seen with the use of thiazide diuretics, but all conditions that impair fluid delivery to the diluting segments decrease the capacity of the diluting segment to excrete a water load and potentiate ADH action and release.

2. **Salt-losing nephritis.** This can occur, albeit rarely given the sodium intake in the average American diet, in patients with chronic renal failure or in patients with relatively preserved glomerular filtration rate but significant interstitial disease such as polycystic kidney disease, medullary cystic disease, or chronic pyelonephritis.

3. **Mineralocorticoid and glucocorticoid deficiency.** Aldosterone is the major Na-conserving hormone and deficiency of this hormone typically results in the impairment of Na conservation. Pure glucocorticoid deficiency is uncommon and is more frequently associated with isovolemic hyponatremia. However, as with hypothyroidism, such individuals behave as though their "effective" circulatory volume is reduced. ADH is cosecreted with corticotropin-releasing factor by the cells in the paraventricular nucleus and cortisol has a negative feedback on both the corticotropin-releasing factor and ADH. With adrenal insufficiency this negative feedback is lost resulting in inappropriate ADH release.

4. **Cerebral salt wasting.** This has been a controversial entity occurring in patients with central nervous system (CNS) disease, particularly in patients with subarachnoid hemorrhage. The syndrome of inappropriate ADH secretion (SIADH) and glucocorticoid deficiency should be excluded prior to considering this diagnosis.

V. EUVOLEMIC HYPONATREMIA. These patients are clinically euvolemic and have no edema. This class of disorders results from nonphysiologic secretion, potentiation, or inappropriate action of ADH.

A. Syndrome of Inappropriate ADH Secretion. This is generally associated with:

1) *Malignancies.* Oat cell carcinoma of the lung, Hodgkin and non-Hodgkin lymphoma, thymoma, and other carcinomas (duodenum, pancreas);

2) *Pulmonary disorders.* Tuberculosis, pneumonia, abscess, asthma, and acute respiratory failure;

3) *CNS disorders.* Tumors, head trauma, subarachnoid or subdural hemorrhage, meningitis, encephalitis, abscess, seizures, psychosis, and delirium tremens;

4) *Drugs.* There are three different mechanisms by which medications can cause SIADH.

   a) *May potentiate ADH action.* Clofibrate, cyclophosphamide, nonsteroidal anti-inflammatory agents, and ADH analogs;

   b) *May stimulate ADH release.* Vincristine, carbamazepine, narcotics, barbiturates, and antidepressants;

   c) *May potentiate ADH action and stimulate its release.* Thiazide diuretics, chlorpropamide, ADH analogs, and rarely nonsteroidal anti-inflammatory agents (NSAIDs).

5) *Other.* Includes transient causes such as general anesthesia, nausea, pain, and stress as well as hereditary causes such as gain-of-function mutations in the ADH (vasopressin) V_2 receptor. 3,4-Methylenedioxymethamphetamine (MDMA), commonly known as ecstasy (E) or molly, is a psychoactive, recreational drug that is a powerful stimulant of ADH.

SIADH is a diagnosis of exclusion. The patient must have no other cause of decreased diluting capacity (thyroid, renal, adrenal, cardiac, or liver disease). The urine is typically hypertonic to plasma but always less than maximally dilute (>100 mOsm/kg H_2O), despite low serum osmolality, and U_{Na} is usually large but always >20 mEq/L. Hypouricemia (<4 mg/dL) is a useful diagnostic clue. The diagnosis is suggested by a less than maximally dilute urine in the presence of plasma hypoosmolality and confirmed by an elevated ADH level.

B. **Hypothyroidism.** Although the mechanism by which hypothyroidism causes hyponatremia is incompletely understood, it is critical to rule out hypothyroidism as a cause of hyponatremia.

C. **"Beer-drinker's Potomania" or "Tea and Toast Syndrome".** These conditions occur in individuals who eat a diet that is poor in solutes and rich in carbohydrates. Such conditions limit the ability to excrete water from ingestion or metabolism due to insufficient dietary osmoles leading to retention of water and hyponatremia. Adequate protein intake or urea administration allows correction of this condition.

D. **Reset Osmostat.** This is most commonly seen in pregnant women and results from downregulation of the central osmoreceptors. ADH release varies appropriately with changes in S_{osm}, but the S_{osm} threshold for ADH release is below normal. S_{Na}, although reduced, remains stable because water excretion is normal.

E. **Psychogenic Polydipsia.** Patients with psychosis can drink sufficient volumes of fluid to exceed their capacity to excrete their water intake, but this is uncommon if renal function is normal. With mild renal insufficiency (CKD 1 to 2), these patients will have an impairment in diluting capacity.

F. **Nephrogenic Syndrome of Inappropriate Antidiuresis.** Nephrogenic syndrome of inappropriate antidiuresis (NSIAD) was first reported in infants who presented with features of SIADH but had nonexistent ADH levels. The defect is a point mutation in the vasopressin receptor causing an activation of the receptor in the absence of ADH. Subsequently this condition has been reported in a family of adults. The vasopressin receptor is X-linked and thus women may be variably affected because of inactivation of the X chromosome.

VI. **HYPERVOLEMIC HYPONATREMIA.** Patients with edema due to congestive heart failure, nephrotic syndrome, and cirrhosis with ascites can have an increased TBW that exceeds the increase in total body sodium. In these patients, a reduced effective circulating volume (from reduced cardiac output or peripheral arterial vasodilation) decreases filtrate delivery to the diluting segment and stimulates ADH release. In the absence of concomitant diuretic use or renal disease, U_{Na} is usually <15 mEq/L, and U_{osm} is >350 mOsm/kg H_2O. Acute or chronic renal failure can cause hyponatremia because renal diluting capacity is reduced.

VII. **CLINICAL PRESENTATION.** Most patients with hyponatremia are asymptomatic. Symptoms generally occur when significant hyponatremia (S_{Na} <125 mEq/L) has evolved in <24 hours (acute hyponatremia). Nausea, vomiting, and headache are common presenting symptoms, but the clinical course can rapidly deteriorate to seizures, coma, and respiratory arrest. Severe acute hyponatremia (S_{Na} <120 mEq/L) developing over <24 hours has a mortality of up to 50%, predominantly due to complications of cerebral edema.

VIII. TREATMENT

A. Acute Versus Chronic Hyponatremia. Correction of hyponatremia in patients who are asymptomatic or who have only subtle neurologic dysfunction (and thus likely have chronic hyponatremia) should be gradual. Chronic hyponatremia in the absence of neurologic signs should be treated primarily with water restriction. However, if there is evidence of neurologic deterioration, cerebral edema, especially if there is evidence that the hyponatremia developed rapidly, the administration of a sodium chloride solution or the administration of an aquaretic agent (both described below) may be necessary, along with admission to an intensive care unit and frequent measurements of S_{Na}. Overzealous correction of S_{Na} in patients with chronic hyponatremia has been associated with the osmotic demyelination syndrome, which can result in flaccid paralysis and death. Although the reasons are not clear, it appears that individual susceptibility to the osmotic demyelination may vary across patient populations. Postmenopausal women appear to be at greater risk for residual neurologic injury.

1. **Symptomatic, euvolemic hyponatremia.** More rapid correction of hyponatremia is indicated if the risks of complications from cerebral edema outweigh the risk of aggressive treatment. Symptoms attributable to acute (<24 to 48 hours) severe hyponatremia may be subtle (lethargy, nausea, vomiting, agitation, hallucinations, weakness, headache) or severe (seizures, coma, Cheyne–Stokes respiration, pseudobulbar palsy). A well-designed treatment regimen to treat symptomatic or severe hyponatremia (S_{Na} <125) should include:

   1) Admission to an intensive care unit for monitoring of electrolytes, blood pressure, neurologic status, renal function, and frequent, every 1 to 2 hours, measurement of S_{Na} during its correction.
   2) For severe, symptomatic (coma or seizures) hyponatremia, administration of 100 mL of 3% NaCl infused over 10 minutes repeated up to three times only as needed to abate symptoms.
   3) Once symptoms have stabilized (usually after a correction of 4 to 6 mmol/L) all replacement fluids should be held, S_{Na} and S_{OSM} remeasured, and a new rate of replacement fluid calculated. For acute hyponatremia the goal is to correct the S_{Na} by no more than 8 mEq/24 hours. For chronic hyponatremia, the goal for S_{Na} correction is 4 to 6 mEq/ 24 hours.
   4) In those who present with an S_{Na} of <120 and whose rate of correction of S_{Na} in 24 hours is over 12 mEq, or over 8 mEq in those at high risk of osmotic demyelination syndrome, solute-free water administration may be necessary to prevent too rapid increase in serum sodium.
   5) Once the S_{Na} has increased above 125 mEq/L, correction can be then carried out by water restriction or with an aquaretic agent.

      It is crucial to ensure that during treatment of hyponatremia, the S_{Na} is increased only to the normal range. Osmotic demyelination syndrome has been correlated both with too rapid correction of S_{Na} and with its overcorrection.

2. **Mild, euvolemic hyponatremia.** Mild hyponatremia, due to SIADH, can usually be treated by water restriction to 1 L/day. The volume of excess water that must be excreted to normalize S_{Na} can be calculated as:

$$\text{Excess water (L)} = \text{current TBW} - \text{normal TBW}$$
$$\text{Current TBW (men)} = 0.6 \times \text{current LBM (women)} = 0.5 \times \text{current LBM}$$
$$\text{Normal TBW} = ([0.6 \times \text{current LBM}] \times \text{current } S_{Na})/\text{normal } S_{Na}$$

When the cause of SIADH is not reversible, aquaretic agents or urea (ure-Na) loading may be used.

3. **Urea.** Urea, although known to be effective as a treatment of hyponatremia for decades, was not widely utilized due to its bitter taste. More recently, a more palatable form of urea, Ure-Na, has become available, over the counter as a medical food, to treat hyponatremia. 15 g of ure-Na equals 250 mOsm and the osmotic load would induce a loss of excess water in SIADH. However, urea may also ameliorate the hyponatremia in SIADH by another mechanism; urea by increasing the inner medullary urea concentration may promote increased sodium chloride reabsorption in the ascending loop of Henle.

4. **Aquaretic agents.** There are two FDA-approved aquaretic agents, conivaptan (Vaprisol) and tolvaptan (Samsca). Conivaptan is a dual AVP V_1 and V_2 receptor antagonist that is only available in an intravenous formulation. Tolvaptan is a selective, oral, competitive AVP V_2 receptor antagonist. These agents lead to a pure water diuresis decreasing urine osmolality without affecting U_{Na} or U_K thus leading to an increase in S_{Na}. Caution should be used with conivaptan because it is metabolized by CYP450 and has a number of drug interactions.

5. **Hypovolemic hyponatremia.** Initial therapy should include:

   1) Discontinuation of diuretics;
   2) Correction of nonrenal fluid losses;
   3) Expansion of the effective circulating volume with 0.9% NaCl to replace one-third of the sodium deficit over 6 hours and the remainder over the next 24 to 48 hours.

   A general estimate of the total body sodium deficit can be calculated as follows:

$$\text{Sodium deficit (mEq)} = 0.6 \times \text{LBM (kg)} \times (140 - S_{Na})$$

6. **Hypervolemic hyponatremia.** Initial therapy should include salt and fluid restriction if the hyponatremia is secondary to reduced renal perfusion in the states of congestive heart failure and cirrhosis. Therapy to improve the underlying disease should be undertaken (e.g., improve and optimize the cardiac output in patients with congestive heart failure). While aquaretic agents appear to be safe for the treatment of severe hypervolemic and euvolemic hyponatremia, their routine use is not recommended.

IX. **HYPEROSMOLAR HYPONATREMIA.** Hypertonic infusions of glucose, mannitol, or glycine can cause shifts of ICF to the extracellular compartment with corresponding reduction in S_{Na}. In the case of hyperglycemia, for every 100 mg/dL glucose greater than 100 mg/dL, S_{Na} will decrease by 1.6 mEq/L.

X. **HYPERNATREMIA (S_{Na} >145 mEq/L).** Hypernatremia is less frequent than hyponatremia but occurs in about 1% of hospitalized elderly patients.

A. Pathophysiology. Hypernatremia implies a relative deficiency of TBW compared with total body sodium, that is, cellular dehydration. Either excessive (solute-free) water loss or excessive sodium retention, such as administration of hypertonic NaCl or $NaHCO_3$, can produce this syndrome. Of note, even patients who are ADH deficient (central diabetes insipidus) can maintain their S_{osm} if they have access to water and can drink because even mild hypertonicity potently stimulates thirst. Thus, hypernatremia requires an impaired thirst mechanism or lack of access to water (either due to mental status changes, restraints, or intubation).

B. Etiology. Hypernatremia can be classified according to the total body sodium content and the state of hydration.

1. Decreased total body sodium. Loss of hypotonic body fluids results in effective circulating volume depletion and hypernatremia. The usual signs of hypovolemia are present: poor skin turgor, postural hypotension, tachycardia, dry mucous membranes, and flat neck veins. Hypotonic fluid losses can occur from:

1) *Extrarenal sources.* Skin or gastrointestinal losses (vomiting, nasogastric suction, osmotic diarrhea) are common. The renal response leads to a high U_{osm} (>800 mOsm/kg H_2O) and a low U_{Na} and U_{Cl} (both <10 mEq/L).

2) *Renal sources.* Hypotonic polyuria can be produced by: (a) diuretics; (b) osmotic diuresis caused by glucose, mannitol, or urea (postobstructive diuresis); or (c) nonoliguric acute tubular necrosis. The urine may be either hypotonic or isotonic, and the U_{Na} is usually >20 mEq/L. More commonly, osmotic agents shift fluid to the extracellular compartment resulting in *hypo*natremia.

2. Normal total body sodium. Loss of (solute-free) water can result in hypernatremia. Evidence of volume contraction is lacking unless the water losses are extreme. The usual causes include:

1) *Extrarenal Water Loss.* Both skin and pulmonary losses of water can result in hypernatremia. In addition, water can be drawn from the extracellular compartment into damaged cells (rhabdomyolysis) with similar consequences. The U_{osm} is high and U_{Na} is a function of sodium intake.

2) *Renal Water Loss.* This more common cause of excess water loss is usually due to partial or complete failure to synthesize or secrete ADH (central diabetes insipidus) or to diminished or absent renal response to its action (nephrogenic diabetes insipidus). These disorders are characterized by an inability to concentrate the urine maximally, the result of both ADH deficiency (or resistance) and reduction of the medullary osmotic gradient by chronic polyuria. Approximately half of the cases of central diabetes insipidus are idiopathic and are usually diagnosed in childhood. Other causes include head trauma, hypoxic or ischemic encephalopathy, and CNS neoplasms. Patients with nephrogenic diabetes insipidus have impaired urinary concentrating ability despite maximal synthesis and release of ADH. Nephrogenic diabetes insipidus results from (a) a failure of the countercurrent mechanism to generate a hypertonic medullary and papillary interstitium or (b) a failure of ADH to increase the water permeability of the collecting duct. Nephrogenic diabetes insipidus (DI) may be congenital but more commonly is acquired. Chronic diseases of the renal medulla (medullary cystic disease, pyelonephritis), poor protein or salt

| TABLE 17.1 | Fluid deprivation test |

(1) During the test, urine output, weight, and vital signs must be strictly monitored to prevent severe volume contraction; weight loss should not exceed 3–5%.

(2) Patients with mild polyuria (<6 L/day) should have fluids withheld the night preceding the test (e.g., 6 PM); patients with severe polyuria (>6 L/day) should be fluid deprived only during the day (e.g., 6 AM) to allow close observation; time to achieve a maximal U_{osm} varies from 4 to 18 h.

(3) S_{osm} should approach 295 mOsm/kg H_2O after fluid deprivation and before ADH administration.

(4) U_{osm} is measured at baseline and hourly until two values vary by <30 mOsm/kg H_2O or 3–5% of body weight is lost.

(5) Five units of subcutaneous aqueous vasopressin or 10 μg of intranasal DDAVP are administered, and 1 h later a final U_{osm} is measured.

intake, hypercalcemia, hypokalemia, various systemic diseases (amyloidosis, multiple myeloma), and numerous medications (demeclocycline, lithium, glyburide) have been implicated as causes of nephrogenic DI.

3. **Increased total body sodium.** This is usually iatrogenic resulting from administration of hypertonic sodium-containing solutions (NaHCO$_3$ given to patients with metabolic acidosis) or from inappropriate repletion of hypotonic insensible fluid losses with 0.9% saline in critically ill patients.

XI. CLINICAL PRESENTATION AND DIAGNOSIS. Signs and symptoms of hypernatremia include lethargy, restlessness, hyperreflexia, spasticity, and seizures, which may progress to coma and death. Patients with central or nephrogenic diabetes insipidus may have profound polyuria and polydipsia. Cerebral dehydration leads to capillary and venous congestion, cerebrovascular tears, venous sinus thrombosis, and subcortical–subarachnoid hemorrhages. Mortality in infants and children is 43% in acute and 7% to 29% in chronic hypernatremia, whereas adults with acute hypernatremia have mortality rates as high as 60%.

Central diabetes insipidus can be distinguished from nephrogenic diabetes insipidus by the fluid deprivation test (Table 17.1) followed by exogenous ADH administration. Patients with severe central diabetes insipidus have baseline S_{osm} and S_{Na} that are high normal, and their urinary concentrating ability improves after ADH administration but not after water deprivation. In patients with severe nephrogenic diabetes insipidus, baseline S_{osm} is also increased, but they fail to respond to either ADH treatment or water deprivation. A more direct approach to distinguish central diabetes insipidus is to measure plasma or urine ADH levels simultaneously with S_{osm} after either fluid restriction or hypertonic saline infusion. Patients with central diabetes insipidus will have subnormal levels of ADH for the level of S_{osm}, whereas patients with nephrogenic diabetes insipidus will exhibit normal or elevated ratios.

XII. TREATMENT

A. Decreased Total Body Sodium. Initially patients should receive isotonic NaCl until the effective circulating volume has been restored. Thereafter, hypotonic solutions (D_5W or 0.45% NaCl) can be used.

B. Normal Total Body Sodium. Pure water loss should be replaced with either enteral or intravenous solute-free water (e.g., D_5W when fully metabolized). The water deficit (WD) can be calculated as follows:

$$WD\ (L) = (0.6 \times current\ LBM) \times ([current\ S_{Na} - 140]/140)$$

Normally the WD should be replaced over 48 hours with frequent monitoring of S_{Na} and S_{osm}. The S_{Na} should decrease by no more than 12 mEq over 24 hours. Faster rates of correction can cause seizures.

The treatment of choice for central diabetes insipidus is intranasal deamino-8-D-arginine vasopressin (DDAVP), a synthetic analogue of ADH, 10 to 20 micrograms twice daily. Therapy for acquired nephrogenic diabetes insipidus should be directed toward the primary disorder. Thiazide diuretics and a low-salt intake will decrease the polyuria.

C. Increased Total Body Sodium. Hypertonic sodium-containing solutions should be discontinued and diuretics administered to promote excretion of the excess salt and water.

XIII. SUGGESTED READINGS

Arieff AI. Hyponatremia associated with permanent brain damage. *Adv Intern Med.* 1987;32: 325–344.

Ayus JC, Wheeler JM, Arieff AI. Postoperative hyponatremic encephalopathy in menstruant women. *Ann Intern Med.* 1992;117(11):891–897.

Decaux G, Vandergheynst F, Bouko Y, et al. Nephrogenic syndrome of inappropriate antidiuresis in adults: high phenotypic variability in men and women from a large pedigree. *J Am Soc Nephrol.* 2007;18(2):606–612.

Ellison DH, Berl T. Clinical practice. The syndrome of inappropriate antidiuresis. *N Engl J Med.* 2007;356(20):2064–2072.

Feldman BJ, Rosenthal SM, Vargas GA, et al. Nephrogenic syndrome of inappropriate antidiuresis. *N Engl J Med.* 2005;352(18):1884–1890.

Marsden PA, Halperin ML. Pathophysiological approach to patients presenting with hypernatremia. *Am J Nephrol.* 1985;5(4):229–235.

Palmer BF. Hyponatraemia in a neurosurgical patient: syndrome of inappropriate antidiuretic hormone secretion versus cerebral salt wasting. *Nephrol Dial Transplant.* 2000;15(2):262–268.

Schrier RW, Gross P, Gheorghiade M, et al. Tolvaptan, a selective oral vasopressin V2-receptor antagonist, for hyponatremia. *N Engl J Med.* 2006;355(20):2099–2112.

Sterns RH. Treatment of severe hyponatremia. *Clin J Am Soc Nephrol.* 2018;13(4):641–649.

Verbalis JG, Berl T. Disorders of water balance. In: Brenner BM, ed. *The Kidney.* Saunders; 2008: 459–504.

18 Potassium Disorders

Charles S. Wingo, I. David Weiner

In healthy individuals, multiple hormones and transporters finely regulate serum potassium concentration (S_K) between 3.5 and 5 mEq/L. However, disorders of S_K are common, may present without symptoms, and can be lethal. Hypokalemia (S_K <3.5 mEq/L) and hyperkalemia (S_K >5.0 mEq/L) can occur from drugs or dietary, hormonal, renal, or gastrointestinal abnormalities. Both conditions are associated with a greater mortality than individuals with normal S_K.

I. **PHYSIOLOGY.** S_K is determined by the balance between K^+ intake, K^+ excretion, and transcellular K^+ shifts. K^+ is present in almost all foods, but the concentration is highest in fruits and vegetables. In general, food higher in NaCl content tends to be lower in K^+ content, and vice versa. Dietary K^+ is almost completely absorbed in the normal gastrointestinal tract. Approximately 90% of potassium intake is excreted in the urine, with the remainder in the stool. Renal K^+ excretion normally determines long-term K^+ balance. However, when diarrhea is present, enteric losses of potassium can be substantial and can lead to hypokalemia. Because potassium is primarily an intracellular cation (only 2% of total body potassium stores are in extracellular fluid), small changes in the balance between intracellular and extracellular compartments can lead to large changes in S_K.

A. **Renal Regulation of Potassium.** Renal potassium excretion reflects the balance between glomerular filtration, tubular reabsorption, and tubular secretion. In contrast to almost all other solutes excreted by the kidneys, potassium transport in the proximal tubule and loop of Henle is not the major regulatory mechanism. Instead, the major mechanism determining K^+ excretion is secretion by the aldosterone-sensitive distal nephron (ASDN). The ASDN comprises the connecting segment, initial collecting tubule, and the collecting duct.

K^+ secretion in the ASDN is linked to Na^+ reabsorption. Na^+ reabsorption involves luminal sodium uptake, via the apical epithelial Na^+ channel (ENaC), which is coupled to basolateral K^+ exit via Na^+-K^+-ATPase. Potassium that enters the cell via Na^+-K^+-ATPase can be secreted into the luminal membrane either coupled to chloride secretion or via apical potassium channels. Magnesium is necessary for normal regulation of apical K^+ channels, and chronic hypomagnesemia may lead to excessive K^+ secretion. During Cl^--depletion metabolic alkalosis significant passive coupled K^+-Cl^- secretion occurs resulting in potassium depletion.

Several physical factors regulate ASDN K^+ secretion. Increased tubular fluid flow, distal sodium delivery, luminal pH, and reduced luminal chloride concentration all stimulate potassium excretion. Most diuretics, except K^+-sparing diuretics, enhance potassium secretion by increasing distal nephron luminal flow and sodium delivery. Thiazide diuretics, when dosed for equal effects on Na^+ secretion, increase K^+ excretion to a greater extent than the loop diuretics; the mechanism is currently incompletely understood. Dietary potassium loading and chronic hyperaldosteronism each stimulate ASDN potassium secretion. The primary acute action of aldosterone is to promote Na^+ retention, but long-term aldosterone stimulation reduces S_K by renal and extrarenal mechanisms. In addition, dietary K^+ intake stimulates K^+ secretion through gastrointestinal potassium sensors that are not fully defined.

The kidney conserves potassium in response to hypokalemia by both decreasing potassium secretion and stimulating potassium absorption. Active potassium reabsorption occurs in the collecting duct by luminal proton-potassium pumps (H^+-K^+-ATPases).

B. **Effect of Acid–Base Disturbances.** Metabolic alkalosis frequently leads to hypokalemia. This is in part, due to an increase in bicarbonate excretion, which increases K^+ excretion to offset the negative charge of bicarbonate (HCO_3^-). Metabolic alkalosis is also associated with conditions that cause hypokalemia, such as primary and secondary aldosteronism. Whether acidosis causes hyperkalemia is somewhat controversial, but the simplest explanation is that some conditions that cause metabolic acidosis, such as diabetic ketoacidosis (DKA) and lactic acidosis associated with tissue ischemia, cause hyperkalemia as a direct effect of the underlying condition, and not as a result of the acidosis. Respiratory acid–base disorders typically have little-to-no effect on serum K^+.

C. **Key Hormones.** Several hormones directly affect S_K. The clinically most important are insulin, catecholamines, and aldosterone. Insulin, β-adrenergic receptor agonists, and aldosterone each stimulate the Na^+-K^+-ATPase present in almost all cells. This leads to redistribution from extracellular to the intracellular compartments and decreases serum K^+. The effect of insulin and β-adrenergic receptor agonists is rapid, within minutes, whereas the effect of aldosterone is slower and requires hours. Aldosterone also has chronic effects on extrarenal and renal transport mechanisms that reduce S_K. Many other hormones can alter K^+ homeostasis, including thyroid hormone, parathyroid hormone, and dopamine, but their effect is not generally large enough, or sufficiently frequent, to lead to common clinical K^+ disorders.

II. HYPOKALEMIA

A. **Pathogenesis.** Hypokalemia develops either due to acute transcellular K^+ shifts, from the extracellular to the intracellular compartments, or from prolonged K^+ losses from the extracellular compartment. Prolonged K^+ losses can result from either inappropriately high renal K^+ excretion or excessive fecal K^+ loss. Excessive urinary K^+ loss is most frequently associated with use of either loop or thiazide diuretics, but may result from other electrolyte disorders, endocrinologic disorders or, very rarely, from genetic disorders. Each of these is exacerbated by a high NaCl diet. With total body K^+ loss, there is a shift of K^+ from intracellular to the extracellular fluid compartments, most notably skeletal muscle, which decreases the magnitude of the change in serum K^+. With chronic K^+ loss, this may result in decreases of total body K^+ deficit of 100 to 500 mmol or more.

B. **Adverse Consequences.** Symptoms from hypokalemia are not common (<5% of patients), but their frequency increases with $S_K < 2.5$ mEq/L, and with rapid decreases in S_K. The most common patient-reported symptom is muscular weakness, which may progress to respiratory failure with severe hypokalemia.

TABLE 18.1	Clinical manifestations of hypokalemia

Cardiac
  Predisposition to digitalis glycoside toxicity
  Ventricular irritability
  Abnormal electrocardiogram (flattened T waves, U waves, ST-segment
    depression)
  Coronary artery spasm
Neuromuscular
  Skeletal (weakness, cramps, tetany, paralysis, and rhabdomyolysis)
Gastrointestinal
  Constipation
  Ileus
Hyperammonemic Encephalopathy
Renal
  Polyuria
  Increased ammoniagenesis
  Increased renal vascular resistance
  Hypertension
  Increased sensitivity of BP to dietary NaCl ingestion
Endocrine
  Decreased insulin sensitivity

Chronic hypokalemia can lead, even in the absence of overt symptoms, to salt-sensitive hypertension and kidney disease. Hypokalemia also frequently leads to metabolic alkalosis, polyuria, and impaired insulin release. In patients with liver disease, hypokalemia can lead to hyperammonemic encephalopathy. Finally, hypokalemia is associated with increased mortality, likely because of increased development of lethal ventricular arrhythmias. Additional symptoms are shown in Table 18.1.

C. Presentation. Because the symptoms associated with hypokalemia are quite non-specific, hypokalemia is typically identified from measurement of serum electrolytes in appropriate patient populations. These populations include individuals with new-onset weakness or respiratory failure, those with hypertension or kidney disease, or individuals who use diuretics. Because hypokalemia may occur in up to 20% of hospitalized patients, serum electrolytes should be a routine component of the assessment of hospitalized patients.

D. Evaluation. Evaluation should focus on the medication history, measurement of serum Mg^{2+}, volume status, and blood pressure. Surreptitious laxative use, diuretic use, or self-induced vomiting may not be readily apparent. Figure 18.1 provides a recommended diagnostic approach and Table 18.2 provides a differential diagnosis. Transcellular shifts should be considered when the onset is acute, and is frequently associated with administration of β-adrenergic agonists, that is, terbutaline in the asthmatic or pregnant patients, insulin in the diabetic, or sudden hypokalemia may have a genetic etiology, such as hypokalemic periodic paralysis. Transcellular shifts are often associated with low urinary K^+ excretion if samples are obtained while the patient is hypokalemic.

Hypokalemia due to decreased total body K^+ can be due to either renal or extrarenal mechanisms. These can be differentiated by assessing urinary K^+

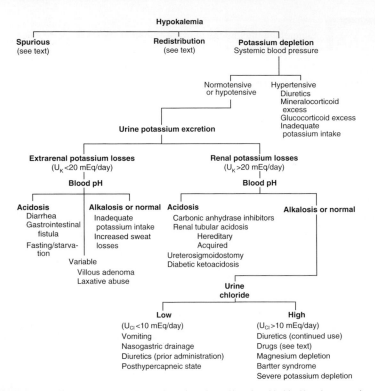

FIGURE 18.1: Diagnostic approach in hypokalemic patients. U_{Cl}, urine chloride; U_K, urine potassium.

excretion, which will be suppressed when due to extrarenal causes (typically <20 mEq/day or <20 mEq/g creatinine). Extrarenal mechanisms usually involve either gastrointestinal K$^+$ losses, such as chronic diarrhea or nasogastric suction, or occasionally from severe and prolonged diaphoresis leading to sweat K$^+$ loss.

Hypokalemia in the hypertensive patient most frequently is due to diuretics, low dietary potassium intake, particularly if associated with high NaCl ingestion, or mineralocorticoid excess (e.g., primary aldosteronism and renal artery stenosis). Cushing syndrome is less frequently associated with hypokalemia. Thiazides and loop diuretics commonly cause hypokalemia, but rarely are sufficient to produce severe hypokalemia (S_K <3.0 mEq/L) in the absence of concomitant factors. Assessment of the AM plasma aldosterone and plasma renin activity should be considered in hypertensive patients with hypokalemia, particularly if they have truly resistant hypertension.

Hypokalemia not associated with diuretics, extrarenal losses, or excessive aldosterone is often due to hypomagnesemia. This is particularly true in patients treated with a proton-pump inhibitor, which frequently leads to hypomagnesemia. Hypomagnesemia can lead to hypokalemia by disrupting regulation of ASDN K$^+$ channels, leading to excessive K$^+$ secretion and ongoing renal K$^+$ losses. Identification and treatment of the hypomagnesemia may be sufficient to correct the hypokalemia.

TABLE 18.2	Differential diagnosis of hypokalemia

Artifactual (high white blood cell count)
Redistribution (cellular shift)
   β-Adrenergic agonists (epinephrine, terbutaline)
   Theophylline toxicity
   Refeeding (hyperalimentation)
   Acute insulin administration
   Periodic paralysis (familial, thyrotoxic, acquired)
   Barium poisoning
   Mineralocorticoid excess (both renal and extrarenal effects, see below)
Intestinal
   Inadequate dietary intake
   Gastrointestinal losses
   Diarrhea and chronic laxative abuse
   Ureterosigmoidostomy (urinary diversion)
   Villous adenoma
   Gastrointestinal fistulas
Renal losses
   Metabolic alkalosis (vomiting, nasogastric drainage)
   Diuretics
   Hypomagnesemia
   Antibiotics/antifungal/chemotherapeutic agents
   Penicillins (e.g., carbenicillin)
   Amphotericin B (renal tubular acidosis)
   Toluene toxicity (glue-sniffing)
   Aminoglycosides
   Cisplatin
   Glucocorticoids (increased cellular potassium loss and increased excretion)
   Mineralocorticoid excess
   Adrenal adenoma or bilateral adrenal hyperplasia
   Glycyrrhizic acid intoxication (natural licorice ingestion)
   Adrenal enzyme–deficiency syndromes
   Renal tubular acidosis (RTA)
   Proximal (type II) RTA
   Distal (type I) RTA
   Acute renal failure syndromes (especially with recovery of renal function and
      diuretic phase of acute tubular necrosis)
   Postobstructive diuresis
   Interstitial nephritis
   Bartter syndrome, Liddle syndrome, Gitelman syndrome
   Acute leukemia (lysozymuria)

Hypokalemia is not commonly associated with muscle weakness. When chronic weakness is present, the hypokalemia is typically associated with total body K^+ depletion. When the weakness is acute, consideration for transcellular K^+ shifts should be considered, and should include consideration of hypokalemic periodic paralysis.

E. Treatment. Treatment of hypokalemia involves consideration of the speed of therapy needed and the magnitude of K^+ replacement that is needed. Hypokalemia associated with ventricular arrhythmias or severe hypokalemia associated with a need for emergent surgery should be aggressively treated, and may necessitate intravenous therapy. In the absence of these conditions, oral therapy is generally preferred, and intravenous therapy should be used only if oral therapy cannot be used.

S_K is not a good indicator of the total body K^+ deficit because of difficulty in quantifying the extent of intracellular K^+ loss. In general, the more prolonged the hypokalemia the greater the total body K^+ deficit.

Potassium replacement with KCl is the mainstay of therapy for hypokalemia and may be done orally or intravenously. Oral replacement over several days is safe and rarely causes hyperkalemia in patients with well-preserved renal function when given in doses up to 120 mEq/day.

Intravenous replacement should be reserved for patients unable to take oral potassium, who have life-threatening conditions (e.g., recurrent ventricular tachycardia, ventricular fibrillation or respiratory failure with severe hypokalemia, paralysis, or digitalis intoxication with arrhythmias), or in those needing correction of the hypokalemia prior to emergent surgery. Rates of up to 10 mEq/h are generally safe; doses of 20 to 40 mEq/h should have continuous EKG monitoring because variable rates of cellular K^+ uptake increase the risk of iatrogenic hyperkalemia developing. Doses up to 40 mEq/h should be given through a central venous catheter because of the risk of tissue necrosis if extravasation occurs; however, *these doses are rarely necessary.* S_K should be checked at least every 2 to 4 hours during high-dose replacement.

Treatment of the underlying condition causing the hypokalemia is central to therapy. If due to diuretics, addition of a K^+-sparing diuretic, for example, amiloride, triamterene, or spironolactone, can be considered. Dietary NaCl restriction typically will decrease the magnitude of diuretic-induced hypokalemia, and addition of medications that inhibit the renin–angiotensin–aldosterone system (RAAS) may be beneficial. Patients with hypertension and hypokalemia should be screened for primary or secondary aldosteronism and have these treated appropriately if identified. Dietary modification to increase intake of high K^+ foods and to decrease dietary NaCl intake is usually beneficial. Hypomagnesemia, if present, should be treated, and proton-pump inhibitors discontinued unless there is an absolute indication for their continued use. If diarrhea is present, then identification of its etiology should ensue, and appropriate therapy initiated. With genetic causes of hypokalemia, for example, Gitelman or Bartter syndrome), multimodality therapy involving oral KCl, K^+-sparing diuretics, and RAAS inhibitors may be needed. However, normalization of S_K in genetic cases may be difficult to achieve. In such cases, the hypokalemia likely reflects abnormally large renal K^+ clearance rather than body K^+ depletion.

III. HYPERKALEMIA

A. Pathogenesis. Hyperkalemia develops either from renal potassium excretion that is insufficient to maintain a normal S_K or in response to transcellular potassium shifts. In the presence of normal renal function, the kidneys possess sufficient capacity to excrete K^+ as to preclude chronic, diet-induced hyperkalemia. However, a significant component of this capacity involves gastrointestinal tract K^+ sensors; this means that intravenous K^+, which does not activate these sensors, can easily lead to possibly lethal hyperkalemia. The other major cause of hyperkalemia involves transcellular shifts of K^+ from intracellular stores into the extracellular compartment. Common causes of hyperkalemia may be an artifact of blood collection, such as hemolysis, which may occur during the phlebotomy procedure or during the extracorporeal handling of the blood sample; intravascular hemolysis typically does not lead to hyperkalemia unless massive. Other common causes of transcellular K^+ shifts include hyperosmolarity, that is, hyperglycemia in DKA, insulin deficiency, and RAAS blockade. Although metabolic acidosis is often said to cause hyperkalemia, acute acidosis by itself typically does not cause acute transcellular K^+ shifts. Instead the hyperkalemia is frequently a consequence of the underlying cause of the acidosis. For example, in DKA, the hyperosmolarity due to hyperglycemia and the associated insulin deficiency are the primary causes of the hyperkalemia, and treatment of the DKA corrects the hyperkalemia. Similarly, in lactic acidosis due to tissue ischemia, the hyperkalemia results from tissue ischemia and cellular K^+ loss. However, the hyperkalemia may be the cause of the acidosis, as in type IV renal tubular acidosis (RTA), through its effects on ammonia metabolism. In this case, correction of the hyperkalemia corrects the acidosis.

Although unusual, pseudohyperkalemia should also be considered in the evaluation of hyperkalemia. Sample hemolysis, discussed above, is the most common cause of pseudohyperkalemia. Other causes are shown in Table 18.3.

| TABLE 18.3 | Causes of hyperkalemia |

Common
    Spurious and improper blood collection technique
    Exercise and ischemic blood drawing
    Pseudohyperkalemia
        Hemolysis
        Leukocytosis
        Thrombocytosis
    Drug-induced hyperkalemia (see Table 18.5)
    Acute or chronic renal disease
    Acidosis and hyperkalemic renal tubular acidosis

Increased cellular release or potassium load
    Tissue necrosis or trauma (rhabdomyolysis, tissue lysis, hematoma)
    Hyperosmolality
    Exogenous potassium administration

Decreased cellular potassium uptake
    Insulin deficiency (e.g., diabetic ketoacidosis)
    Aldosterone deficiency or blockade (see Table 18.5) (acquired and hereditary forms)
    β-Adrenergic blockers (e.g., propranolol)
    Digitalis poisoning

Redistribution and Uncommon
    Hyperkalemic periodic paralysis, succinylcholine
    Familial hyperkalemia
    Arginine and lysine administration
    Fluoride intoxication
    Hyperkalemic hypertensive syndromes (pseudohypoaldosteronism type 2)

TABLE 18.4	Electrocardiographic findings in hyperkalemia

Peaking or tenting of T waves
Flattening of P waves
Prolongation of PR interval
Bradycardia, nodal rhythm
Widening of QRS complex (to sine wave)
Ventricular fibrillation, asystole, or both

B. **Adverse Consequences**. The major consequence of hyperkalemia is due to its effects on the cardiac conduction system. Hyperkalemia decreases SA nodal arrhythmogenicity, slows conduction, and alters repolarization. Altered ventricular repolarization leads to the development of "peaked" T waves; this should involve changes in all leads, and if present on isolated leads of a 12-lead electrocardiogram should not be misconstrued as evidence of cardiac effects of hyperkalemia. The combination of these cardiac effects can lead to progressive bradycardia, AV nodal blockade, QRS prolongation, and the development of ventricular fibrillation.

Chronic hyperkalemia has its major adverse effect on systemic acid–base homeostasis, leading to metabolic acidosis. This occurs because hyperkalemia impairs multiple components of ammonia metabolism, the primary component of net acid excretion. Because chronic metabolic acidosis can accelerate progression of chronic kidney disease (CKD), induce muscle atrophy, impair glucose sensitivity, and alter bone mineralization, and is associated with increased mortality, correction of the hyperkalemia and the resultant metabolic acidosis is indicated.

C. **Presentation**. In general, the symptoms of hyperkalemia are nonspecific. Instead, recognition of this disorder relies on recognizing its association with decreased kidney function, that is, CKD, with specific drugs, and in specific clinical circumstances, such as DKA. Diagnosis depends on appropriate measurement of S_K. It is critical to recognize that *life-threatening hyperkalemia can be silent*, so evidence of EKG changes (see Table 18.4) should be treated emergently, because progression to ventricular fibrillation may be rapid and the time course can be unpredictable.

D. **Evaluation**. If hyperkalemia is severe, such as $S_K \geq 6.5$ mmol/L, a 12-lead electrocardiogram should be obtained urgently for evidence of cardiac conduction deficits described above, while confirmatory whole blood or plasma K is obtained. If present, emergent therapy should be initiated (see below). Comparison to prior EKGs when the patient was normokalemic is most useful.

Next, eliminate spurious hyperkalemia. Extracorporeal hemolysis should be explicitly noted in the laboratory report. If hemolysis is identified, the sample should be redrawn, preferably through a large-bore needle (to avoid hemolysis) and without prolonged tourniquet time for repeat analysis prior to any specific therapy. Either plasma potassium (heparinized tube) or whole blood potassium (arterial blood gas instrument) are preferred for confirmatory testing.

Second, consider the possibility of pseudohyperkalemia. The white blood cell and platelet count should be evaluated. Pseudohyperkalemia frequently occurs from potassium released during clotting when the platelet count is $>1,000,000/mm^3$ or the white blood cell count is $>200,000/mm^3$. Even platelet

TABLE 18.5	Drug-induced hyperkalemia

Common
  Potassium-sparing diuretics (amiloride, triamterene)
  Nonsteroidal anti-inflammatory drugs
  Cyclosporine and tacrolimus
  Mineralocorticoid receptor blockers
  Heparin
  Angiotensin-converting enzyme inhibitors and angiotensin II receptor blockers
  Pentamidine
  Sulfamethoxazole-trimethoprim (high dose)
Uncommon
  β-Adrenergic antagonists
  Succinylcholine
  Digitalis poisoning

counts between $500,000/mm^3$ and $1,000,000/mm^3$ are associated with a significant incidence of hyperkalemia. In such cases, the discrepancy between S_K and plasma potassium values may exceed 1.0 mEq/L. Rarely, pseudohyperkalemia may also be due to "leaky" erythrocytes of either acquired (infectious mononucleosis) or hereditary etiology.

In the absence of pseudohyperkalemia or potassium redistribution (Table 18.3), an S_K above the normal range (5.0 to 5.3 mEq/L for most laboratories) is commonly due to drugs (Table 18.5), renal disease, or metabolic acidosis. Hyperkalemia is frequently observed when renal function is severely compromised, that is, stage IV CKD, but can be seen in stage III CKD, particularly in patients treated with multiple RAAS inhibitors. Diabetes mellitus, particularly if CKD is present, increases the risk of hyperkalemia. Less common causes of diminished renal potassium clearance include defective adrenal mineralocorticoid production and rare genetic causes such as hyperkalemic hypertensive syndrome (pseudohypoaldosteronism type II or Gordon syndrome).

Patients with adrenal cortical insufficiency with combined glucocorticoid and mineralocorticoid deficiency, that is, Addison disease, may exhibit mild degrees of hyperkalemia, but impairment of renal sodium conservation is usually the predominant clinical finding. In contrast, hyporeninemic hypoaldosteronism with preserved glucocorticoid function is common in patients with CKD, particularly with concomitant diabetes mellitus. The hyporeninemic hypoaldosteronism reflects underlying volume expansion. Treatment with mineralocorticoid analogs should be avoided because they may accelerate the progression of the underlying CKD and worsen the volume expansion.

Table 18.6 lists laboratory and diagnostic tests that are helpful in establishing the etiology of hyperkalemia.

E. **Treatment.** Hyperkalemia can be life threatening because of its effects on cardiac conduction. If EKG changes of hyperkalemia are observed, emergent therapy should be instituted. Drug therapy for the acute treatment of hyperkalemia is listed in Table 18.7. Simultaneous use of several or all of these measures may be indicated if EKG abnormalities exist. It is important to recognize that only K^+-binding resins and dialysis remove potassium from the body; other treatments should be considered as temporary measures.

TABLE 18.6	Laboratory and diagnostic tests to evaluate hyperkalemia

Urinalysis
Bladder catheterization or ultrasound
Renal ultrasound
Electrocardiogram
Urine and serum electrolytes
Serum creatinine and blood urea nitrogen
Arterial blood gases and pH
White blood cell count
Platelet count
Hematocrit (if low, may indicate chronic kidney disease)

Intravenous calcium is the most rapid way to reverse the cardiac effects of hyperkalemia. It has a rapid onset of action (~0.5 to 2 minutes), but its cardio-protective effects may last only 30 to 60 minutes. A second dose may be given if no resolution of EKG changes is seen. Slower infusions should be given with EKG monitoring in patients on digitalis to prevent both symptoms of hyper-calcemia and myocardial digitalis toxicity.

Insulin stimulates cellular potassium uptake and is the second most rapid way to treat hyperkalemia (onset of action in 15 to 30 minutes). Ten units of reg-ular insulin given intravenously will reliably decrease S_K in 10 to 20 minutes and should be accompanied by glucose ($D_{50}W$ 1 ampule), except in hyperglycemic patients. Effects of insulin and glucose last 4 to 6 hours and can be repeated every 20 minutes as needed to reverse EKG changes. However, these effects depend on sustained insulin action and the hyperkalemia frequently recurs if other measures are not implemented.

β-Adrenergic receptor agonists can reduce S_K by stimulating cellular K^+ uptake. Nebulized albuterol, 10 to 20 mg (two to eight times the usual nebulized dose), has an onset of action in 30 minutes and can decrease S_K by up to 1 mEq/L. The major limitation of β-agonist therapy is tachycardia and arrhythmias.

The use of $NaHCO_3$ (1 to 2 ampules intravenously) should be reserved for patients with frank acidosis who have preserved renal function because its effect is likely limited solely to increasing renal K^+ excretion. Due to its hypertonicity, $NaHCO_3$ may precipitate volume overload or it may lead to hyperosmolarity, which itself can worsen hyperkalemia. Of note, intravenous $NaHCO_3$-containing solutions should not be given in the same intravenous line as calcium to prevent precipitation of calcium carbonate.

Definitive therapy of hyperkalemia usually involves K^+ removal from the body. This may be accomplished by either diuretic therapy, if renal function is preserved, with enteric K^+-binding resins, or with dialysis.

Diuretics are often effective in the long-term therapy of hyperkalemia but should not be relied upon with acute or with life-threatening hyperkalemia. Thiazide diuretics, when dosed for equivalent effect on Na^+ excretion as loop diuretics, produce greater urinary K^+ excretion, and often can be the first line of diuretic therapy. Because the effectiveness of both loop and thiazide diuretics decreases as GFR decreases, higher doses are needed in patients with CKD.

Enteric K^+-binding resins are effective at removing K^+ for many patients. Treatment options include sodium polystyrene sulfate (SPS, Kayexalate),

TABLE 18.7	Drug therapy for hyperkalemia

Drug	Dose	Onset of action (min)	Duration of action	Comments
Calcium gluconate or chloride	10–30 mL (10% solution) IV	1–3	30–60 min	Should be initial therapy for life-threatening hyperkalemia with EKG changes. May need repeat treatments.
Insulin/Glucose	5–10 U regular insulin with 25 g glucose (repeat every 40–60 min)	15–30 min	4–6 h	Glucose may not be needed if severe hyperglycemia is present. If CKD is present, monitor glucose levels because of possible hypoglycemic response.
Albuterol	10 mg nebulized	30 min	2–4 h	May cause tachycardia and/ or ventricular arrhythmias.
Patiromer (Veltassa)	8.4–25.2 g/day orally	4–6 h	12–24 h	Should not be used for life-threatening hyperkalemia because of delayed onset of action.
Sodium zirconium cyclosilicate (Lokelma)	10 g tid for up to 48 h Dose range: 5 g orally every other day	4–6 h	12–24 h	Should not be used for life-threatening hyperkalemia because of delayed onset of action.
Sodium polystyrene sulfate (Kayexalate)	Oral 30–60 g with 70% sorbitol, or enema, 60–120 g	4–6 h	6–12 h	Use is associated rarely with colonic injury and bowel necrosis

patiromer, and sodium zirconium cyclosilicate. All are effective for chronic hyperkalemia treatment, and there is insufficient data to compare relative effectiveness at present. However, patiromer and sodium zirconium cyclosilicate do not cause diarrhea of oral SPS/sorbitol preparations and may be better tolerated. These medications rely on K+ binding in the gastrointestinal tract, and the effect may be delayed for several hours. They should not be relied upon in the therapy of acute hyperkalemia with cardiac effects.

Hemodialysis is an effective method of potassium removal when hyperkalemia is complicated by volume overload, acidosis, and renal failure. Potassium can be removed at a rate of 25 to 30 mEq/h with hemodialysis, whereas peritoneal dialysis can remove 10 to 15 mEq/h. Rapid removal can be problematic in cases of digitalis intoxication because the rapid reduction in S_K can precipitate the effects of digitalis toxicity. The use of a bath dialysate less than 2 mEq/L should generally be avoided because the rate of potassium removal is only marginally better than a 2 mEq/L K^+ dialysate and has the true risk of provoking life-threatening hypokalemia if not monitored closely. Continuous renal replacement therapy does not rapidly remove K^+ and should not be used for life-threatening hyperkalemia; it is effective for chronic hyperkalemia without cardiac effects, however.

Some hyperkalemic patients treated with hemodialysis, particularly diabetics, exhibit rapid increases in S_K to hyperkalemic values even without exogenous K^+ administration or acute cellular lysis (such as with rhabdomyolysis or tumor lysis syndromes). Such individuals represent a particular challenge and their hyperkalemia likely reflect defects in extrarenal K^+ homeostasis. Attention to glucose control, acid–base balance, their medications (see Table 18.5), as well as dietary K^+ intake, may allow improvement or correction of the hyperkalemia.

IV. SUGGESTED READINGS

Allon M, Copkney C. Albuterol and insulin for treatment of hyperkalemia in hemodialysis patients. *Kidney Int.* 1990;38(5):869–872.

Blumberg A, Roser HW, Zehnder C, et al. Plasma potassium in patients with terminal renal failure during and after haemodialysis; relationship with dialytic potassium removal and total body potassium. *Nephrol Dial Transplant.* 1997;12(8):1629–1634.

Blumberg A, Weidmann P, Ferrari P. Effect of prolonged bicarbonate administration on plasma potassium in terminal renal failure. *Kidney Int.* 1992;41(2):369–374.

Mount DB, Zandi-Nejad K. Disorders of potassium balance. In: Taal MW, Chertow GM, Marsden PA, et al., eds. *The Kidney.* 9th ed. Elsevier; 2012:640–688.

Weiner ID, Linas SL, Wingo CS. Disorders of potassium metabolism. In: Freehally J, Johnson RJ, Floege J, eds. *Comprehensive Clinical Nephrology.* 5th ed. Saunders; 2014:118.

Wingo CS, Weiner ID. Approach to the patient with hypo-/hyperkalaemia. In: Turner N, ed. *Oxford Textbook of Clinical Nephrology.* 4th ed. Oxford University Press; 2015:p1–p44.

19 Acid–Base Disorders

I. David Weiner, Charles S. Wingo

INTRODUCTION

An acid–base disorder implies that the quantity of acid and base in extracellular fluid is abnormal. The presence of an acid–base disorder always indicates one or more underlying disease process whose identification and treatment are likely to lead to substantial clinical benefit.

I. DEFINITIONS

A. Acidemia and Alkalemia. Acidemia is the presence of an abnormally low blood pH, that is, <7.36, and alkalemia is the presence of an abnormally high blood pH, that is, >7.44. Either indicates an acid–base disorder.

Blood pH is determined by blood HCO_3^- and pCO_2 concentrations, as shown:

$$pH = 6.1 + log\ \frac{[HCO_3^-]}{0.03 \times pCO_2} \tag{1}$$

All acid–base disorders have an abnormality in either the blood HCO_3^- or pCO_2 and sometimes in both. If they change in a parallel direction, that is, both increase or both decrease, these effects partially, or completely, offset each other and result in a smaller change in pH. When they change in opposite directions, the effect is a greater pH change than explainable by either one alone.

B. Acidosis and Alkalosis. *Acidosis* is a process that decreases the pH. It involves either decreased blood HCO_3^- or increased pCO_2. *Alkalosis* is a process that increases the pH. It involves either increased blood HCO_3^- or decreased pCO_2.

Both acidosis and alkalosis are defined further by whether they result from metabolic or respiratory disorders. Metabolic disorders lead to an abnormal blood HCO_3^- whereas respiratory disorders lead to an abnormal pCO_2. Thus, acidemia is the result of either metabolic acidosis ($\downarrow HCO_3^-$) or respiratory acidosis ($\uparrow pCO_2$), and alkalemia is the result of either metabolic alkalosis ($\uparrow HCO_3^-$) or respiratory alkalosis ($\downarrow pCO_2$).

C. Compensatory Response. Acid–base homeostasis is so critical to health that backup systems compensate, usually incompletely, for any acid–base disturbance. For example, acidemia stimulates brain-stem respiratory centers, that increase ventilation and CO_2 elimination, thereby decreasing pCO_2, that minimizes the acidemia. This response occurs within seconds. Acid–base disorders also alter renal net acid excretion that changes the blood HCO_3^- but this requires 4 to 5 days for completion.

D. Primary Acid–Base Disorders. This combination of acid–base disorders and their compensatory responses results in six primary acid–base disorders shown in Table 19.1.

TABLE 19.1	Primary acid–base disorders

Name	Primary abnormality	Compensation	Magnitude of compensation
Metabolic acidosis	HCO_3^- ↓	Secondary respiratory alkalosis	$\Delta pCO_2 \sim 0.7$ mm Hg per 1 mmol/L ΔHCO_3^-. Minimum pCO_2 8–12 mm Hg
Metabolic alkalosis	HCO_3^- ↑	Secondary respiratory acidosis	$\Delta pCO_2 \sim 1.0$–1.5 mm Hg per 1 mmol/L ΔHCO_3^-. Maximum $pCO_2 \sim 55$ mm Hg
Acute respiratory acidosis	pCO_2 ↑	Minimal change in blood HCO_3^-	$\Delta HCO_3^- \sim 1$ mM per 10 mm Hg ΔpCO_2
Chronic respiratory acidosis	pCO_2 ↑	Secondary metabolic alkalosis	$\Delta HCO_3^- \sim 4$ mM per 10 mm Hg ΔpCO_2
Acute respiratory alkalosis	pCO_2 ↓	Minimal change in blood HCO_3^-	$\Delta HCO_3^- \sim 2$ mM per 10 mm Hg ΔpCO_2
Chronic respiratory alkalosis	pCO_2 ↓	Secondary metabolic acidosis	$\Delta HCO_3^- \sim 4$–5 mM per 10 mm Hg ΔpCO_2

II. EVALUATION OF THE PATIENT WITH AN ACID–BASE DISORDER. Evaluating an acid–base disorder requires the assessment of both blood chemistry and blood gas measurements. Blood gas measurements should use arterial samples but if impractical, a venous blood gas ideally using a central venous or pulmonary artery catheter sample may substitute. If peripheral venous blood is sampled, the tourniquet should be released ~1 minute before sampling to minimize artifacts from tourniquet-induced tissue ischemia. Tissue CO_2 production from venous blood samples increases the pCO_2 by 4 to 5 mm Hg, and decreases the pH by 0.03 to 0.05 pH units but the HCO_3^- is generally maintained. Arterial measurements are the "gold standard."

III. METABOLIC ACIDOSIS

A. Pathophysiology. There are four fundamental mechanisms that can cause metabolic acidosis:

1) either exogenous acid loads or endogenous acid production are increased;
2) extracellular fluid dilution by rapid administration of intravenous solutions that do not contain alkali or alkali precursors (e.g., 0.9% saline);
3) impaired renal net acid excretion that prevents matching with endogenous acid production (e.g., CKD and renal tubular acidosis (RTA); and,
4) bicarbonate loss via the gastrointestinal tract (e.g., diarrhea, fistula).

B. Clinical Presentation. Acute metabolic acidosis usually is associated with symptoms of the underlying disease. Thus, nausea, vomiting, and abdominal pain are frequent with diabetic ketoacidosis (DKA), whereas alcohol abuse, nausea, and vomiting are frequent with methanol or ethylene glycol poisoning. In contrast, chronic metabolic acidosis is generally associated with nonspecific signs and symptoms, such as recurrent kidney stones, hypoalbuminemia, osteomalacia, or osteoporosis in adults and "failure-to-thrive" in children. The respiratory compensation to metabolic acidosis increases the depth and rate of breathing (Kussmaul respiration).

Metabolic acidosis should be considered in all patients with CKD since decreased net acid excretion causes metabolic acidosis and its correction may slow the progression of CKD.

C. Laboratory Analysis. Evaluating the "anion gap (AG)" can distinguish (1) and (2) from (3) and (4), above. AG is calculated using the following formula:

$$AG = [Na^+] - ([Cl^-] + [HCO_3^-]) \tag{2}$$

The normal AG is often stated to be 3 to 11 mM but varies by laboratory.

Albumin functions as an unmeasured anion that contributes to the AG. Accordingly, hypoalbuminemia decreases the expected AG. When hypoalbuminemia is present, the formula for calculating a "corrected anion gap (AG$_{Corr}$)" is:

$$AG_{corr} = AG + 2.5 \times \left(4.0 - \left[Albumin \left(\tfrac{g}{dl}\right)\right]\right) \tag{3}$$

D. Non–Anion Gap Metabolic Acidosis. Metabolic acidosis with an AG in the normal range is termed "non–AG metabolic acidosis." The most common causes are diarrhea, chronic kidney disease, and RTA. With chronic diarrhea, bicarbonate and metabolic alkali precursors, such as organic anions, are lost in the stool and decrease serum bicarbonate levels. Although the kidneys will attempt to correct the ensuing metabolic acidosis by increasing net acid excretion, this process is insufficient to fully restore the serum bicarbonate. With CKD and RTA, the kidneys' inability to generate sufficient net acid excretion leads to non–AG metabolic acidosis.

This difference in the response of net acid excretion facilitates the differentiation of the cause of metabolic acidosis. Urine ammonia is the predominant component of net acid excretion. It is increased with chronic diarrhea, but not with CKD or RTA. Unfortunately, most clinical laboratories only measure urinary ammonia in 24-hour urine collections. For a rapid semiquantitative assessment, ammonia excretion can be calculated as either the "urine anion gap (UAG)" or the "urine osmole gap (UOG)." The formulas used are:

$$UAG = [Na^+]_U + [K^+]_U - [Cl^-]_U \tag{4}$$

$$UOG = Osm_U - (2 \times \{[Na^+]_U + [K^+]_U\}) + \frac{UUN\left(\tfrac{mg}{dl}\right)}{2.8} + \frac{[Glucose]_U}{18} \tag{5}$$

These formulas are based on ammonium (NH$_4^+$) being present in sufficient amounts in nonrenal causes of chronic metabolic acidosis such as diarrhea, typically >100 mmol/L, that it is identifiable as an unmeasured cation and an unmeasured osmole (see Table 19.2).

1. Renal tubular acidosis. RTA is divided into three forms: Type I or distal RTA, type II or proximal RTA, and type IV or hyperkalemic RTA (Table 19.3). The relative frequency is type IV > type I > type II.

■ *Type IV RTA*

This presents typically as mild metabolic acidosis with hyperkalemia. Because the kidneys possess robust K$^+$ excretory mechanisms, almost all patients with type IV RTA have decreased renal function, either CKD or AKI, or are being treated with medications that lead to hyperkalemia (see Chapter 18). Hyperkalemia causes the metabolic acidosis by decreasing ammonia-dependent net acid excretion. In rare patients, the underlying cause of the hyperkalemia

| T A B L E
19.2 | Assessment of UAG and UOG |

UAG—urine anion gap

Measurement (mmol/L)	Interpretation	Diagnosis
>20	Net acid excretion is not increased	CKD or RTA
−20−+20	Not sufficiently predictive of actual net acid excretion	Should not be interpreted
<−20	Increased net acid excretion	Diarrhea

Limitations: less accurate in the presence of CKD, ketoacidosis, glue-sniffing, partially treated type II RTA, D-lactic acidosis, and 5-oxoproline toxicity.

UOG—urine osmole gap

Measurement (mOsm/kg H_2O)	Interpretation	Diagnosis
<150	Net acid excretion is not increased	CKD or RTA
150–200	Not sufficiently predictive of actual net acid excretion	Cannot be interpreted
>200	Increased net acid excretion	Diarrhea

Limitations: Inappropriately elevated in the presence of methanol or ethylene glycol intoxication, or if either fomepizole or mannitol has been administered. Can be suppressed in either highly concentrated or highly dilute urine.

is primary adrenal insufficiency requiring treatment with both glucocorticoids and mineralocorticoids. However, for patients with hyperkalemia and CKD, treatment of mineralocorticoid deficiency, if present, with mineralocorticoids should be avoided since this typically causes hypertension, which accelerates CKD progression. Correction of the hyperkalemia, with a combination of dietary modification, alkali therapy, diuretics, and enteric K^+-binding resins, will likely to correct the metabolic acidosis. Persistent metabolic acidosis in patients with CKD after correction of the hyperkalemia may indicate concomitant CKD-dependent metabolic acidosis.

| T A B L E
19.3 | Typical presenting characteristics of different forms of RTA |

Type	[K^+]	[HCO_3^-], mmol/L	Urine pH (untreated)	Urine pH (alkali-treated patient)	Nephrolithiasis
I (distal)	Low	5–20	≥6.5	≥6.5	Frequent
II	Low or low-normal	15–20	≤6	>6.5	Rare
IV	High to high-normal	15–22	6	6	Rare

■ *Type I RTA*

This presents with hypokalemia, non–AG metabolic acidosis, and a spontaneously alkaline urine pH (≥7). In adults, this typically is an acquired condition, whereas in children it may have a genetic etiology. A more common acquired etiology is autoimmune disease, most frequently Sjögren syndrome. Less common are hypercalciuric conditions that lead to medullary nephrocalcinosis and resultant type I RTA. Common acquired causes include carbonic anhydrase inhibitors or medications that inhibit carbonic anhydrase, such as topiramate. In children, genetic causes of distal RTA can be either autosomal dominant or recessive. Children with genetic type I RTA often present with failure-to-thrive.

■ *Type II (proximal) RTA*

This is the least common RTA. When associated with glycosuria, aminoaciduria, and hypophosphatemia with hyperphosphaturia, it is termed Fanconi syndrome. Type II RTA without Fanconi syndrome is termed isolated type II RTA. In adults, type II RTA is typically an acquired disease, with monoclonal light chain disease and medications as the most common etiologies. Medications include acetazolamide and topiramate, which can cause isolated type II RTA, and tenofovir and ifosfamide, which can cause Fanconi syndrome. Cystinosis is a genetic disease leading to intrarenal cysteine accumulation and type II RTA.

■ *Treatment*

Treating RTA involves treating the underlying disease process, when this can be accomplished, followed by alkali administration, if required. The dose of oral alkali therapy depends on the type of RTA but is typically 0.5 to 1.5 mmol/kg/day for type I and type IV RTA, and as much as 15 mmol/kg/day for type II RTA. Na^+-alkali salts are used for type IV RTA, whereas a combination of Na^+- and K^+-salts are used for type I and type II RTA, which are associated with hypokalemia. Na^+-salts include $NaHCO_3$ and Na-citrate, and K^+-salts include K-citrate. For patients requiring both Na^+- and K^+-alkali administration, Na^+-K^+-citrate can be used.

2. **Diarrhea and enteric fluid loss.** Prolonged enteric fluid loss can cause metabolic acidosis because enteric fluids often contain HCO_3^-. A negative history does not exclude this diagnosis because some patients have surreptitious cathartic usage. The demonstration of increased net acid excretion, using the urine tests outlined above, in a patient with a non–AG metabolic acidosis should strongly suggest this diagnosis. Treatment is based on treating the underlying cause.

3. **Glue-sniffing.** This is an unusual cause of non–AG metabolic acidosis. Although this was initially thought to be a cause of type I RTA, the metabolic acidosis may instead result from the inhaled toluene being metabolized to hippuric acid, which causes the metabolic acidosis.

E. **Anion-Gap Metabolic Acidosis.** The diagnosis of AG metabolic acidosis indicates the presence of excessive acids other than HCl in the extracellular fluid. The most common are lactic acid, ketoacids, and retained phosphates and sulfates in CKD. Lactic acidosis occurs with tissue ischemia, but may be a side effect of metformin therapy. Ketoacidosis can occur with uncontrolled hyperglycemia (DKA), starvation, chronic ethanol abuse, or as a complication of SGLT-2 inhibitors. Exogenous acids that can cause AG metabolic acidosis include metabolites of methanol and of ethylene glycol, 2-oxoproline, and acetylsalicylic acid in overdose. Table 19.4 shows a mnemonic (GOLD MARK) for the differential diagnosis of AG metabolic acidosis.

| TABLE 19.4 | Mnemonic for anion-gap metabolic acidosis |

GOLD MARK

Letter	Name	Information
G	Glycols	Ethylene glycol (antifreeze) and propylene glycol (used as food additive and as a solvent in intravenous solutions). May require emergency therapy.
O	5-Oxoproline	Acetaminophen metabolite. May accumulate with chronic acetaminophen use.
L	L-Lactic acid	Tissue ischemia or metformin toxicity (MALA; metformin-associated lactic acidosis).
D	D-lactic acid	Short-gut syndrome, particularly after oral carbohydrate loads. Occasionally with propylene glycol ingestions and in DKA.
M	Methanol	Present in "wood alcohol." Metabolites (formic acid) can cause blindness. May require emergency therapy.
A	Aspirin	Acetylsalicylic acid, excessive ingestion
R	Renal failure	Accumulation of anions, such as, but not limited to, phosphate and sulfates
K	Ketoacidosis	DKA, starvation or alcoholic ketoacidosis, and as complication of SGLT-2 inhibitor therapy

Prompt evaluation of AG metabolic acidosis is essential because it may be life threatening. Lactic acidosis should prompt rapid investigation into causes of tissue ischemia, including sepsis, and aggressive optimization of blood volume and blood pressure. Metformin-associated lactic acidosis (MALA) can be fatal, and may require urgent hemodialysis to remove retained metformin. Methanol and ethylene glycol intoxication may progress rapidly to irreversible complications. Prompt consultation with a poison-control center and a nephrologist is required.

F. **Alkali Therapy for Metabolic Acidosis.** The place of alkali therapy for metabolic acidosis is controversial. We recommend the treatment paradigm of the recent BICAR-ICU trial for acute metabolic acidosis that reported acute alkali therapy improves mortality in patients with severe metabolic acidosis (pH <7.20 with HCO_3^- <20 mmol/L) providing they also have AKIN stage 2 or 3 AKI. The treatment used was intravenous $NaHCO_3$, 500 mmol/L, at rates up to 1,000 mL/24 h, to obtain pH >7.30.

Chronic metabolic acidosis increases the rate of CKD progression and induces muscle atrophy, bone demineralization, and insulin resistance that, in randomized controlled clinical trials, can be reversed with alkali therapy. Importantly, the side effects associated with NaCl intake, such as increased BP, volume overload, and proteinuria, do not occur with $NaHCO_3$ administration. Thus, aggressive therapy for chronic metabolic acidosis, particularly in patients with CKD, may be warranted, with a target bicarbonate concentration of 23 to 27 mmol/L.

IV. RESPIRATORY ACIDOSIS

A. **Pathophysiology.** Respiratory acidosis reflects impaired respiratory CO_2 excretion. It typically results from impaired alveolar ventilation, but may occur when increased alveolar fluid accumulation impairs pulmonary capillary to alveolar CO_2 movement.

B. **Clinical Presentation.** Acute respiratory acidosis is frequently associated with the sensation of being short-of-breath, reflecting an acute underlying disturbance in alveolar ventilation. However, when impaired respiratory drive results from either respiratory muscle weakness or from CNS sedation, possibly related to medications, the patient may be asymptomatic, or even somnolent. In severe respiratory acidosis, accumulated CO_2 may lead to CNS suppression, termed "CO_2 narcosis." Chronic respiratory acidosis, in contrast, typically has few-to-no specific symptoms until the pCO_2 increases to ~80 mm Hg or higher when it may lead to CO_2 narcosis.

C. **Differentiation of Acute From Chronic Respiratory Acidosis.** Untreated acute respiratory acidosis can progress rapidly to complete respiratory failure and the patient's demise, whereas chronic respiratory acidosis typically is not an immediate concern. This differentiation is based on the history and the degree of compensation (see Table 19.1).

D. **Acute Respiratory Acidosis.** The most common causes of acute respiratory acidosis include asthma and exacerbations of chronic obstructive pulmonary disease (COPD). Less common causes include severe alveolar fluid accumulation, either from pulmonary edema or multilobar pneumonia. Rarely, it can be caused by muscle weakness due to electrolyte disturbances, such as hypokalemia and hypophosphatemia, or a tension pneumothorax. However, medication-induced respiratory drive suppression, such as from narcotic analgesics, is a frequent cause. Emergency treatment of the underlying causes should be instituted and if not rapidly effective, or if hypoxemia is present, urgent intubation and mechanical ventilation should be considered.

E. **Chronic Respiratory Acidosis.** Chronic respiratory acidosis reflects long-standing impairment of respiratory CO_2 elimination that often results from decreased alveolar surface area, as occurs with COPD, interstitial lung disease, or emphysema or chronic neurologic or mechanical disorders, such as Guillain–Barré syndrome, amyotrophic lateral sclerosis (ALS) or obesity–hypoventilation syndrome. Identification of chronic respiratory acidosis should prompt an investigation and treatment of the underlying etiology. Intubation and mechanical ventilation should be avoided if possible unless the underlying etiology can be treated.

V. METABOLIC ALKALOSIS

A. **Pathophysiology.** Metabolic alkalosis indicates the presence of either acid loss greater than the kidneys can balance through urinary HCO_3^- excretion or impaired renal HCO_3^- excretion. There are two primary mechanisms of acid loss. The first is gastric fluid loss, which has a pH as low as 2. This may result either from recurrent vomiting or from naso/orogastric suctioning, particularly if medications to inhibit gastric acid secretion, for example, proton pump inhibitors, are not being used. Simultaneous intravascular volume depletion may contribute. The urine is a second source of acid loss, in the form of net acid excretion. Hypokalemia and hyperaldosteronism, whether primary or secondary, increase net acid excretion and can contribute to metabolic alkalosis.

Kidneys have a robust capacity to excrete alkali. Therefore, a metabolic alkalosis frequently indicates impaired renal alkali excretion. One common cause of impaired renal alkali excretion is impaired renal function, either from AKI or CKD. If the GFR is intact, renal alkali excretion requires Cl^- for exchange with HCO_3^- in the collecting ducts. Thus, conditions that impair distal Cl^- delivery, such as intravascular volume depletion or congestive heart failure, also impair the kidneys' ability to excrete HCO_3^- and contribute to metabolic alkalosis.

B. **Laboratory Analysis.** Laboratory evaluation of metabolic alkalosis begins with an assessment of GFR and urine Cl^-. A decreased GFR impairs the ability to excrete alkali. A urine Cl^- below 20 mmol/L is inadequate for the collecting duct Cl^- delivery to support urinary HCO_3^- excretion; this condition is termed "chloride-responsive metabolic alkalosis." Treatment with 0.9% NS is often effective. When urine Cl^- is not suppressed, it is termed "chloride-unresponsive metabolic alkalosis."

C. **Cl^--Responsive Metabolic Alkalosis.** Cl^--responsive metabolic alkalosis implies metabolic alkalosis with either total body Cl^- deficiency or maximal stimulation of "proximal" Cl^- reabsorption. The development phase frequently involves gastric acid loss from vomiting or naso/orogastric suctioning. Alternatively, volume depletion can cause metabolic alkalosis by concentrating the extracellular HCO_3^- in a smaller fluid volume, as with diuretic therapy. This is termed "contraction alkalosis."

Cl^--responsive metabolic alkalosis is "maintained" when collecting duct Cl^- delivery is sufficiently low to prevent Cl^- for HCO_3^- exchange for urinary HCO_3^- secretion as in total body volume depletion or severe congestive heart failure where there is sufficient stimulation of proximal tubule, loop of Henle, and distal convoluted tubule NaCl reabsorption with little-to-no delivery to the collecting duct. Treatment of the underlying etiology is appropriate.

D. **Cl^--Unresponsive Metabolic Alkalosis.** This implies ongoing acid loss greater than the renal alkali excretory capacity either from gastric fluid losses or renal acid excretion. Both hypokalemia and hyperaldosteronism, whether primary or secondary, stimulate renal net acid excretion. Treatment involves treating the underlying condition.

E. **Acid Therapy of Metabolic Alkalosis.** Treating metabolic alkalosis with acid administration is not generally recommended. Rarely, acetazolamide may be used, but the resulting potassium loss requires careful monitoring.

VI. RESPIRATORY ALKALOSIS

A. **Pathophysiology.** Respiratory alkalosis occurs when hyperventilation increases CO_2 excretion, leading to decreased pCO_2 and increased pH. Variations in endogenous CO_2 production lead to parallel changes in respiratory CO_2 elimination, and do not cause respiratory acid–base disorders.

B. **Clinical Presentation.** Acute alkalosis may lower the ionized calcium sufficiently to lead to oral or limb paresthesias or to carpopedal spasm. Increased vascular reactivity can lead to dizziness and lightheadedness, chest pain, and dyspnea, and rarely to seizures or mental confusion. Chronic respiratory alkalosis, in contrast, typically does not cause specific symptoms.

C. **Laboratory Analysis.** The metabolic compensation to chronic respiratory alkalosis leads to suppressed blood HCO_3^- concentration that minimizes the pH change, whereas the compensation to acute respiratory alkalosis is much smaller. Table 19.1 summarizes these differences.

D. Acute Respiratory Alkalosis. Acute respiratory alkalosis results from acute hyperventilation as occurs during anxiety, panic, and pain. Acute hypoxemia, whether from a pulmonary embolus, asthma exacerbation, or acute ascent to a high elevation, can also stimulate ventilation. In general, identification and treatment of underlying cause(s) is appropriate.

High-altitude illness, which ranges from mild forms with headache, malaise, and anorexia, to life-threatening pulmonary or cerebral edema, may be due in part to acute respiratory alkalosis. Treatment with acetazolamide, which increases renal alkali excretion and thus minimizes the alkalemia, may be helpful in mild cases. However, treatment of high-altitude illness requires further measures.

E. Chronic Respiratory Alkalosis. Chronic respiratory alkalosis indicates chronically increased ventilation leading to increased CO_2 elimination from pregnancy, acute or chronic liver disease, and living at high altitudes. Treatment is not necessary. However, chronic respiratory alkalosis is associated with compensatory metabolic acidosis. Therefore, it is important to establish that the primary acid–base disorder is chronic respiratory alkalosis.

VII. RECOGNITION OF MULTIPLE SIMULTANEOUS PRIMARY ACID–BASE DISORDERS. Many patients may have more than a single primary acid–base disorder. Two approaches should be used to analyze this possibility.

First, the appropriate respiratory response to any metabolic acidosis or metabolic alkalosis involves a compensation that counterbalances the metabolic disorder. The absence of this respiratory compensation (see Table 19.1) indicates that a primary respiratory acid–base disorder is also present.

Second, the presence of an "AG" indicates an AG metabolic acidosis is present, even if the blood HCO_3^- is normal. If changes in the blood HCO_3^- do not parallel the magnitude of the AG change, the patient may have a simultaneous AG metabolic acidosis and either non–AG metabolic acidosis or metabolic alkalosis. An example is chronic respiratory acidosis and chronic compensatory metabolic alkalosis that develops AG metabolic acidosis from lactic acidosis, which may have resulted from acute mesenteric ischemia. Previous blood HCO_3^- measurements may be helpful if available.

VIII. SUGGESTED READINGS

Jaber S, Paugam C, Futier E, et al. Sodium bicarbonate therapy for patients with severe metabolic acidaemia in the intensive care unit (BICAR-ICU): a multicentre, open-label, randomised controlled, phase 3 trial. *Lancet.* 2018;392(10141):31–40.

Mehta AN, Emmett JB, Emmett M. GOLD MARK: an anion gap mnemonic for the 21st century. *Lancet.* 2008;372(9642):892.

Raphael KL. Metabolic acidosis in CKD: core curriculum 2019. *Am J Kidney Dis.* 2019;74(2):263–275.

20 | Calcium, Phosphorus, and Magnesium Disorders

Jogiraju V. Tantravahi

I. NORMAL CALCIUM HOMEOSTASIS

A. **Introduction.** Calcium acts as a co-factor in several important intracellular and extracellular processes. Skeletal muscle contraction and the excitation-contraction of cardiac myocyte contraction require calcium as a co-factor. Among other processes, the generation of the coagulation cascade requires calcium. Bone is the largest reservoir for calcium, and bone calcium and extracellular calcium exist in equilibrium. Because of the importance of calcium in so many homeostatic functions, calcium balance is tightly regulated by the coordinated actions of the kidney, the gastrointestinal system, and the endocrine system. This section includes a review of calcium stores, gastrointestinal absorption of calcium, endocrine regulation of calcium balance, and the renal regulation of calcium.

B. **Calcium Stores and Dietary Calcium.** The human body contains between 1,000 mg and 1,200 mg calcium. Greater than 99% of total body calcium stores are sequestered in bone. Of the remaining 1%, most of the calcium is extracellular. Intracellular or cytoplasmic free calcium stores range between 50 and 100 nmol/L. Extracellular calcium stores range between 2.25 and 2.65 mmol/L, or 9.0 and 10.6 mg/dL. Approximately 55% of extracellular calcium is bound to either protein (mainly albumin) or complexed to other macromolecules and the remaining ~45% of extracellular calcium is free and ionized.

While hormonally regulated bone reabsorption can maintain the calcium level, only dietary calcium intake can replenish body calcium stores. For every 1,000 mg of calcium ingested, 400 mg are absorbed through the gastrointestinal tract. Calcium absorbed through the gastrointestinal tract is in equilibrium with several body calcium pools, including bone and extracellular fluid. Up to 200 mg of calcium are excreted back into the gastrointestinal tract and up to 200 mg of calcium are excreted in the urine. Gastrointestinal absorption of calcium occurs through paracellular and transcellular pathways. The active form of vitamin D, 1,25-dihydroxycholecalciferol, or calcitriol directly facilitates transcellular calcium transport and indirectly facilitates calcium transport by the paracellular pathway. After binding to the vitamin D receptor, calcitriol induces the expression of the calcium channel TRPV6, calbindin D, and the Ca^{2+}-ATPase leading to increased active transport of calcium across the enterocyte basolateral membrane.

C. **Endocrine Regulation of Calcium Balance.** Calcitriol and parathyroid hormone (PTH) are the most important endocrine regulators of calcium balance. Calcitriol synthesis begins with photochemical conversion, within the skin, of 7-dehydrocholesterol to cholecalciferol, also known as vitamin D_3. Cholecalciferol then undergoes two sequential hydroxylation steps. The first of these, 25-hydroxylation, occurs in the liver and is not rate limiting and measurement

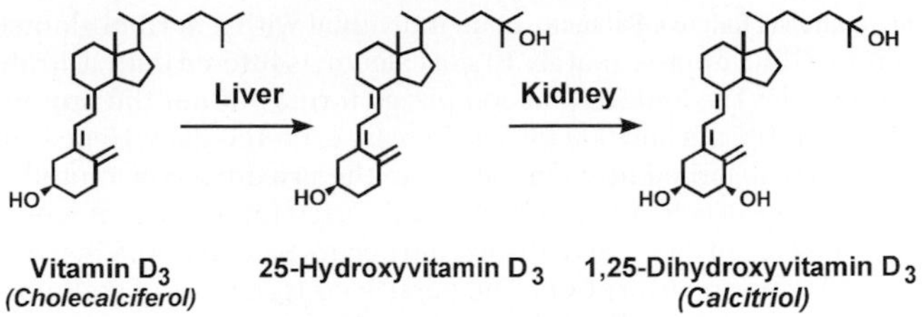

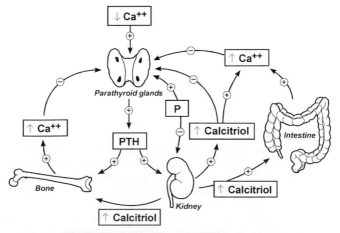

Vitamin D₃   **25-Hydroxyvitamin D₃**   **1,25-Dihydroxyvitamin D₃**
(Cholecalciferol)   *(Calcitriol)*

FIGURE 20.1: Biosynthesis of vitamin D.

of 25-hydroxycholecalciferol levels has been accepted as a surrogate marker of total body vitamin D stores. The second, rate-limiting hydroxylation, occurs in the kidney, where 25-hyroxycholecalciferol undergoes modification to 1,25-dihydroxycholecalciferol or calcitriol. Calcitriol exerts most of its influence on calcium homeostasis within the gastrointestinal tract and bone. However, within the kidney, calcitriol does facilitate calcium reabsorption in the distal nephron. Calcitriol also regulates its own synthesis by suppressing 1-α-hydroxylase and leading to a stimulation of the enzyme 24-hydroxylase, which converts 25-hydroxycholecalciferol to the inactive 24,25-dihydroxycholecalciferol (Figure 20.1).

PTH is a polypeptide hormone synthesized and secreted by the chief cells of the parathyroid gland. PTH synthesis and release are controlled at the level of transcription and post-transcription. Hypocalcemia is a profound stimulus for PTH release. The calcium-sensing receptor (CaSR) responds to variations in the serum calcium leading to changes in PTH secretion. In response to hypocalcemia, PTH is released from its stores and transcription of the PTH gene increases. PTH affects calcium regulation in several ways. PTH directly stimulates bone resorption, increases calcitriol synthesis by inducing expression of 1-α-hydroxylase, and PTH, such as calcitriol, facilitates calcium reabsorption in the distal nephron (Figure 20.2).

FIGURE 20.2: Parathyroid hormone (PTH) feedback loop.

D. Renal Regulation of Calcium Balance. In an individual with a normal glomerular filtration rate (GFR), approximately 10 g of calcium is filtered daily. Ultrafilterable calcium includes the ionized and complexed forms but not the protein-bound form. Between 100 mg and 300 mg calcium are excreted daily. Hence, up to 99% of calcium is reabsorbed in the nephron. In the proximal convoluted tubule, a small percentage of calcium is actively transported under the influence of PTH. However, the bulk of calcium reabsorption occurs passively and in parallel with sodium and water reabsorption. The passive co-transport of sodium and calcium is important clinically. In hypercalcemic states, volume expansion with saline corrects the extracellular fluid deficit, caused by hypercalcemia-induced osmotic diuresis, and facilitates calcium excretion and correction of hypercalcemia. However, among individuals predisposed to nephrolithiasis, high sodium intake with resulting hypercalciuria may increase the frequency of kidney stone formation.

While there is no transport of calcium in the thin ascending loop of Henle, up to 20% of the filtered calcium load is reabsorbed in the thick ascending loop of Henle. This calcium reabsorption occurs primarily through a paracellular pathway, although there is some transcellular reabsorption. Two ion transporters, the apical Na^+-K^+-$2Cl^-$ cotransporter (NKCC2) and the renal outer medullary potassium (K^+) (ROMK) channel generate the electrochemical gradient necessary for paracellular transport. PTH increases calcium transport by increasing paracellular permeability. High calcium states activate the CaSR leading to decreased paracellular permeability and calciuria. Paracellular calcium transport can be inhibited by administration of a loop diuretic, as loop diuretics inhibit action of the NKCC2 transporter. With inhibition of the NKCC2 transporter, an electrochemical gradient favoring paracellular transport cannot be established, and calciuria ensues. Loop diuretic therapy combined with saline expansion is an important therapeutic maneuver in the management of severe hypercalcemia. The final 5% to 10% of calcium reabsorption occurs in the distal convoluted tubule in an energy-requiring transcellular pathway.

II. HYPERCALCEMIA

A. False and True Hypercalcemia. False hypercalcemia occurs with an increase in plasma proteins, including albumin, leading to an increase in total serum calcium with no change in ionized calcium levels, and is not clinically relevant. True hypercalcemia results from an increase in the plasma ionized concentration and hypercalcemia should be confirmed by measuring an ionized calcium level. Hypoalbuminemia can mask a diagnosis of hypercalcemia. For every 1 g/dL decrease in the serum albumin, the expected serum calcium level should be adjusted downward by between 0.8 mg/dL and 1 mg/dL.

B. Causes of Hypercalcemia. The most important causes of hypercalcemia are listed in Table 20.1. In general, the causes of hypercalcemia can be classified as PTH dependent, vitamin D dependent, or paraneoplastic. The most common causes of hypercalcemia are hyperparathyroidism (usually primary) and malignancy-associated causes. Familial hypocalciuric hypercalcemia (FHH) is an autosomal dominant condition that presents with asymptomatic hypercalcemia. PTH levels are normal or slightly elevated and vitamin D levels are suppressed. The diagnosis can be made by measuring the urine calcium to creatinine clearance ratio in a 24-hour urine sample. FHH patients have hypocalciuria with most patients excreting less than 200 mg/day. In addition, the urine calcium to creatinine ratio is less than 0.01. Conversely, patients with primary

TABLE 20.1	Causes of hypercalcemia

Hyperparathyroidism
Primary hyperparathyroidism
Tertiary hyperparathyroidism

Neoplastic diseases
Hematopoietic neoplasms, including multiple myeloma (osteoclastic-activating factor causing release of calcium) and lymphoma (nonrenal calcitriol production)
Solid tumors, including breast cancer and prostate cancer (osteoclastic-activating factor causing release of calcium) and solid tumors elaborating PTH-related peptide

Granulomatous diseases
Granulomatous diseases including sarcoidosis, mycobacterial infections, and fungal infections (nonrenal calcitriol production)

Endocrinopathies
Pheochromocytoma, hyperthyroidism

Vitamin intoxication
Hypervitaminosis D, hypervitaminosis A

Genetic
Familial hypocalciuric hypercalcemia, Gitelman syndrome

Miscellaneous
Immobilization
Drug therapy (lithium, thiazide diuretics)
Milk alkali syndrome (ingestion of calcium salts)

hyperparathyroidism have a urine calcium to creatinine clearance ratio greater than 0.02.

C. **Treatment of Symptomatic Hypercalcemia.** Symptomatic hypercalcemia presents in several ways. The severity of symptoms worsens if hypercalcemia develops rapidly. Renal manifestations include acute kidney injury, polyuria, and nephrolithiasis. Gastrointestinal symptoms include nausea and vomiting. Other systemic symptoms include bone pain and cardiac conduction system abnormalities. The most concerning symptoms are neurologic and include lethargy, encephalopathy, and coma. Table 20.2 lists the significant symptoms caused by hypercalcemia.

The treatment of symptomatic hypercalcemia should be based on the underlying cause. However, in nearly every case, treatment should begin with volume expansion with isotonic saline. Once the patient's volume deficit has been treated, brisk calciuresis can be achieved with a high dose of a loop diuretic. Severe symptomatic hypercalcemia can be treated with mithramycin or calcitonin. Mithramycin causes thrombocytopenia and liver function abnormalities, so toxicity limits its use. Calcitonin effectively reduces the serum calcium, but tachyphylaxis occurs quickly. Bisphosphonate therapy, even in patients with chronic kidney disease, is the standard of care for maintaining a normal calcium level following conservative therapy. As seen in Table 20.1, hypervitaminosis D can develop from vitamin D intoxication, granulomatous diseases such as sarcoidosis and tuberculosis, and from malignancy. Patients who develop hypercalcemia from hypervitaminosis D respond well to treatment with glucocorticoids or ketoconazole (an inhibitor of renal and extrarenal calcitriol

TABLE 20.2	Signs and symptoms of hypercalcemia and hypocalcemia

Mild hypercalcemia
Asymptomatic progressing to nausea, vomiting, constipation, polydipsia, polyuria, and volume depletion
Moderate hypercalcemia
Bone pain, pseudogout, acute kidney injury, nephrolithiasis (if chronic), depression, impaired cardiac conduction and arrhythmia, depression, psychosis
Severe hypercalcemia
Soft tissue calcification (if chronic), acute kidney injury, neuropsychiatric symptoms including somnolence, encephalopathy, amnesia, stupor, and coma
Acute hypocalcemia
Paresthesias, hypotension, QT prolongation, atrioventricular block, ventricular fibrillation, tetany, seizures
Chronic hypocalcemia
Depression, cataracts, brittle nails, dry skin

synthesis). In cases refractory to all medical therapy, hemodialysis can effectively reduce the serum calcium. Bisphosphonate therapy and calcimimetics effectively reduce the calcium concentration in patients with asymptomatic hypercalcemia and, in particular, in patients with primary hyperparathyroidism.

III. HYPOCALCEMIA

A. False and True Hypocalcemia. As with hypercalcemia, hypocalcemia can present as either false or true. Hypoalbuminemia accounts for nearly every instance of false hypocalcemia. True hypocalcemia results from a decrease in the serum-ionized calcium concentration with the measurement of the ionized calcium confirming the diagnosis.

B. Causes of Hypocalcemia. The most important causes of hypocalcemia are listed in Table 20.3. As with hypercalcemia, the main causes of hypocalcemia are PTH dependent (lack of PTH) and vitamin D dependent (lack of vitamin D).

TABLE 20.3	Causes of Hypocalcemia

Vitamin D deficiency
Vitamin D deficiency from sunlight deprivation, decreased intake, or decreased absorption
Decreased calcitriol formation (chronic kidney disease, type 1 vitamin D–dependent rickets)
Resistance to calcitriol action (type 2 vitamin D–dependent rickets)
Vitamin D deficiency from hypoparathyroidism
Miscellaneous
Acute pancreatitis
Hypomagnesemia
Hungry bone syndrome

In addition, hypocalcemia can result from sequestration as with pancreatitis, tumor lysis syndrome, hungry bone disease, or rhabdomyolysis. Hypocalcemia from hypoparathyroidism is accompanied by hyperphosphatemia. Hypocalcemia from vitamin D deficiency is accompanied by low or normal phosphorus levels.

C. **Treatment of Symptomatic Hypocalcemia.** Similar to hypercalcemia, the symptoms of hypocalcemia depend on the rapidity of their development and the severity of the deficit. There are no renal manifestations of hypocalcemia. The most common symptoms are neurologic and musculoskeletal. The most common symptoms are listed in Table 20.2. Familiar clinical manifestations include twitching of facial muscles in response to tapping the facial nerve (Chvostek sign) and carpal spasm caused by forearm ischemia from inflating a blood pressure cuff (Trousseau sign).

In the rare case of respiratory alkalosis-induced hypocalcemia, a strategy for retaining carbon dioxide should be used. Severe hypocalcemia manifesting with tetany or seizures should be treated with bolus calcium gluconate (preferred over calcium chloride, as the chloride salt can cause skin necrosis with extravasation). To maintain the calcium level over an extended period, a continuous calcium infusion should be used. Up to 24 g of calcium gluconate can be mixed in 1 L of 5% dextrose in water or normal saline and continuously infused. Hypomagnesemia causes hypocalcemia by inducing resistance to PTH action and diminishing PTH secretion. Hence, hypomagnesemia should be corrected concurrently with calcium therapy. Chronic hypocalcemia, which is usually asymptomatic, can be managed with oral calcium supplementation and vitamin D.

IV. NORMAL PHOSPHORUS HOMEOSTASIS

A. **Phosphorus Stores and Dietary Phosphorus Intake.** The human body contains between 560 mg and 850 mg of phosphorus, or between 1% and 1.5% of fat-free mass. Phosphorus is in equilibrium among several compartments, including bone, the extracellular fluid, nucleic acids, phospholipids, and other intracellular compartments. Up to 85% of phosphorus is complexed with calcium in bone. Up to 14% of phosphorus is intracellular, with the free intracellular phosphate concentration at approximately 4.3 mg/dL. Serum phosphorus species make up at most 1% of the total body phosphorus stores. Still, the serum phosphate concentration is maintained with a range of 2.5 mg/dL and 4.5 mg/dL. Dietary phosphorus intake varies between 700 mg and 2,000 mg daily. Between 60% and 75% of dietary phosphorus is absorbed in the small intestine.

B. **Endocrine Regulation of Phosphorus Balance.** Most of the endocrine regulation of phosphorus balance occurs within the kidney. Insulin facilitates phosphorus transport across cell membranes through ubiquitous phosphate transporters. Within the gastrointestinal tract, phosphorus is absorbed through transepithelial and paracellular routes. In the small intestine, the type 2 sodium-phosphorus transporter (Na-Pi) NPT2a mediates transepithelial phosphorus transport. Several hormones are thought to influence both paracellular and transepithelial phosphorus absorption, including insulin-like growth factor 1, growth hormone, insulin, thyroid hormone, and calcitriol. Calcitriol has been shown to increase expression of NPT2a, enhancing intestinal phosphorus absorption.

C. **Renal Regulation of Phosphorus Balance.** The maintenance of extracellular phosphate homeostasis depends almost entirely on the kidney. As will be discussed in another section, chronic kidney disease causes significant impairments in normal phosphorus homeostasis. Phosphorus is freely filtered at the glomerulus. In individuals with normal renal function, between 3,700 mg and 6,100 mg are filtered daily. Net renal excretion varies between 600 mg and 1,500 mg daily, demonstrating tubular reabsorption of between 75% and 85% of the daily filtered load. Approximately 85% of tubular reabsorption occurs proximally. Reabsorption is an energy-dependent process that requires sodium. Three Na-Pi transporters (NPT2a, NPT2c, PiT-2) are expressed in the apical membrane of proximal tubular cells. Using the electrochemical energy derived from sodium transport, the phosphate transporters move phosphorus from the luminal fluid into the cell and eventually the peritubular capillaries. Trivial phosphorus reabsorption occurs in the loop of Henle, distal convoluted tubule, and collecting duct.

Metabolic and hormonal inputs affect renal phosphorus absorption. Ingestion of a high-phosphorus diet causes removal of Na-Pi transporters. Dietary phosphorus restriction leads to insertion of Na-Pi transporters, enhancing phosphorus reabsorption. PTH decreases renal phosphorus reabsorption and enhances phosphaturia by decreasing the number of Na-Pi transporters. Glucocorticoids and estrogens induce phosphaturia by their effects on Na-Pi transporter abundance. Thyroid hormone increases Na-Pi transporter abundance and facilitates increased phosphorus reabsorption. Calcitriol increases proximal tubular reabsorption of phosphorus, although the effect of calcitriol on PTH and calcium may have indirect effects on phosphorus reabsorption.

Fibroblast growth factor-23 (FGF-23) has been proposed as a master controller of phosphorus metabolism. FGF-23 is produced by osteoblast in response to hyperphosphatemia. FGF-23, in conjunction with the kidney-produced Klotho protein, binds to the FGF receptor 1. These interactions lead to FGF-23–directed decrease in Na-Pi transporter activity and decreased expression of 1-α-hydroxylase, the rate-limiting step in calcitriol formation. Deletion of the FGF-23 gene or the Klotho gene causes hyperphosphatemia, calcitriol toxicity, and vascular calcification.

D. Causes of Hyperphosphatemia. An algorithm for the evaluation of hyperphosphatemia and hypophosphatemia is given in Figure 20.3. The causes of hyperphosphatemia are given in Table 20.4. The most common causes include chronic kidney disease, lytic states such as tumor lysis syndrome or rhabdomyolysis, hypoparathyroidism, or from treatment-induced causes. Acute

TABLE 20.4	Causes of hyperphosphatemia

Reduced renal phosphorus excretion
Acute kidney injury
Chronic kidney disease

Hypoparathyroidism syndromes
Hypoparathyroidism (idiopathic, iatrogenic)
Type 1 and 2 pseudohypoparathyroidism

Increased phosphorus supply
Vitamin D intoxication, excessive intake of phosphorus salts through oral, intravenous, or rectal routes

Cellular shift
Hemolysis, rhabdomyolysis, malignant hyperthermia, tumor lysis

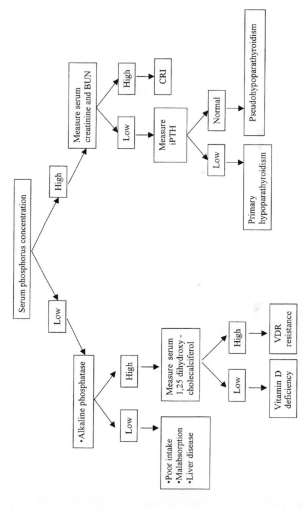

FIGURE 20.3: Workup of hypocalcemia. BUN, blood urea nitrogen; CRI, chronic renal insufficiency; iPTH, intact parathyroid hormone; VDR, vitamin D receptor.

hyperphosphatemia can induce hypocalcemia. Chronic hyperphosphatemia, particularly in chronic kidney disease causes pruritus, vascular calcification, soft tissue calcification, and calcific uremic arteriolopathy.

E. **Treatment of Hyperphosphatemia.** Acute hyperphosphatemia should be treated by increasing urinary phosphorus excretion with volume expansion. If renal excretion cannot be increased because of acute kidney injury (as with profound rhabdomyolysis or tumor lysis syndrome), prolonged high-flux hemodialysis effectively removes phosphorus. Dextrose and insulin promote intracellular phosphorus transport. Chronic hyperphosphatemia, most often seen with chronic kidney disease, requires interruption of gastrointestinal absorption with an oral phosphate binder. Common preparations include calcium acetate, sevelamer carbonate, lanthanum carbonate, and iron-containing phosphate binders.

F. **Causes of Hypophosphatemia.** The causes of hypophosphatemia are given in Table 20.5. The most common causes include vitamin D deficiency, hyperparathyroidism, malnutrition, refeeding syndrome or enhanced renal excretion from inherited causes, acquired Fanconi syndrome, or oncogenic hypophosphatemic osteomalacia. In the latter condition, mesenchymal tumors secrete phosphatonins such as FGF-23 (among other proteins) causing phosphorus wasting. Individuals with mild hypophosphatemia are asymptomatic. Severe hypophosphatemia can cause muscle weakness to the point of respiratory distress, rhabdomyolysis, and hemolysis. In states of chronic hypophosphatemia, bone mineralization is impaired.

G. **Treatment of Hypophosphatemia.** Severe hypophosphatemia (serum phosphorus less than 1 mg/dL) should be treated with intravenous sodium phosphate (up to 24 mmol). Otherwise, oral phosphorus replacement with high phosphorus containing foods such as dairy products (skim milk, cheese) will effectively treat the phosphorus deficit. Phosphorus salts, such as potassium phosphate or a combination of sodium and potassium phosphate can be used to treat phosphorus deficiency.

TABLE 20.5	Causes of hypophosphatemia

Excess urinary phosphorus loss from increased renal excretion
Hyperparathyroidism
Vitamin D deficiency
Oncogenic hypophosphatemic osteomalacia from mesenchymal tumors
Extracellular volume expansion
Glucocorticoid therapy
Acquired renal tubular defects
Decreased renal tubular phosphate reabsorption
Rickets
Fanconi syndrome (idiopathic, congenital, acquired)
Decreased gastrointestinal phosphorus absorption
Malnutrition
Starvation (chronic alcoholism)
Vitamin D deficiency
Cellular shift
Hyperventilation, cellular synthesis, cellular metabolism

V. CALCIUM AND PHOSPHORUS DYSREGULATION IN CHRONIC KIDNEY DISEASE

A. Adaptive Mechanisms to Preserve Calcium and Phosphorus Homeostasis in Chronic Kidney Disease. Even a modest reduction in the GFR results in several electrolyte abnormalities, including hypocalcemia and hyperphosphatemia. Alterations in serum calcium and phosphorus levels result in hyperparathyroidism, an increase in FGF-23 levels, and a reduction in calcitriol levels. The changes in calcium and phosphorus homeostatic hormones mainly facilitate phosphorus excretion in early chronic kidney disease. Calcium levels are maintained by increased bone turnover.

B. Maladaptive Calcium and Phosphorus Homeostasis in Advanced Chronic Kidney Disease. As the GFR falls, several concurrent processes occur. Despite the development of hypocalcemia, calcitriol production falls because of increased PTH levels. Increased FGF-23 levels inhibit 1-α-hydroxylation of 25-hydroxycholecalciferol. Therefore, restoration of calcium balance is not restored through gastrointestinal or renal absorption but rather through bone resorption. Hyperphosphatemia stimulates PTH and FGF-23 production. In the early stages of chronic kidney disease, PTH and FGF-23-Klotho act as potent phosphatonins. As outlined above, the decrease in calcitriol levels will also decrease renal calcium absorption. As the GFR continues to fall, the kidney becomes less responsive to phosphatonins. Worsening hyperphosphatemia results in still higher PTH levels. The combination of hyperparathyroidism and decreased calcitriol action results in osteitis fibrosa, a condition of increased bone turnover and decreased bone mass. FGF-23 levels continue to increase as the GFR falls. The pathogenic role of FGF-23 in renal bone disease in patients with advanced chronic kidney disease has yet to be determined.

C. Treatment of Dysregulated Calcium and Phosphorus Homeostasis in Chronic Kidney Disease. As the GFR worsens, phosphorus excretion decreases despite high levels of phosphatonins. Therefore, phosphate binder therapy is necessary to decrease the serum phosphorus level. With a decrease in the phosphorus level, the PTH level will fall, leading to decreased bone turnover. However, with decreased bone turnover and decreased calcitriol levels, hypocalcemia will result. Therefore, patients with advanced chronic kidney disease will require some form of pharmacologic vitamin D therapy. Calcimimetic therapy has become an important tool in the management of severe hyperparathyroidism. Calcimimetics correct hyperphosphatemia but can cause hypocalcemia. The hypocalcemia can be corrected with calcium supplementation, the addition of pharmacologic vitamin D therapy, or both. As the pathogenic role of FGF-23 in renal osteodystrophy remains unclear, no therapies targeted at renal FGF-23 metabolism are in clinical practice.

VI. NORMAL MAGNESIUM HOMEOSTASIS

A. Magnesium Stores and Dietary Magnesium Intake. Magnesium is the second most abundant intracellular cation. Several cellular processes, including DNA replication, protein synthesis, and cardiac excitability require magnesium as a co-factor. The average adult has 24 g of magnesium, of which 99% is intracellular. Within the intracellular compartment, 90% is bound and 10% is free. The serum magnesium concentration lies between 1.8 mg/dL and 2.4 mg/dL. Up to 30% of extracellular is bound to albumin. Between 10% and 15% of extracellular magnesium is complexed into anions, leaving up to 55% of extracellular magnesium as ionized and free. As with calcium and phosphorus, the magnesium pool is in equilibrium between bone, the gastrointestinal tract, the kidney, and the extracellular space. Adults ingest an average of 300-mg magnesium daily.

Magnesium absorption in the gastrointestinal tract varies depending on the magnesium intake, with gastrointestinal absorption falling to 25% of daily ingested load in high-magnesium diets and increasing to 70% of the daily ingested load in magnesium-depleted diets. In the small intestine and colon, magnesium is absorbed via transcellular and paracellular pathways. The transient receptor potential melastatin (TRPM) cationic channels TRPM6 and TRPM7 facilitate transcellular transport. Transcellular transport increases in low magnesium states. Vitamin D enhances magnesium absorption.

B. **Renal Regulation of Magnesium Balance.** In states of normal renal function, the daily filtered magnesium varies between 2,000 mg and 2,500 mg. The normal kidneys excrete approximately 100-mg magnesium daily. Only 10% to 30% of magnesium is reabsorbed in the proximal tubule by a paracellular pathway presumably linked to sodium gradient–driven water transport. Between 40% and 70% of magnesium is reabsorbed in the thick ascending loop of Henle by a paracellular route. Paracellular transport requires generation of a lumen-positive transepithelial voltage generated by the NKCC2 transporter, the ROMK channel, and selective paracellular divalent cation transport by claudin 16 and claudin 19. Because the NKCC2 transporter action is necessary to facilitate paracellular transport, loop diuretics cause urinary magnesium wasting. A trivial amount of magnesium is reabsorbed in the distal nephron through the TRMP6 channel. Magnesium restriction, PTH, aldosterone, and amiloride increase magnesium absorption. Several medications, including loop diuretics, thiazide diuretics, aminoglycosides, tacrolimus, and chemotherapeutic agents cause urinary magnesium wasting. Several congenital conditions, including Bartter syndrome and Gitelman syndrome also cause magnesium wasting.

C. **Causes, Symptoms, and Treatment of Hypermagnesemia.** The causes of hypermagnesemia are given in Table 20.6. Mainly, hypermagnesemia is caused by decreased urinary excretion or increased gastrointestinal absorption of magnesium-containing medications such as laxatives or antacids. High-dose continuous magnesium therapy given for the treatment of preeclampsia causes iatrogenic hypermagnesemia. At magnesium levels greater than 3.0 mg/dL, deep tendon reflexes are lost. As the levels increase, abnormal cardiac conduction, hypotension, and respiratory paralysis may occur. Treatment of hypermagnesemia consists of withdrawal of exogenous magnesium and intravenous administration of calcium gluconate.

TABLE 20.6	Causes of hypermagnesemia

Increased magnesium load
Pharmacologic magnesium therapy, including high-dose intravenous magnesium infusion in women with preeclampsia
Excess use of magnesium-containing medications, including antacids, oral purgatives, or enemas
Decreased renal excretion
Acute kidney injury, chronic kidney disease
Miscellaneous
Familial hypocalciuric hypercalcemia
Adrenal insufficiency

TABLE 20.7	Causes of hypomagnesemia

Increased urinary losses not related to drug therapy
Bartter syndrome
Gitelman syndrome
Hypercalcemia
Isotonic volume expansion
Glycosuria and diabetic ketoacidosis
High urinary output states not related to diuretic therapy, such as the polyuric
  phase of acute kidney injury
Increased urinary losses related to drug therapy
Loop and thiazide diuretics
Aminoglycosides
Amphotericin B
Trisodium phosphonoformate (Foscarnet)
Antineoplastic agents, particularly cis-platinum
Calcineurin inhibitors including cyclosporine and tacrolimus
Decreased gastrointestinal absorption
Malabsorption syndromes
Short gut syndrome
Purgative use
Prolonged proton pump inhibitor use
Decreased intake
Malnutrition, as in chronic alcohol use
Miscellaneous
Acute pancreatitis

D. Causes, Symptoms, and Treatment of Hypomagnesemia. The causes of hypomagnesemia are given in Table 20.7. The most common causes of hypomagnesemia include malabsorption either from gastrointestinal diseases or from malnutrition, miscellaneous causes such as acute pancreatitis, or increased renal losses from drugs or congenital causes. Because hypomagnesemia is often accompanied by hypokalemia and hypocalcemia, symptoms attributable to magnesium deficiency solely are difficult to discern. Many symptoms seen with hypocalcemia, such as carpopedal spasm, tetany, seizure, tremor, and weakness are seen with hypomagnesemia. Symptomatic hypomagnesemia should be treated with intravenous magnesium sulfate. Chronic asymptomatic hypomagnesemia can be treated with magnesium salts. Unfortunately, these preparations are poorly tolerated because they cause diarrhea.

VII. SUGGESTED READINGS

Blaine J, Chonchol M, Levi M. Renal control of calcium, phosphate, and magnesium homeostasis. *Clin J Am Soc Nephrol.* 2015;10:1257–1272.

Kestenbaum B, Houllier P. Disorders of calcium, phosphate, and magnesium metabolism. In: Feehally J, Floege J, Tonelli M, et al. eds. *Comprehensive Clinical Nephrology.* 6th ed. Elsevier; 2019.

Disease of the Urinary Collecting System

21

Renal Stone Disease

Muna T. Canales, Benjamin K. Canales

Renal stone disease affects millions of individuals worldwide and is associated with significant morbidity. Costs attributed to management and care of patients with stone disease in the United States exceeded $10 billion in the year 2006. Several surgical and medical therapeutic options exist for management of stone disease such as extracorporeal shock wave lithotripsy (ESWL), ureteroscopy, endoscopic percutaneous extraction, and medical expulsive therapy (MET). Although such therapies have improved our ability to treat the acute passage of renal stones, many individuals benefit from preventive therapy given the chronic and recurrent nature of renal stone disease.

I. **EPIDEMIOLOGY.** Renal stone disease leads to over 1 million emergency room visits annually. Nearly one in eleven Americans reports a history of stone disease. The peak incidence among men is age 40 to 60 years and, among women, age 20 to 50 years. In general, male sex, White race, older age, obesity, and diabetes mellitus are associated with higher prevalence of renal stone disease. Also, in the southeastern United States, the prevalence of nephrolithiasis is approximately twice as high as in the rest of the country. This is thought to be related to the warmer climate, which can lead to increased insensible fluid loss and reduced urine output.

Renal stone disease is frequently recurrent. In the absence of preventive treatment, the recurrence rate after the initial episode is over 60% at 5 years. Prevention can significantly reduce the morbidity and expense of this disease because the vast majority of these patients have an identifiable metabolic cause for their stones.

II. **PATHOPHYSIOLOGY OF STONE FORMATION**
A. **Stone Composition.** Renal stones are composed nearly entirely of mineral (>95%). Mineral crystals can be found within the urine of almost all humans. Crystalluria is thought to be a natural, physiologic response to water conservation and mineral homeostasis. Instead of being bound and excreted harmlessly in the urine as occurs in nonstone formers, crystals nucleate and aggregate in stone formers initiate a cascade of events that culminate in stone formation. Because the most common stone-forming crystalloids contain calcium, it is not surprising that nearly 80% of renal stones consist of calcium either bound to oxalate (~35% of stones), phosphate (~8% of stones), or a mixture of both calcium oxalate and calcium phosphate (~35%). Pure uric acid stones account for 10% of all stones, while struvite stones (or "infection stones") composed of magnesium ammonium phosphate crystals account for about 9% (Table 21.1). Cystine stones, a result of an autosomal recessive disorder leading to impaired

			Urinary risk factors	Visible by
Mineral type	**Frequency**[a]	**Crystal morphology**	**and associations**	**x-ray?**
Calcium oxalate monohydrate	35–70%	"Dumbbell"	Hyperoxaluria > Hypercalciuria	Yes
Calcium oxalate dihydrate		"Envelope"	Hypercalciuria > Hyperoxaluria	Yes
Calcium phosphate	8–20%	Blunt-ended needles or prisms, often in clumps	Hypercalciuria Hypocitraturia Urine pH >7	Yes
Uric acid	10%	Rhomboid or lemon-shaped, sometimes yellow or reddish-brown	Urine pH <5.5 Metabolic syndrome	No
Struvite	9%	"Coffin lids"	Recurrent UTI with urea-splitting bacteria; pH >7	Yes
Cystine	1%	Hexagonal	Cystinuria: Homozygous recessive gene for cystine transport	Yes

TABLE 21.1 Frequency, morphology and key pearls by stone type

[a]Frequency present in a kidney stone. May occur in combination with other stone types.

proximal tubular resorption of dibasic amino acids, are a rare (1%) but significant cause of nephrolithiasis.

B. Urinary Environment. Several factors interact to cause these stone-forming crystalloids to come out of solution in the urine. The most important include (a) *supersaturation* of the crystalloids in the urine, meaning the crystalloids are present in a concentration that is too high for them to dissolve; (b) the presence of *promoters* defined as physical or chemical stimuli that promote stone formation; and (c) a deficiency of *inhibitors* of stone formation in the urine. The presence of just one of these factors may not be sufficient to cause stone formation. Instead, a combination of factors may be necessary to ultimately lead to the stone-forming event.

Considering the principle of supersaturation, and the effect of promoters and inhibitors, major risk factors for stone formation can be placed in three categories:

1. *Factors that increase supersaturation*
   - low urinary volume
   - high urinary excretion of stone-forming minerals (i.e., calcium, uric acid, oxalate)
2. *Promoters of stone formation*
   - abnormal urinary pH (i.e., uric acid and cystine stones are more likely to form in acidic urine, whereas struvite and calcium phosphate stones are more likely to form in alkaline urine)
   - a nidus for crystal precipitation (i.e., sodium urate crystallization promotes calcium oxalate deposition on the sodium urate crystals and speeds the rate of stone formation)
3. *Lack of Inhibitors*
   - a deficiency of inhibitors of stone formation, such as citrate and Mg^{2+} (citrate binds Ca^{2+} and Mg^{2+} binds oxalate)

C. Identifiable Causes of Stone Formation. Approximately 97% of all patients with renal stones will have one or more identifiable causes of stone formation. Beyond low urine volumes, the most common contributing factors include hypercalciuria, hyperoxaluria, hypocitraturia, hyperuricosuria, and infection.

Hypercalciuria is the most common metabolic abnormality identified among renal stone formers. Excessive urinary calcium excretion leads to the supersaturation of urine with calcium and the subsequent development of calcium oxalate (most commonly dihydrate form) and/or calcium phosphate (if alkaline urine) stones. In most cases, hypercalciuria is idiopathic, familial, and affected by diet. Idiopathic hypercalciuria can be classified into subtypes of absorptive (i.e., gut absorbs excess calcium), resorptive (i.e., increased bone turnover leads to increased renal-filtered load of calcium) or renal "leak" (i.e., decreased renal calcium reabsorption). However, *the distinction between mechanisms has little bearing upon treatment.* Excessive dietary intake of sodium can contribute to increased urinary calcium excretion. The associated volume expansion reduces sodium reabsorption in the loop of Henle, which, in turn, reduces calcium reabsorption in this segment and leads to increased urinary calcium excretion. Secondary causes of hypercalciuria are less common and include primary hyperparathyroidism and disorders of vitamin D excess such as sarcoidosis.

Hyperoxaluria is only moderately more common among stone formers than nonstone formers. Indeed, most patients with calcium oxalate stones excrete normal amounts of urinary oxalate. Higher urinary oxalate levels combine with urinary calcium to raise the supersaturation of the urine for calcium oxalate and thus increase calcium oxalate stone formation (most commonly monohydrate form). Sources of oxalate in the body include gastrointestinal absorption (~30%) and endogenous production through hepatic metabolism of glycine, glycolate, hydroxyproline, vitamin C, and other substances (~70%). A rare cause of hyperoxaluria is primary hyperoxaluria, an inborn error of glyoxylate metabolism leading to overproduction of oxalate. Patients typically present early in life though a small subset are identified in adulthood after presentation with stone disease or genetic testing of an affected family member. However, genetic causes of hyperoxaluria are uncommon. Hyperoxaluria is more frequently due to increased gut absorption. This may occur related to intake of foods with high oxalate content such as spinach, peanuts, or chocolate. In addition, gastrointestinal disorders associated with fat malabsorption, such as Crohn disease, gluten-sensitive enteropathy, or gastrointestinal bypass surgery, may lead to hyperoxaluria—this is termed *enteric hyperoxaluria*. Oxalate is typically excreted in the stool when it is bound to a divalent cation such as Ca^{2+}. In the unbound form, oxalate is absorbed primarily in the colon and excreted in the urine. In enteric hyperoxaluria, reduced availability of Ca^{2+} due to chelation of divalent cations by the high stool fat content leaves oxalate unbound and free to be absorbed.

Hypocitraturia is a risk factor for calcium stone formation. Citrate is an important inhibitor of stone formation due to its ability to complex urinary calcium, theoretically preventing its incorporation into calcium-based stones. Hypocitraturia may be due to conditions that either increase endogenous acid production, such as excessive dietary protein intake, or increase base loss, such as chronic diarrhea. Recently, the carbonic anhydrase inhibitors topiramate and zonisamide, popular medications used to treat migraine headaches, have been associated with increased risk of calcium phosphate stones in part through generation of mild renal tubular acidosis leading to hypocitraturia and alkaline urine.

Hyperuricosuria is ironically a more significant risk factor for calcium oxalate rather than uric acid stone formation. With respect to calcium oxalate stone risk, uric acid crystals may serve as a nidus on which calcium oxalate crystals deposit, leading to increased calcium oxalate stone growth. For pure uric acid stones, the impact of hyperuricosuria on stone formation is dwarfed by the role of urine pH. The solubility of uric acid is strongly pH dependent as uric acid crystals form at low pH (acid urine). Thus, even at very low urine uric acid concentrates but at low pH, uric acid crystals may form. Conversely, even with very high urine uric acid excretes, at sufficiently high urine pH (an alkaline urine), no uric acid crystals will form. Conversely, even with very high urine uric acid excretes, at sufficiently high urine pH (alkaline urine), no uric acid crystals will form.

Infection with urea-splitting bacteria, such as Proteus, some Klebsiella species and others can lead to increased formation of magnesium ammonium phosphate stones also known as struvite stones. Bacterial urease hydrolyzes urinary urea to ammonia in a reaction that consumes a proton, thereby increasing both urinary ammonia and pH. At high urine pH, magnesium, phosphate, and ammonium form struvite which is insoluble and can rapidly grow in size until it fills the collecting system, forming the classic "staghorn" calculus. Bacteria are frequently incorporated into the growing struvite stone, leading to difficulty sterilizing the urine.

III. CLINICAL PRESENTATION

A. Symptomatic. *Severe, intense pain* is the most common presentation of renal stone disease. Pain is sudden in onset although it may increase over a period of hours to a peak in some individuals. It may be either steady or colicky and patients classically squirm, unable to find a comfortable position. *Pain most commonly occurs when the stone has moved out of the renal pelvis and is moving through the ureter and remaining in the urinary tract.* An obstructing or partially obstructing stone in the renal pelvis or upper ureter is characteristically associated with flank and abdominal pain. Stones either in the middle or lower third of the ureter typically cause pain that radiates downward to the inguinal ligament and into the urethra or testicle and penis. When stones are present in the portion of the ureter within the bladder wall, they may cause dysuria and frequency. Nausea and vomiting frequently accompany the pain and may contribute to the development of dehydration. Many affected individuals characterize the pain as the worst they have ever experienced.

Hematuria, gross and microscopic, may occur as a result of local trauma to the epithelium of the renal pelvis or bladder from the stones.

Infection within the stone may lead to recurrent urinary tract infections and, if accompanied by obstruction or partial obstruction, requires emergent decompression.

Obstruction of the renal pelvis or ureter may occur. Untreated obstruction, even if partial, can lead to irreversible loss of renal function, particularly if lasting longer than 4 weeks.

B. Asymptomatic. *Incidentally* found stones may be discovered on abdominal radiography or computed tomography (CT) imaging or during follow-up imaging in known stone formers.

Microscopic hematuria may be the only manifestation of stone disease and, in the asymptomatic patient, usually associated with stones in the renal pelvis or parenchyma.

IV. DIAGNOSIS. Key diagnostic steps in the setting of acute stone event should include:

History should emphasize diet, lifestyle factors, medication use, familial disorders, and the presence or absence of previous renal stones.

Urinalysis usually reveals either gross or microscopic hematuria. If pyuria is present, then infection should be excluded by urine culture and clinical picture. Crystalluria may permit a presumptive identification of stone type (Table 21.1). However, only freshly voided, warm urine should be used for examinations. When urine is cooled, the solubility of dissolved crystalloids decreases, possibly leading to their precipitation and an incorrect diagnosis.

Radiologic studies are key to the evaluation of the symptomatic stone former. Noncontrast spiral CT scan of the abdomen and pelvis is the gold standard test to diagnose urinary tract stones, identifying both radiopaque and radiolucent calculi with a sensitivity and specificity of >96%. A plan abdominal radiograph may show radiopaque stones (80% of all stones) containing either calcium, struvite, or cysteine, but may miss radiolucent uric acid stones. Ultrasound is useful in identifying hydronephrosis but has poor sensitivity for stone detection.

Crystallographic stone analysis. Patients should strain their urine through a filter until the stone is passed to obtain the stone for crystallographic analysis of its composition.

V. MANAGEMENT. The management of renal stone disease should be divided into two components: treatment of *acute stone passage*, and the *chronic management* after pain, obstruction, and/or infection is treated.

A. Acute Management. Once other conditions such as appendicitis, cholecystitis, and pyelonephritis are excluded as the cause of the patient's symptoms, pain control is essential. Rapid pain control is best achieved with ketorolac tromethamine or parenteral narcotics. Intravenous volume repletion will assist both in decreasing symptoms related to volume depletion and in increasing urine output, which may aid in the passage of the renal stones. If infection is suspected, either because of the presence of fever and leukocytosis or pyuria and bacteriuria on urinalysis, empirical antibiotics should be started. In general, all patients should have their urine cultured.

In most patients, the acute renal colic can be managed in an outpatient setting. Indications for admission and surgical intervention include: (a) any degree of bilateral urinary obstruction; (b) solitary kidney; (c) fever and/or urinary tract infection with obstruction; (d) intractable nausea and vomiting; (e) pain not controlled by oral analgesics; and (f) a stone unlikely to spontaneously pass based upon size and location. A stone within the distal ureter is more likely to pass compared with a stone in the more proximal ureter. As a rough guide for the percent likelihood of spontaneous stone passage based upon size up to 10 mm, use the following formula: ([10 − Stone size in millimeters] × 10%).

Most renal stones pass spontaneously. Although the utility of it has been questioned in recent randomized trials, MET (or tamsulosin 0.4 mg by mouth daily until stone passage or definitive therapy) should be utilized for all patients with stones located in the distal ureter. Tamsulosin, a selective α-blocker, is thought to work by relaxing ureteral smooth muscle and facilitating stone passage, particularly for stones >5 mm in size. Stones that do not pass spontaneously or require intervention can be approached with a variety of techniques that include ESWL, ureteroscopy with stone basket manipulation and/or laser lithotripsy, and endoscopic percutaneous extraction. In industrialized countries, open or laparoscopic stone surgery is reserved for failed endoscopic procedures, unreasonably large stone burdens, or in the setting of renal ectopia or complex collecting system.

B. Chronic Management. The chronic management of renal stone disease is based upon two observations. First, renal stone disease may be the initial presentation of an underlying systemic disease that may cause morbidity or mortality unrelated to the stone disease if not identified. Second, over 60% of patients with renal stone disease will develop at least one recurrence. Of those, many will develop frequent recurrences that can become an economic burden, substantially lower quality of life and increase risk of chronic kidney disease.

Exclude an underlying systemic disease. The first goal of the chronic management of renal stone disease is to exclude an underlying systemic disease that may predispose to stone formation. This assessment begins with a detailed history. On laboratory data, patients with hypercalcemia, whether overt or borderline, should have an ionized calcium and a parathyroid hormone (PTH) level measured to exclude the presence of primary hyperparathyroidism. If PTH is suppressed, non–PTH-mediated cause of hypercalcemia, such as sarcoidosis, should be considered. Patients with hypokalemic, non–anion-gap metabolic acidosis should have the urine pH and urine anion gap measured to determine whether they have distal renal tubular acidosis. Inflammatory bowel disease and gout are generally suspected based on a typical history, although the presence of hyperuricemia may be helpful (though not required) in the diagnosis of gout. Inborn errors of metabolism that cause renal stones are frequent causes of stones in children. These include cystine stones in cystinosis, glycine stones in hyperglycinuria, uric acid stones in Lesch–Nyhan syndrome, and oxalate stones in primary hyperoxaluria. Congenital distal renal tubular acidosis may also be present in children and is frequently associated with impaired growth or failure to thrive.

Prevention of Recurrence. The second component of the chronic management of renal stone disease is prevention of recurrence. Recall that >60% of initial stone formers will recur by 5 years and that a metabolic etiology can be found in almost 97% of these patients. For the first-time stone former, particularly those without family history of stone disease, a detailed history to exclude intake of medications or diet/lifestyle that may predispose to stone formation (i.e., high-sodium diet, calcium supplementation, carbonic anhydrase inhibitors) and a limited metabolic evaluation consisting of serum calcium, phosphorus, uric acid, a basic metabolic profile, and urinalysis with urinary cystine measurement are adequate. For the recurrent stone former or for those first-time stone formers who would be high risk for complications should they recur, targeted therapy should be based upon the automated analysis of calcium, oxalate, uric acid, citrate, pH, total volume, creatinine, sodium, magnesium, and phosphorus in a 24-hour urine specimen. The 24-hour urine collection should be performed at least 4 to 6 weeks after the acute stone-forming event for the sole purpose of allowing the patient to return to their normal daily life, providing the most accurate snapshot of dietary habits. Information from the 24-hour urine can be used to identify factors to address with diet and medical therapy, and to monitor adherence to such therapies (Table 21.2).

- *Low urine volume* should be increased to greater than 2 L/day. Higher urine volumes prevent recurrence by decreasing the concentration of crystalloids. Most beverages are acceptable to achieve this goal, though sugar-sweetened drinks should be avoided.
- *Hypercalciuria* should be treated by measures that decrease urinary calcium excretion. First, underlying causes of hypercalcemia such as primary hyperparathyroidism or other causes should be investigated and treated if present. If hypercalcemia is not present, dietary modification including a sodium-restricted diet (<2,300 mg/day sodium) that avoids high animal protein intake should be advised. Thiazide and thiazide-like diuretics may also be used to decrease urinary calcium excretion and reduce stone recurrence rates. Potassium citrate may be added to this regimen should thiazide-related hypokalemia or hypocitraturia ensue. Sodium citrate is usually avoided because the sodium content can increase urinary calcium excretion.
- *Hyperoxaluria* is treated by addressing the underlying cause whenever possible. In general, hyperoxaluria is managed with a low-oxalate diet. Fat malabsorption, which increases enteric permeability to oxalate, should be treated aggressively with a low-fat diet, high-dose calcium citrate supplementation (2 g/day), bile acid sequestrants, and low-oxalate diet. If marked hyperoxaluria greater than 5 to 10 times the upper limit of normal is identified, evaluation for primary hyperoxaluria related to genetic defects in oxalate metabolism should be undertaken.
- *Hyperuricosuria* can be treated by measures that either increase the solubility of uric acid or decrease the production of uric acid. Alkalinization

TABLE 21.2   Summary of urinary factors contributing to renal stone formation and approach to treatment

Abnormality	Stones formed	Dietary and environmental contributing factors	Treatment
Hypercalciuria	Calcium-based	High dietary sodium High dietary animal protein	Sodium restriction Moderate animal protein Thiazide diuretics
Hypocitraturia	Any	Diarrhea (gastrointestinal alkali loss) Hypokalemia Renal tubular acidosis	Potassium citrate
Low urine volume	Any	Low intake Occupational gastrointestinal losses	Target urine output >2 L/day
Hyperuricosuria	Calcium oxalate >> uric acid	Hyperuricemia High-purine diet	Low-purine diet Allopurinol
Hyperoxaluria	Calcium oxalate	High-oxalate diet Low-calcium diet Malabsorptive state (such as gastric bypass)	Low-oxalate diet Dietary calcium Address malabsorption: Bile acid resin, low-fat diet, high-dose calcium with meals

of urine (target pH > 6.0) markedly increases the solubility of uric acid and should be first-line therapy for uric acid stone formers. Potassium citrate is effective because oral citrate can cause a mild metabolic alkalosis and subsequent alkalinization of the urine. For calcium oxalate stone formers with documented hyperuricosuria and normocalciuria, allopurinol 300 mg daily decreases the production of uric acid and can lower calcium oxalate stone recurrence up to 50%.

■ *Hypocitraturia* is treated with oral potassium citrate. As noted above, citrate ingestion leads to mild metabolic alkalosis, thus increasing urinary citrate excretion. Potassium citrate is often needed at up to 40 to 60 mEq/day, in divided doses, but gastrointestinal upset sometimes complicates adherence to potassium citrate. Liquid and crystal formulations that can be added to a favorite drink may enhance adherence.

In the case of infection-related stones, the 24-hour urine is less helpful. Treatment of the underlying infection is key and, ultimately, surgical intervention is required for definitive therapy. Appropriate antibiotics should be administered based upon the results of urine culture and sensitivity, accompanied by a referral to urology for removal. Because the offending bacteria can become incorporated into the stone matrix, prolonged antibiotic treatment (even in the presence of negative urine culture) may be required if complete surgical removal is not possible. Acetohydroxamic acid, a urease inhibitor, may be helpful in slowing stone growth.

VI. SUGGESTED READINGS

Borghi L, Meschi T, Amato F, et al. Urinary volume, water and recurrences in idiopathic calcium nephrolithiasis: a 5-year randomized prospective study. *J Urol.* 1996;155(3):839–843.

Borghi L, Schianchi T, Meschi T, et al. Comparison of two diets for the prevention of recurrent stones in idiopathic hypercalciuria. *N Engl J Med.* 2002;346(2):77–84.

Chandhoke PS. Evaluation of the recurrent stone former. *Urol Clin North Am.* 2007;34(3):315–322.

Curhan GC. Epidemiology of stone disease. *Urol Clin North Am.* 2007;34(3):287–293.

Ettinger B, Tang A, Citron JT, et al. Randomized trial of allopurinol in the prevention of calcium oxalate calculi. *N Engl J Med.* 1986;315(22):1386–1389.

Moe OW. Kidney stones: pathophysiology and medical management. *Lancet.* 2006:367(9507): 333–344.

Park S, Pearle MS. Pathophysiology and management of calcium stones. *Urol Clin North Am.* 2007;34(3):323–334.

Rule AD, Lieske JC, Pais VM. Management of kidney stones in 2020. *JAMA.* 2020;323(19):1961–1962.

Scales CD, Smith AC, Hanley JM, et al. Urologic Diseases in America Project. Prevalence of kidney stones in the United States. *Eur Urol.* 2012;62(1):160–165.

22

Urinary Tract Infections

Michael Lipkowitz

Urinary tract infection (UTI) is a common clinical problem. A UTI is *complicated* if it is associated with an increased risk of serious complications or treatment failure (e.g., congenital malformations, obstruction, stones, presence of a foreign body, or immune deficiency states). Whether a UTI is complicated or not determines the therapy and the follow-up.

I. **EPIDEMIOLOGY.** In the United States, at least 250,000 episodes of acute pyelonephritis occur annually. Acute cystitis accounts for more than 10 million outpatient encounters per year and recurs in about 30% of healthy women with normal urinary tracts. There is a peak in incidence in women aged 14 to 24, and after the peak incidence increases with age. The incidence of symptomatic UTI in adult men <50 years of age is much lower. Complicated UTI occurs in 2 to 3 million patients/y, of which >80% are catheter associated.

II. **RISK FACTORS.** UTIs are more common in women. The exceptions are those associated with congenital malformation in early childhood and obstruction, which occurs more frequently in males.

III. **PATHOGENESIS**

A. **Bacterial Factors.** More than 95% of UTIs result from the ascension of uropathogens from the external genitalia. The remainder are due to the hematogenous dissemination of organisms such as *Staphylococcus aureus*, *Pseudomonas aeruginosa*, and *Salmonella typhi* (Table 22.1). UTIs in women are often due to the colonization of the vaginal introitus and the periurethral area. Once within the bladder, bacteria may multiply and ascend to the ureters, especially if there is vesicoureteral reflux to the kidneys. Most UTIs are due to *Escherichia coli*, especially serogroups (called *uropathogenic strains*) 01, 02, 04, 06, 07, 075, and 0150, which possess virulence factors that facilitate their adhesion to uroepithelium.

B. **Host Factors.** The presence of lactobacilli in the normal vaginal flora prevents colonization. This environment is disrupted by the use of spermicidals and menopause, thereby increasing the risk of recurrent UTIs. Sexual activity introduces pathogens into the bladder, where they adhere to uroepithelial cells and cause infection. Incomplete bladder emptying predisposes to UTI. Within the kidney, the medulla is most susceptible to infection.

IV. **CLINICAL PRESENTATION AND DIAGNOSIS.** UTI syndromes range from asymptomatic bacteriuria (ASB) to life-threatening, tissue-invasive infections associated with shock and multiple organ failure. Symptoms are not closely related either to the presence of bacteriuria or to the site of infection. Pyuria is suggestive of UTI. Urinary leukocyte esterase activity and urinary nitrite may be used as

TABLE 22.1	Bacterial etiology of urinary tract infections (UTIs)

| | Frequency in UTIs (%) | |
Organisms	Uncomplicated	Complicated
Gram-negative organisms		
Escherichia coli	70–80	50–65
Klebsiella spp.	1–2	5–10
Proteus mirabilis	1–2	2–17
Citrobacter spp.	<1	5
Enterobacter spp.	<1	2–10
Pseudomonas aeruginosa	<1	2–19
Other (*including Candida* sp.)	<1	6–20
Gram-positive organisms		
Enterococci	5–10	7–11
Coagulase-negative staphylococci (*Staphylococcus saprophyticus*)	5–10	2–5
Group B streptococci	<1	1–4
Staphylococcus aureus	<1	1–2
Other	<1	2

a screening test, but >10 leukocytes/mm^3 in unspun urine has a better correlate with infection. In contrast, the examination of spun urine for leukocytes has high false-positive and false-negative results. A Gram stain of unspun urine showing one or more organisms per oil immersion field correlates with the presence of >10^5 bacteria/mL.

The cornerstone of diagnosis is a quantitative urine culture. Significant bacteriuria refers to >10^5 colony-forming units (CFUs)/mL of a single uropathogen. However, 20% to 30% of true, symptomatic bacterial UTIs in women that respond to appropriate treatment have lesser counts. Therefore, in a symptomatic woman, a lower cutoff improves the test sensitivity.

V. MAJOR URINARY TRACT INFECTION SYNDROMES

A. **Asymptomatic Bacteriuria.** ASB is broadly defined as a positive urine culture in an asymptomatic patient. In asymptomatic women, the presence of two consecutive cultures with >10^5 CFU/mL of the same bacterial species in clean-catch voided urine specimens establishes this diagnosis. In men, a single positive specimen suffices. In any asymptomatic patient, a single catheterized urine specimen showing >10^2 CFU/mL of one bacterial species is enough to establish the diagnosis of ASB. ASB is common and generally benign. ASB may be associated with pyuria in elderly patients. Treatment is generally not warranted, except in high-risk patient groups that include pregnant patients, renal transplant recipients, those undergoing genitourinary procedures, and in neutropenic patients.

B. **Acute, Uncomplicated Cystitis or Urinary Tract Infection in Women.** Acute, uncomplicated cystitis or UTI in women is characterized by burning on urination, dysuria, frequency, and/or suprapubic pain without fever or costovertebral tenderness. Acute dysuria in a young, sexually active woman is usually caused

T A B L E 22.2	Commonly used oral regimens for acute, uncomplicated cystitis	

Drug and dose	Interval	Duration (days)
First line		
Nitrofurantoin (Macrobid), 100 mg	q12h	5
Trimethoprim-sulfamethoxazole, 160/800 mg	q12h	3
Fosfomycin 3g	Once	1
Second line (beta lactam)		
Amoxicillin clavulanate, 500 mg	q12h	5–7
Cefpodoxime proxetil, 100 mg	q12h	5–7
Cefixime, 400 mg	q24h	5–7
Third line (fluoroquinolone)		
Ciprofloxacin, 250 mg	q12h	3
Ciprofloxacin, 500 mg extended release	q24h	3
Levofloxacin, 250 mg	q24h	3

by acute cystitis, acute urethritis from *Chlamydia trachomatis*, *Neisseria gonor-rhoeae*, or *Herpes simplex*, or vaginitis caused by *Candida* spp. or *Trichomonas vaginalis*. The presence of pyuria favors acute cystitis and urethritis. However, definitive diagnosis requires the finding of significant bacteriuria in a mid-stream urine specimen. In these circumstances, $>10^3$ CFU/mL should be used because this increases the sensitivity from 50% to 80% and retains a specificity of 90%. However, urine cultures are generally not necessary in uncomplicated acute cystitis.

Treatment depends on the assessment of the risk of multidrug-resistant (MDR) organisms. Risk of MDR is high if any of the following in the last 3 months:

Culture of an MDR bacteria on urine isolate
Use of trimethoprim-sulfamethoxazole (TMP-SMX), fluoroquinolone (FQ) or third-generation cephalosporin
Inpatient health facility stay (e.g., hospital, long-term care)
Travel to region with high rate of MDR

Three-day regimens (Table 22.2) are preferred for the treatment of acute, uncomplicated cystitis. Single-dose regimens are less effective. Nitrofurantoin must be given for at least 5 days. Current recommendations suggest nitrofuran-toin or TMP-SMX, (although resistance rates are rising) and fosfomycin (often held in reserve for MDR strains). The second-line therapy is now beta-lactam antibiotics, with FQs as a third line given increasing resistance and the risk of tendon/aneurysm rupture, etc. Routine follow-up cultures should be under-taken only when infection persists or recurs within 2 weeks, when a longer course (10 to 14 days) with an agent based on sensitivities should be prescribed. A recurrence after 2 weeks should be treated as a new episode of UTI.

C. **Recurrent, Acute, Uncomplicated Cystitis in Women.** Most recurrent, acute, uncom-plicated cystitis episodes in women are due to reinfection with the same uropathogen. The first prevention step should be postcoital voiding, avoiding spermicides, and local or systemic estrogen replacement in postmenopausal women. The next step should be imaging studies to detect a sequestered focus of infection or a complicating structural or functional disorder. Structural disorders (stricture, etc.) may need to be treated to hasten improvement or prevent recurrence. These may respond to an extended course (4 to 6 weeks) of TMP-SMX or an FQ. Prophylaxis should be considered for women who experience two or more symptomatic infections within 6 months or three or more over 12 months. Women with less frequent episodes should also be offered prophylaxis if these episodes cause disability or significant discomfort. Effective strategies include:

- low-dose, long-term prophylaxis with either TMP-SMX (40/200-half a single strength tablet daily or 3×/wk) or a Nitrofurantoin (50 mg BID or 100 mg daily)
- a single dose of the above agents given after coitus; and a single dose at the onset of symptoms of UTI

Other maneuvers such as cranberry juice, probiotics, and D-mannose have not been clearly proven to be effective.

D. Acute Urethral Syndrome in Women. Acute urethral syndrome in women is similar to acute, uncomplicated UTI but has a smaller number (10^2 to 10^4 CFU/mL) of usual uropathogens or infection with *Chlamydia trachomatis*. Pyuria is almost always present. Because vaginitis may present similarly, vaginal examination and cultures should be performed and appropriate treatment provided. Those with dysuria who lack pyuria or do not respond to antimicrobials should be managed symptomatically.

E. Acute, Uncomplicated Pyelonephritis in Women. Symptoms of acute, uncomplicated pyelonephritis in women range from a mild illness to septic shock and renal failure. These patients can have fever, chills, flank pain, nausea and vomiting, and costovertebral tenderness. Symptoms of cystitis are variable. A Gram stain of the urine sediment should guide empiric therapy. A urine culture should always be performed, and $>10^4$ CFU/mL uropathogens is positive in >95% of patients.

Outpatient therapy (Fig. 22.1) with oral agents, usually an FQ, is safe and effective in selected patients, but in areas with high FQ resistance, should be preceded by IV infusion of a long-acting β-lactam. It can be instituted after initial stabilization in the emergency department (Table 22.3). Indications for hospitalization include inability to maintain oral hydration or to take medications, severe illness with high fevers, severe pain and debility, noncompliance, and uncertainty about the diagnosis. For gram-positive organisms, therapy with ampicillin or amoxicillin/clavulanic acid, or vancomycin in patients with penicillin allergy, is appropriate. However, these infections are usually caused by gram-negative bacilli. An FQ, a β-lactam/aminoglycoside combination, or a broad-spectrum β-lactam (e.g., imipenem, ceftazidime, ceftriaxone, or piperacillin/tazobactam) are all appropriate (Table 22.4). Once sepsis is controlled and the patient is afebrile, oral therapy with an FQ or TMP-SMX or other agent depending on culture results should be given for 14 days. Failure to obtain a response within 72 hours should trigger a search for a complicating problem such as a stone, obstruction, or poor bladder emptying. Nitrofurantoin should not be used to treat pyelonephritis, as it does not achieve therapeutic tissue levels. Follow-up cultures should be done only if symptoms recur.

F. Urinary Tract Infection in Pregnancy. UTI in pregnancy is associated with premature labor and delivery, increased fetal loss, and prematurity. Routine screening and treatment of ASB are standard practice at the first prenatal visit. Further

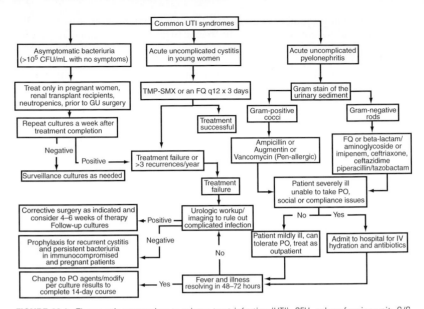

FIGURE 22.1: Therapeutic approaches to urinary tract infection (UTI). CFU, colony-forming unit; C/S, culture and sensitivity; dx, diagnosis; FQ, fluoroquinolone; GU, genitourinary; TMP-SMX, trimethoprim-sulfamethoxazole.

screening is needed in women at high risk for infection (e.g., presence of urinary tract anomalies, hemoglobin S, or preterm labor). Treatment is similar to that for nonpregnant women with acute, uncomplicated UTI with a short-term course. However, sulfonamides should be avoided in the first trimester and near term because of the risk of kernicterus in the newborn, and FQs affect fetal cartilage development. Nitrofurantoin, ampicillin, and cephalexin are safe. Pregnant women with overt pyelonephritis should be admitted for parenteral therapy with β-lactam and aminoglycosides. Suppressive therapy is recommended for women with persistent bacteriuria (>2 positive urine cultures). Nitrofurantoin (50 to 100 mg orally at bedtime) for the duration of the pregnancy or cephalexin (250 to 500 mg orally at bedtime) may be used. A culture should be obtained 1 week after completion of therapy and repeated monthly.

TABLE 22.3 Commonly used oral agents for uncomplicated pyelonephritis

Drug and dose	Interval	Duration (days)
Fluoroquinolones	q12h	7–10
Ciprofloxacin, 500 mg	q12h	7–10
Gatifloxacin, 400 mg	q12h	7–10
Levofloxacin, 500 mg	q12h	7–10
Trimethoprim-sulfamethoxazole, 160/800 mg	q12h	10–14
Amoxicillin-clavulanate, 875/125 mg	q12h	10–14

TABLE 22.4	Commonly used parenteral regimens for acute, uncomplicated pyelonephritis	

Drug and dose	Interval
Ceftriaxone, 1–2 g	q24h
Cefepime, 1 g	q12h
Ciprofloxacin, 200–400 mg	q12h
Gatifloxacin, 400 mg	q24h
Levofloxacin, 250–500 mg	q24h
Gentamicin, 3–5 mg/kg (±ampicillin)	q24h
Gentamicin, 1 mg/kg (±ampicillin)	q8h
Ampicillin, 1 g (+gentamicin)	q6h
Trimethoprim-sulfamethoxazole, 160/800 mg	q12h
Aztreonam, 1 g	q8–12h
Ampicillin/sulbactam, 1.5 g	q6h
Piperacillin/tazobactam, 3.375 g	q6–8h

Note: See text for duration.

G. **Urinary Tract Infection in Men.** UTIs in men are usually associated with obstruction from congenital disorders in the young and acquired disorders in the old. In men <50 years of age, anal intercourse, lack of circumcision, intercourse with a woman colonized with uropathogens, and acquired immunodeficiency syndrome with a CD4 count of <200/mm^3 are important risk factors. Men without one of these risk factors, and especially those who have recurrent infections, should undergo a urologic evaluation and an intensive treatment course (minimum of 4 to 6 weeks). UTI in men usually represents tissue invasion of the prostate or kidney, or both, and should be treated for at least 14 days. Recurrent infection often indicates a sequestered focus within the prostate that is difficult to eradicate due to poor antimicrobial penetration, presence of prostatic calculi, or prostatic enlargement causing bladder neck obstruction.

H. **Complicated Urinary Tract Infections.** Complicated UTIs involve a wide variety of structural and functional defects of the urinary system with a wide range of organisms. Antibiotic resistance is common and mandates an individualized approach to therapy. Acutely septic patients should receive broad-spectrum antibiotic combinations until definitive bacteriologic data are available. If it is possible to correct an underlying structural defect, a shorter course of antibiotics (7 to 14 days) should be used to control the symptoms, and a prolonged 4- to 6-week course should be used if such correction is not possible. Catheter-related infection is the most common cause of complicated UTI. Prevention should include avoidance of a catheter when possible, sterile insertion, prompt removal, and use of a closed collecting system—intensive adherence to these principles via nursing-driven protocols can dramatically reduce incidence. Prophylactic systemic antimicrobials are not indicated except in pregnant women or patients undergoing urologic procedures who require short-term catheterization. If an infection occurs, catheters should be removed if possible and subsequent urine culture obtained before treatment, which should be adjusted depending on culture results. When the catheter can't be removed, it should be exchanged and culture obtained from the new catheter followed by antibiotic therapy.

Patients with spinal cord injuries who require catheter bladder drainage are predisposed to recurrent UTIs. Pyuria and significant bacteriuria ($>10^5$ CFU/mL) are usually present, and common antibiotic resistance necessitates parenteral antibiotics. Intermittent catheterization is recommended but treatment of ASB with prophylactic antibiotics is not.

Emphysematous pyelonephritis is necrotizing pyelonephritis with gas-forming *E. coli*, *Klebsiella pneumoniae*, *P. aeruginosa*, or *Proteus mirabilis*. Most cases occur in patients with diabetes and are associated with obstruction. Computed tomography (CT) shows gas within the renal parenchyma. Emergency nephrectomy and broad-spectrum antibiotics lower the mortality from 75% to 20%.

In patients with adult polycystic kidney disease, clinical differential diagnosis of UTI is usually acute pyelonephritis or cyst infection and can be difficult to establish. Most antibiotics do not penetrate the cyst; therefore, lipid-soluble drugs such as ciprofloxacin or TMP-SMX are used. If urine cultures are negative, a cyst infection is most likely, in which case treatment should be continued for 4 to 6 weeks. In cysts >3 cm in diameter on CT scan, drainage is recommended.

Another rare entity seen in patients with recurrent UTIs, especially in the presence of nephrolithiasis, is xanthogranulomatous pyelonephritis. Patients have typical symptoms of pyelonephritis, as well as anorexia, weight loss, and a palpable mass on examination, which is easily confirmed by a CT scan. It closely mimics renal cancer, but pathology reveals an inflammatory and necrotic mass. Treatment is antibiotics and nephrectomy.

I. **Candidal Infections of the Urinary Tract.** Candidal infections of the urinary tract are common in patients with diabetes, with indwelling catheters, or in patients receiving corticosteroids or broad-spectrum antibiotics. The first step is to correct these factors where possible. If candiduria persists, systemic antifungal therapy is recommended. Fluconazole (200 to 400 mg/day) is effective against *Candida albicans* and *Candida tropicalis*, but not against *Candida krusei* or *Candida glabrata*, which should be treated with low-dose amphotericin (10 mg/day) plus flucytosine (100 mg/kg/day) in divided doses for 14 days. Patients who require an indwelling catheter may receive amphotericin or nystatin bladder rinses via a three-way catheter. However, this has an efficacy of only approximately 50%.

J. **Urinary Tract Infection in Kidney Transplant.** UTI is common after transplant occurring in more than 25% of patients, and is associated with acute T-cell–mediated rejection, allograft dysfunction or loss, and death. Most centers screen by culture for asymptomatic bacteriuria for the first 3 months and if present treat as for uncomplicated cystitis, although there is no strong evidence to define the length of the screening/treatment period. Acute cystitis without symptoms of complicated disease such as allograft pain and tenderness, fever, presence of stents, etc., is treated similarly to uncomplicated UTI above, although cultures are usually performed. Complicated UTI is treated with broad-spectrum parenteral antibiotics covering both gram-positive and gram-negative organisms until culture results are available to guide therapy.

VI. SUGGESTED READINGS

Anger J, Lee U, Ackerman AL, et al. Recurrent uncomplicated urinary tract infections in women: AUA/CUA/SUFU guideline. *J Urol.* 2019;202(2):282–289. doi:10.1097/JU.0000000000000296

Ariza-Heredia EJ, Beam EN, Lesnick TG. Urinary tract infections in kidney transplant recipients: role of gender, urologic abnormalities, and antimicrobial prophylaxis. *Ann Transplant.* 2013:18:195–204. doi:10.12659/AOT.883901

Carreno JJ, Tam IM, Meyers JL, et al. Longitudinal, nationwide, cohort study to assess incidence, outcomes, and costs associated with complicated urinary tract infection. *Open Forum Infect Dis.* 2019;6(11):ofz446. doi:10.1093/ofid/ofz446

Chu CM, Lowder JL. Diagnosis and treatment of urinary tract infections across age groups. *Am J Obstet Gynecol.* 2018;219(1):40–51. doi:10.1016/j.ajog.2017.12.231

Flores-Mireles AL, Walker JN, Caparon M, et al. Urinary tract infections: epidemiology, mechanisms of infection and treatment options. *Nat Rev Microbiol.* 2015;13(5):269–284. doi:10.1038/nrmicro3432

Gupta K, Hooton TM, Naber KG, et al. International clinical practice guidelines for the treatment of acute uncomplicated cystitis and pyelonephritis in women: a 2010 update by the Infectious Diseases Society of America and the European Society for Microbiology and Infectious Diseases. *Clin Infect Dis.* 2011;52(5):e103–e120. doi:10.1093/cid/ciq257

Hypertension

23 Approach to the Hypertensive Patient

Christopher S. Wilcox

Hypertension is a level of blood pressure (BP) that, when lowered by antihypertensive treatment, predicts a net benefit to the patient for protection from cardiovascular, cerebrovascular, or renal diseases. A BP consistently above 140/90 mm Hg previously was considered sufficient to diagnose hypertension. However, epidemiologic studies report an increased development of cardiovascular disease (CVD) and stroke at levels of BP above 120/80 mm Hg and risk rises log-linearly with systolic blood pressure (SBP) above 120 mm Hg. Moreover, results from the SPRINT and ACCORD trials described below have prompted a reevaluation (see Table 23.1). Although absolute CVD risk rises with age and associated CVD, chronic renal disease (CKD), and diabetes mellitus (DM), the current guidelines that have been based on solid results from randomized controlled clinical trials have led to one set of BP goals regardless of associated risk.

It is important to measure the BP correctly (Table 23.2).

I. INCIDENCE. The incidence of hypertension is approximately 5% in young adults, 50% by age 50 years, and 80% by age 80. It is increased in those with DM or CKD.

II. RISKS. Hypertension increases the risk of many common conditions (Table 23.3). It is one of the several factors that increase the risk of CVD and stroke (Table 23.4). Hypertension accelerates the decline in renal function in patients with diabetic nephropathy and those with CKD and proteinuria >1 g daily. These patients should normally receive an angiotensin-converting enzyme inhibitor (ACEI) or an angiotensin receptor blocker (ARB).

Hypertension accelerates the decline in cognitive function in patients with dementia, the decline in cardiac function in those with congestive heart failure (CHF), and the progression of left ventricular hypertrophy (LVH) in those affected and the decline in renal function in those with diabetic nephropathy or proteinuric CKD but optimum BP targets are not changed for these conditions.

III. CLASSIFICATION. Each patient with hypertension should be classified according to the severity (Table 23.3), the pathologic type (Table 23.5), and the cause (see Chapter 20).

Treatment of borderline hypertension is generally nonpharmacologic. Treatment of stage 1 normally can be delayed during evaluation, but stage 2 requires treatment within days.

Isolated systolic hypertension in the young implies a high cardiac output and rapid left ventricular ejection. This responds well to beta-adrenoceptor blockade. Isolated systolic hypertension is common in the elderly, in whom it results from the loss of elasticity in the arteries and arterioles and from aortic

TABLE 23.1	Categorization of BP for the diagnosis of hypertension and its severity in the United States

BP category	SBP (mm Hg)	DBP (mm Hg)
Normal	<120	<80
Elevated	120–129	<80
Hypertension		
• Stage 1	130–139	80–89
• Stage 2	140–159	90–99
• Stage 3	>160	>100

If SBP and DBP fall into two separate categories, the higher category is used.
See JNC8: Whelton PK, Carey RM, Aronow WS, et al. 2017 ACC/AHA/AAPA/ABC/ACPM/AGS/APhA/ASH/ASPC/NMA/PCNA Guideline for the prevention, detection, evaluation, and management of high blood pressure in adults: executive summary: a report of the American College of Cardiology/American Heart Association Task Force on Clinical Practice Guidelines. *Hypertension*. 2018;71(6):1269–1324.

TABLE 23.2	Measurement of office BP

1. Patient resting, seated for 3–5 min with feet on the floor
2. Maintain a quiet and calm environment
3. Select a cuff whose bladder length covers >80% of the arm
4. Position the arm at the level of the heart
5. Take 2 or more readings and average them
6. Take the BP in both arms. Report the higher value
7. With auscultation, use Korotkoff phase I (appearance) and V (disappearance for SBP and DBP
8. Deflation rate should be 2–3 mm Hg per second

After JNC8 (see legend to Table 23.1).

TABLE 23.3	Risks of untreated hypertension

Aortic aneurysm
Cerebrovascular accident
Coronary artery disease
Chronic renal insufficiency (notably nephrosclerosis)
Congestive cardiac failure
Dementia
Myocardial infarction
Peripheral vascular disease

T A B L E **23.4**	Factors that increase risk of cardiovascular disease

African-American ethnicity
Age[a]
Atherosclerosis at any site
Chronic renal failure
Coincident arterial disease
Diabetes mellitus[a]
Dyslipidemia (raised LDL or triglyceride, low HDL)[a]
Endothelial dysfunction
Family history of myocardial infarction below age 50 y[a]
Hypertension[a]
Hyperhomocysteinemia
Hyperuricemia
Inflammation (raised C-reactive protein)
Left ventricular hypertrophy[a]
Microalbuminuria
Obesity/underactivity
Previous target organ injury[a]
Raised plasma levels of asymmetric dimethyl arginine
Smoking[a]

[a]Major independent risk factor.

atherosclerosis. This results in a rapid progression of the left ventricular ejection pressure wave down the aorta and a rapid "ricochet" shock wave from stiffened arterioles. This return wave is transmitted back to the ascending aorta where it can summate with the cardiac contraction to yield a sharp increase in SBP.

Hypertension in the elderly carries an unfavorable prognosis for myocardial infarction and especially for stroke. It responds well to diuretics. Hypertension is classified by pathology and causes:

A. **Pathologic Type.** Benign hypertension is usually asymptomatic and progresses slowly (Table 23.5). Malignant hypertension accounts for <1% of all hypertension. The hallmarks are stage 2 or 3 hypertension (Table 23.1) with grade IV funduscopic changes of papilledema, retinal hemorrhages, and exudates (Table 23.6), accompanied by headache and often by fluctuating neurologic signs caused by increased intracranial pressure and patchy cerebral ischemia. Untreated, malignant hypertension can progress to seizures, fixed neurologic deficits, coma, and death. Patients usually have proteinuria, hematuria, and active urinary sediment. They may progress over weeks or months to renal failure. Some have microangiopathic hemolytic anemia, circulating schistocytes and dysfunction of other organs.

B. **Cause.** Essential hypertension encompasses about 95% of patients who have no discernible cause. Most (70%) have a family history of hypertension, which usually presents between age 20 and 55 years.

Secondary hypertension is described in Chapter 24.

IV. ETIOLOGIC FACTORS IN ESSENTIAL HYPERTENSION

A. **Genetic Factors.** The probability of hypertension is increased if one parent is hypertensive. Many genes are responsible but each individually carries only a

T A B L E 23.5	Pathologic type of hypertension	
	Benign	**Malignant**
Onset	Gradual, ages 20–55	Sudden
Progression	Slow over years	Rapid over weeks
Vascular pathology	Medial hypertrophy	Myointimal proliferation and fibrinoid necrosis
Kidney pathology	Nephrosclerosis and atrophy	Ischemia and hemorrhagic microinfarction
Funduscopic changes	Arterial narrowing and tortuosity	Hemorrhages and exudates; usually papilledema
Renal failure	Absent or slowly progressive	Rapidly progressive often with proteinuria or active urinary sediment

small increased risk except for those regulating sodium transport or aldosterone secretion (see Chapter 16).

B. Diet. Excessive intake of the following dietary constituents is associated with increased BP: sodium chloride, caffeine, and alcohol (more than two drinks per day). Lower BP is associated with high intakes of calcium and potassium.

A DASH diet (Dietary Approaches to Stop Hypertension) lowers BP. It has a high content of calcium, magnesium, and potassium and is based on fruits, nuts, grains, vegetables, low-fat dairy products, white meat, and fish.

C. Renin–Angiotensin–Aldosterone System. Approximately 40% of hypertensive patients have low renin values. This includes many African Americans, the elderly, and those with chronic renal insufficiency. They often have salt-sensitive

T A B L E 23.6	Funduscopic changes in hypertension				
Class	Arterial to venous ratio[a]	Focal arteriolar spasm[b]	Hemorrhages and exudates	Papilledema	Arteriolar light reflex
Normal	3:4	none	0	0	Fine yellow line; blood column
Grade 1	1:2	none	0	0	Broad yellow line; blood column
Grade II	1:3	2:3	0	0	Broad "copper wiring" line; no blood
Grade III	1:4	1:3	+	0	Broad "silver wire" line; no blood
Grade IV	Fine	Obliteration	+	+	Fibrous cords; no blood

[a]Ratio of arterial to venous diameters.
[b]Ratio of diameter of regions of spasm to more proximal segments.

hypertension. Approximately 10% of hypertensives have high renin values. They are often young, White patients. The remarkable effectiveness of ACEIs, ARBs and mineralcorticosteroid receptor antagonists (MRAs) testifies to the importance of the renin–angiotensin–aldosterone (RAAS) in hypertension. However, to be fully effective, especially in patients with low-renin hypertension, these drugs should be combined with a salt-restricted diet and a diuretic.

D. **Sympathetic Nervous System.** Plasma levels of norepinephrine and epinephrine are normal or mildly elevated in most hypertensive patients. However, a subgroup has increased sympathetic tone (hyperdynamic circulation, raised heart rate, elevated catecholamines). Baroreceptor function is impaired in the elderly and those with extensive atherosclerosis who have elevated catecholamines and wider BP fluctuations.

E. **Renal Function.** Early in hypertension, the renal blood flow is reduced, while the glomerular filtration rate is maintained. The ensuing rise in filtration fraction promotes renal salt retention by the proximal tubule. Renal function deteriorates in a minority of hypertensive patients and creates a vicious cycle, whereby a decline in renal function impairs salt excretion, which raises BP and perpetuates further renal damage. African Americans have more organ damage for a given level of hypertension and are much more likely to develop nephrosclerosis and renal insufficiency. This has been related to a mutation in the gene for apolipoprotein A1 that is frequent only in those of African descent (see Chapter 6).

F. **Lifestyle.** BP is increased by pain, emotion, anxiety, obesity, and smoking but is reduced by exercise.

V. **CLINICAL PRESENTATION OF HYPERTENSION.** There are no specific symptoms associated with hypertension. Headache occurs in severe or malignant hypertension. It is usually occipital, throbbing, and present on awakening. Initial examination of all hypertensive patients should include measurements of BP and pulse while the patient is lying down and after 2 minutes of standing. An orthostatic fall in BP implies blocked cardiovascular reflexes (e.g., drugs, such as alpha-receptor blockers, autonomic neuropathy or pheochromocytoma in which the heart rate does not increase on standing) and/or volume depletion. Initially, the BP should be measured in both arms and the timing of femoral and radial pulses correlated (marked differences in pulse pressure or a delayed femoral pulse suggests severe aortic atherosclerosis or coarctation). The BP of children or adolescents should be measured in the arm and the leg to exclude coarctation of the aorta. The fundi should be examined (Table 23.6) for hypertensive or atherosclerotic changes. More severe changes imply prolonged duration and a worse prognosis.

VI. **QUESTIONS TO ANSWER IN EACH HYPERTENSIVE PATIENT.** Key questions should be addressed in each patient suspected of hypertension (Table 23.7).

1. Does the patient have hypertension? Several measurements of BP are necessary because patients are often anxious at the first visit (Table 23.2). They should take their BP regularly at home with an automated device. The BP records should be written down and brought to each clinic visits. The self-recorded BP should be checked against a clinic measurement to ensure accuracy. "White coat" or "office" hypertension is an elevated BP in the clinic but not in the home setting. It is seen in 30% of hypertensive patients. It is associated with a higher probability of subsequent hypertension and a modest increase in LVH. It does not need urgent treatment but should prompt

TABLE 23.7	Questions to answer in each hypertensive patient

Does the patient have hypertension?
What is the severity of hypertension?
Is hypertension benign or malignant?
Is there a secondary cause?
Has there been organ damage?
Are there modifiable dietary or lifestyle factors?
What are the coincident risk factors for cardiovascular disease?
Are there specific drug indications or contraindications?

arrangement for regular BP checks. A more precise diagnosis of white coat hypertension, and a more accurate definition of the true BP burden and response to treatment, requires an ambulatory 24-hour BP monitor (ABPM). This can assess whether the BP dips during sleep at night. "Nondipping" hypertension is associated with target organ damage and is an adverse finding that should prompt more aggressive treatment and follow-up. The following can overestimate BP: fear, pain, anxiety, a rigid arterial wall (checked by palpation at wrist during BP measurement), or a large arm (use a large cuff) (Table 23.2).

2. What is the severity of hypertension? See Table 23.1.
3. Is hypertension benign or malignant? See Table 23.5.
4. Is there a secondary cause? See Chapter 24.
5. Has there been organ damage? Assess the impact on the heart (heart failure, hypertrophy, extra heart sounds, pulmonary rales, a raised jugular venous pressure), kidney (proteinuria, microalbuminuria, hematuria, azotemia, reduced creatinine clearance), vessels (peripheral pulses and bruits, abdominal aneurysms), and fundi (see Table 23.6).
6. Are there modifiable dietary or lifestyle factors? Assess the level of salt intake from measurements of 24-hour renal sodium excretion. (Measure creatinine excretion to assess the adequacy of collection, which should be 15 to 25 mg/kg.) Patients on a "no added salt" diet should achieve a daily sodium excretion of 120 to 150 mmol (equals 120 to 150 mEq) or less. More than two alcoholic drinks daily raises the BP. Aerobic, moderate exercise >30 minutes, five times weekly reduces BP and cardiovascular risk. A DASH diet reduces BP independent of weight reduction.
7. What are the coincident risk factors for CVD? See Table 23.4.
8. Are there specific drug indications or contraindications? See chapters on individual drugs.

VII. ROUTINE LABORATORY TESTS (SEE CHAPTER 1). Assessment of end-organ function and secondary causes are detailed in Table 23.8.

VIII. SPECIAL INVESTIGATIONS. The following have value in selected patients.
A. Computed Tomography or Renal Ultrasound. Computed tomography or renal ultrasound is indicated when the kidneys are palpated on examination (suggesting polycystic kidney disease or tumor) or anatomic abnormalities of the collecting system are suspected (patients with recurrent urinary tract infection, unexplained pyuria or hematuria, symptoms of prostatism, or previous renal stone

T A B L E **23.8**	Tests for patients diagnosed as hypertensive

Urinalysis (protein, glucose, and blood; microscopy if dip is abnormal)
Electrolytes, calcium, blood urea nitrogen, and serum creatinine
Blood sugar and lipid profile (repeat fasting if abnormal with HbAlc)
Electrocardiogram (echocardiogram if abnormal)
24-h urine for sodium excretion, creatinine clearance, and microalbumin excretion
For more severe hypertension or those with a family history of early cardiovascular disease:
    Plasma renin activity and serum aldosterone concentration
    Plasma metanephrines
    Echocardiogram

Note: These routine tests may not detect patients with some secondary causes such as renovascular hypertension.

disease). Renal ultrasound is used to detect renal size (decreased in renal parenchymal disease), urinary tract obstruction, or renal cystic disease.

B. Radionuclide Scanning. Radionuclide scanning is described in Chapters 2 and 24.

C. Renal Arteriography. Aortography and selective renal arteriography are the definitive procedures for visualizing renal artery stenosis (see Chapters 2 and 24). They are also valuable in the workup of classic-type polyarteritis nodosa (for demonstration of renal aneurysms) and in the diagnosis of renal infarction or tumor. A digital subtraction arteriogram decreases the dye load and the risk of contrast-induced nephropathy in patients with impaired renal function or DM.

IX. SUGGESTED READING

Whelton PK, Carey RM, Aronow WS, et al. 2017 ACC/AHA/AAPA/ABC/ACPM/AGS/APhA/ASH/ASPC/NMA/PCNA Guideline for the prevention, detection, evaluation, and management of high blood pressure in adults: executive summary: a report of the American College of Cardiology/American Heart Association Task Force on Clinical Practice Guidelines. *Hypertension.* 2018;71(6):1269–1324.

24 Urgent, Emergent, Resistant and Secondary Forms of Hypertension

Christopher S. Wilcox

I. DEFINITIONS. A *hypertensive crisis* is the point at which the management of an acutely elevated blood pressure (BP) is decisive for the outcome. The level of BP is less important than the extent of end-organ damage. *Hypertensive urgency* denotes a sudden rise in BP without an acute deterioration in the function of a critical organ. Typically, the BP can be lowered in the ward or clinic with oral antihypertensive agents over a few hours or days, with arrangement for clinic follow-up. *Hypertensive emergency* denotes a sudden rise in BP with an acute deterioration in function of a critical target organ. The BP should be lowered (not to the normal range) in minutes or hours under close monitoring in an intensive care unit. Clinical disorders of hypertensive emergencies and their initial management are shown in Tables 24.1 and 24.2. *Severe hypertension* denotes a BP >160/110 mm Hg, but the patient is asymptomatic, the rise in BP is gradual, and there are no retinal hemorrhages or papilledema. Severe hypertension can be treated in the clinic under supervision. *Resistant hypertension* denotes a failure to reach goal BP despite adhering to appropriate doses of a three-drug regimen that includes a diuretic. *Secondary hypertension* denotes hypertension with a specific cause.

II. HYPERTENSIVE EMERGENCIES AND URGENCIES

A. Epidemiology, Etiology, and Pathogenesis. Essential hypertension and all secondary forms can give rise to a hypertensive crisis. Many patients have renal parenchymal or renovascular disease.

The pathophysiology of a hypertensive emergency remains incompletely understood. An abrupt rise in vascular resistance and activation of the renin–angiotensin–aldosterone (RAA) system are key features. Endothelial damage from a severe and abrupt elevation in BP decreases autoregulatory responses and promotes vasoconstriction and renal ischemia while an abrupt natriuresis leads to pressure-induced volume depletion that activates the RAA system further. A vicious cycle can develop into malignant hypertension when a sharp increase in BP causes endothelial damage and fibrinoid necrosis of arterioles and capillaries leading to worsening renal ischemia, renin release, and hypertension. This can require saline infusion and cessation of diuretic therapy.

Autoregulation of renal and cerebral vessels normally maintains a stable blood flow during variations of mean arterial pressure (MAP) within the physiologic range of approximately 75 to 120 mm Hg (generally equivalent to a systolic blood pressure (SBP) of 90 to 180 mm Hg). If the MAP abruptly exceeds

TABLE 24.1   Hypertensive emergencies, therapies, and BP goals

Emergency	Drug of choice	BP target (mm Hg)
Aortic dissection	Beta blocker plus nitroprusside	SBP 120 in 20 min[a]
Myocardial infarction	Nitroglycerin, nitroprusside	
Left ventricular failure	Nitroglycerin, nitroprusside	
Hypertensive encephalopathy	Nitroprusside	25% reduction over 2–3 h[a]
Catecholamine excess:		
• Pheochromocytoma	Phentolamine	To control paroxysm
• Clonidine withdrawal	Clonidine	10–20% over 1–2 h
Eclampsia or preeclampsia	MgSO$_4$, hydralazine, methyldopa	Usually <90 DBP
Ischemic stroke		Do not reduce the BP in early phase
Hemorrhagic stroke	Nitroprusside, labetalol	SBP 140–160 in 1 h[a]

[a]If tolerated.

this limit, the capillary pressures and flows increase. In the brain, this leads to capillary hypertension, hyperemia, disruption of the blood–brain barrier, cerebral edema, and microhemorrhage. In the kidney, there is patchy ischemia and necrosis in glomerular capillaries, leading to the escape of red blood cells into tubular fluid, the appearance of red blood cell casts, and generalized capillary hypertension leading to proteinuria. Patients with long-standing hypertension develop a compensatory vascular hypertrophy and a shift in the autoregulation curve toward higher levels of MAP. This can provide protection from hypertensive encephalopathy, even when the BP exceeds 220/110 mm Hg but may make

TABLE 24.2   Parenteral drugs used to treat hypertensive emergencies

Agent	Dosage (IV)	Onset (min)	Peak (min)	Duration	Comments
Hydralazine	0.5–1.0 mg/min	1–5	10–80	3–6 h	
Nitroglycerin	5–100 µg/min	1–2	2–5	5 min	Reduces pre- and postload
Nitroprusside[a]	0.25–10 µg/kg/min	1	1–2	5 min	Nitrovasodilator
Esmolol	250–500 µg/min bolus, then 50–100 µg/kg/min	1	5	15 min	β1-blocker
Labetalol	20 mg then 0.5–2 mg/min	5	10	3–6 h	α1/β-blocker
Nicardipine	5–15 mg/h	5–10	45	50 h	CCB
Phentolamine	0.5–1 mg/min	1	5	10 min	α-blocker

[a]Thiocynate accumulates over 2 days or earlier in patients with reduced GFR and can cause severe toxic reactions. Light sensitive. CCB, calcium channel blocker.

them prone to cerebral ischemia and syncope during modest reductions in BP. By contrast, cerebral autoregulation can be exceeded in a previously normotensive patient, even at a BP of 160/100 mm Hg as can occur in acute glomerulonephritis or eclampsia. Thus, the context and the rate of rise of BP can be more important than the level of BP achieved.

B. **Clinical Manifestations of Hypertensive Crisis and Patient Evaluation.** The manifestations of a hypertensive crisis are those of end-organ dysfunction. *Malignant hypertension* is characterized by BP >160/100 mm Hg, retinal hemorrhages, and papilledema. Azotemia, proteinuria, circulating schistocytes, and microangiopathic hemolytic anemia can occur. *Hypertensive encephalopathy*, which occurs during malignant hypertension, is characterized by a reversible alteration in the level of consciousness, with headache, vision changes (including blindness), and seizures. If untreated, this can progress to cerebral hemorrhage, coma, and death.

Patients should be questioned concerning their use of medications, including monoamine oxidase inhibitors, cocaine, amphetamines, and recent clonidine withdrawal. Careful funduscopic examination is mandatory to detect the presence of arterial hemorrhages and papilledema (see Table 23.5). Investigations should include complete blood cell count, serum electrolytes, blood urea nitrogen, creatinine, urinalysis, electrocardiogram, and chest x-ray to assess end-organ damage. A peripheral blood smear can detect schistocytes that imply endothelial damage. Appropriate drug screening should be considered. Computed tomography (CT) or magnetic resonance imaging (MRI) scans are required in those with an abrupt onset of focal neurologic signs or decreased consciousness. The MRI scan of patients with hypertensive encephalopathy shows edema of the parieto-occipital white matter, which is termed *posterior leukoencephalopathy*. Investigations for secondary causes of hypertension are usually deferred until the crisis is resolved.

C. **Management.** The goal of treatment of a hypertensive emergency is to decrease the BP sufficiently to prevent or limit end-organ damage. This must be balanced against the dangers of hypoperfusion and ischemia of vital organs. The BP should be lowered within minutes in patients with hypertensive emergencies by using parenteral agents. However, the MAP normally should not be lowered by >25%, or the diastolic blood pressure (DBP) reduced <100 to 110 mm Hg, within the first 2 hours. Rarely should the goal be to achieve a normal BP within hours. Special caution is necessary in patients with preexisting neurologic or cardiac dysfunction and in the elderly. The selection of a drug to reduce the BP in a controlled and predictable manner depends on the clinical condition and the end-organ damage (Table 24.1). Monitoring of arterial pressure and other parameters in the intensive care unit is required for patients with a hypertensive emergency. Sodium nitroprusside is reliable and safe in many settings and provides optimal minute-to-minute control of BP but requires intra-arterial monitoring. It carries a risk of thiocyanate toxicity when infused at high rates for >24 to 48 hours, especially in patients with renal or hepatic impairment. Another intravenous (IV) drug that has slightly slower onset and offset times is labetalol (a combined alpha- and beta-adrenergic receptor blocker). Volume depletion should be anticipated in patients with malignant hypertension or adrenergic crisis, who may require saline infusion. Diuretics should be used cautiously, if at all, in patients with emergency hypertension, except in those with pulmonary edema or renal failure. The drugs used to treat hypertensive emergencies are outlined in Table 24.2.

The BP of patients with a hypertensive urgency may be lowered to target levels over several hours or days with oral agents such as an angiotensin-converting enzyme inhibitor (ACEI), an angiotensin-receptor blocker (ARB), clonidine, labetalol, or a calcium channel blocker (CCB). However, short-acting dihydropyridines, such as nifedipine, have caused an abrupt or severe fall in BP, leading to permanent neurologic damage in some patients. Therefore, these drugs should be avoided. Patients should be followed up in the clinic after achieving the target BP. Thereafter, they should be given careful instruction for BP measurement and drug therapy, usually including a diuretic.

D. Management in Specific Settings

1. **Hypertensive encephalopathy.** Sodium nitroprusside is preferred because it allows rapid onset and tight control of BP. Although it is a vasodilator, the sharp fall in BP is usually sufficient to reduce the cerebral capillary pressure and thereby improve cerebral edema. Loop diuretics activate the RAA and can induce hypovolemia and hypotension and should be used cautiously. Intra-arterial monitoring is required. The BP should be decreased during the first hour by a maximum of 25% or to a DBP of 100 to 110 mm Hg. A higher target is desirable in patients with preexisting or evolving fixed neurologic deficits. Any neurologic deterioration should prompt a search for alternative or additional causes, such as a new stroke and a consideration of allowing the BP to increase somewhat to determine if that improves the neurologic function. Clonidine should be avoided because of its central depressant action.

2. **Hypertensive cerebral hemorrhage.** The optimal treatment is uncertain. Reducing BP has been shown to reduce further bleeding but may result in ischemia, especially in patients with subarachnoid hemorrhage complicated by vasospasm. Therapy with IV sodium nitroprusside or labetalol is often required for acute intracerebral hemorrhage with SBP >170 mm Hg. The early target SBP is usually 140 to 160 mm Hg. In contrast, IV antihypertensive therapy is generally withheld in patients with subarachnoid hemorrhage in the early stages because of concern for worsening zonal cerebral ischemia, unless hypertension is severe (DBP >130 mm Hg). Nimodipine is a parenteral CCB that decreases vasospasm and improves outcome in patients with subarachnoid hemorrhage. It should be used cautiously to obviate hypotension, especially in patients receiving diuretics.

3. **Hypertension and cerebral ischemia.** Many patients have a temporary increase in BP after an acute thrombotic stroke. Because cerebral autoregulation is impaired in the ischemic penumbra, antihypertensive therapy should not normally be instituted in the acute phase after an ischemic stroke, unless the BP is extremely high and thrombolytic therapy is required.

4. **Acute aortic dissection.** Acute aortic dissection requires complete initial blockade of cardiac (beta$_1$)-adrenergic receptors to reduce the cardiac rate and contractility, and thereby to reduce the shear stress on the aortic wall. Esmolol given IV is a good choice. Verapamil is an alternative in patients with bronchospasm. Vasodilators, such as sodium nitroprusside should be used only after complete beta blockade since, if given alone, they increase the cardiac rate and contractility, and increase the shear force on the aortic wall that may extend the dissection despite a fall in BP.

5. **Hypertension with myocardial ischemia.** Nitroglycerine is the drug of choice. It improves coronary perfusion, reduces myocardial stretch and energy metabolism, and reduces preload. Parenteral labetalol or beta blockers

are useful. Sodium nitroprusside and direct vasodilators cause reflex tachycardia and may worsen ischemia and should be avoided.

6. **Hypertension with left ventricular failure.** Hypertension with left ventricular failure should be treated with IV nitroglycerin and furosemide, which can be combined with sodium nitroprusside to control hypertension. When given parenterally, loop diuretics can cause venodilatation, which, together with the diuresis, reduces the cardiac preload. However, venodilatation is not seen in patients who are established on oral loop diuretic therapy or in those receiving ACEIs or nonsteroidal anti-inflammatory agents. ACEIs are often useful, but beta-adrenergic blockers should be avoided in the acute phase because of the risk of worsening bronchospasm or reducing cardiac output.

7. **Preeclampsia and eclampsia.** Parenteral therapy is reserved for patients with SBP >180 mm Hg or DBP >110 mm Hg. Timely delivery of the fetus is the only cure. Before this, the DBP should not be lowered excessively, or <90 mm Hg, because the uteroplacental blood flow is not autoregulated. Indeed, any reduction in maternal BP can induce fetal distress. Hydralazine is the traditional choice, but labetalol and nicardipine are alternatives. Magnesium sulfate is used as prophylaxis for seizures. Sodium nitroprusside may be toxic to the fetus, and ACEIs cause nephrotoxicity to the newborn. These agents should be avoided (see Chapter 25).

8. **Perioperative hypertension.** Perioperative hypertension increases the risk of bleeding especially in those with arterial anastomoses, myocardial ischemia, and stroke. Sodium nitroprusside provides excellent BP control. Esmolol and labetalol are used to lower BP further and to limit reflex tachycardia.

9. **Sympathetic crises.** Pheochromocytoma, sympathomimetic drugs (e.g., cocaine, amphetamine, phencyclidine), a combination of a monoamine oxidase inhibitor with tyramine-containing foods, or abrupt discontinuation of treatment with a short-acting central sympatholytic agent (e.g., clonidine): all can cause abrupt, severe, adrenergically mediated hypertension. The first step is to reintroduce clonidine, if that is the culprit. An alpha-adrenergic antagonist, such as phentolamine, is rational. Monotherapy with beta-adrenergic blockers evokes unopposed alpha-adrenergic vasoconstriction and may paradoxically worsen the hypertension. Therefore, beta-adrenergic blockers should not be used until alpha-adrenergic blockade is achieved. Alternatively, labetalol or carvedilol provide combined alpha and beta blockade.

10. **Renal insufficiency.** Renal insufficiency can be a cause or a consequence of accelerated or malignant hypertension. Labetalol and sodium nitroprusside can be used in combination with diuretics to control hypertension in patients with volume overload, pulmonary edema, or resistant hypertension. ACEIs are drugs of first choice for patients with scleroderma renal crisis or malignant hypertension. However, ACEIs or ARBs should be used with caution in the management of patients with bilateral renal artery stenosis (RAS) or stenosis of a single (e.g., transplanted) functioning kidney as they may precipitate an acute fall in GFR. Because autoregulation is impaired or absent in patients with malignant hypertension or renal insufficiency, any drug that lowers the BP may reduce the GFR, at least in the short term and increase the serum creatinine concentration by up to 20%. With restoration of a normal BP, renal autoregulation and hemodynamics improve, and the elevated serum creatinine usually returns to baseline.

TABLE 24.3	Causes of drug-resistant hypertension

Pseudoresistance:
   "White coat" or "office" hypertension
   Inappropriate use of regular-sized cuff in obese subjects
   Nonadherence to drug therapy or diet
   Inadequate drug dose or inappropriate drug combination
   Absent or inadequate diuretic therapy
   Excess salt intake
   Kidney disease
Drug induced:
   Nonsteroidal anti-inflammatory agents (NSAIAs)
   Cyclooxygenase-2 inhibitors
   Cocaine, amphetamines, other illicit drugs
   Sympathomimetics (decongestants, anorectics)
   Oral contraceptives, adrenal steroids
   Cyclosporine and tacrolimus
   Erythropoietin
   Licorice and some chewing tobaccos
   Some over-the-counter supplements (e.g., ephedra)
Associated conditions:
   Obesity and sleep apnea
   Excessive alcohol intake
   Secondary hypertension

Parenteral drugs used for emergency hypertension are reviewed in Table 24.2.

III. RESISTANT HYPERTENSION. After confirming good compliance, the clinician should exclude secondary causes of hypertension and "white coat" or "office hypertension." This requires the patient to record their home BPs twice daily, or the use of an ambulatory BP monitor. An automated, unobserved BP can be measured in the clinic, if available.

Causes of drug-resistant hypertension are shown in Table 24.3. Subtle volume overload is the most common cause of resistant hypertension. It is especially common in patients with renal impairment or those receiving aggressive vasodilator therapy. Dietary salt restriction and appropriate doses of diuretics are required. The most common cause of drug-resistant hypertension is the failure to use a diuretic or the use of a diuretic in an adequate dose. The PATHWAY trial evaluated the antihypertensive effects of add on drugs given to resistant patients and reported that spironolactone was the most effective agent.

IV. SECONDARY HYPERTENSION. Estimates of the percentage of hypertensive patients with a secondary cause vary widely (Table 24.4). Some diseases are accompanied by an increased prevalence of hypertension, notably diabetes mellitus and chronic kidney disease (CKD) (see Chapter 6) but are not considered causes of secondary hypertension. The prevalence of secondary hypertension increases substantially among patients with severe and drug-resistant hypertension and

TABLE 24.4 Secondary causes of hypertension	
Cause	**Approximate prevalence (%)**
Renovascular disease	1–10
Primary aldosteronism	1–20
Thyroid disease	0.5
Pheochromocytoma	<0.2
Cushing syndrome	<0.2
Drug related	0.1–1.0

should be considered in all whose BP is not controlled while taking three or more medications. A selective screening to limit expensive testing is mandated by the low prevalence of many secondary causes. Screening tests must be highly sensitive (few false negatives) to avoid failing to diagnose a form of hypertension that may be curable or require specific therapy.

A. Renovascular Hypertension

1. **Definition and causes.** RAS is the narrowing (usually >75% to be functionally significant) of one or both renal arteries or their branches. Renovascular hypertension is less common than RAS. It is hypertension that is improved or cured by correction of an RAS. Ischemic nephropathy is chronic renal insufficiency caused by RAS that is often bilateral or accompanied by renal functional impairment, such as nephrosclerosis, in the contralateral kidney. The most common cause of renovascular hypertension is an atherosclerotic plaque in the proximal 1 cm of renal artery (osteal lesion) (Table 24.5). Fibromuscular dysplasia of the renal arteries does not usually progress or cause renal arterial thrombosis, and therefore rarely causes ischemic nephropathy, although rare subgroups can be progressive (Table 24.6).

2. **Pathophysiology.** Renal hypoperfusion releases renin from the juxtaglomerular cells of the afferent arteriole. Renin generates angiotensin II that raises BP by many means including vasoconstriction and salt retention. Patients with bilateral RAS or stenosis of a transplanted or solitary kidney cannot mount a pressure natriuresis. Their BP is dependent on body fluids and requires treatment with a reduced salt intake and diuretics. They can experience episodes of "flash" pulmonary edema caused by overfilling of the bloodstream. Acute or recurrent pulmonary edema in a hypertensive and

TABLE 24.5 Causes of renovascular hypertension	
Lesions intrinsic to kidney or its blood vessels	**Extrinsic lesions**
Atherosclerosis	Urinary tract obstruction
Fibromuscular dysplasia	Abdominal aortic aneurysm
Vasculitis	Emboli
Renal cysts	Renal capsular hematoma

TABLE 24.6	Comparison of atherosclerotic and fibromuscular renal artery stenosis	

Feature	Atherosclerosis	Fibromuscular dysplasia
Proportion of cases (%)	80	20
Age of onset	After 55 y	Adolescence onward
Gender	Both	Female to male, 10:1
Site of lesion	Usually osteal	Distal renal artery or branch
Radiologic appearance	Single lesion	Often multiple, short lesions
Progression	Usual	Rare
Arterial occlusion/thrombosis	Over time	Rare
Atherosclerosis elsewhere	Common	Less common
Renal failure	Over time	Rare

azotemic patient suggests this diagnosis. The natural history of untreated atherosclerotic renovascular diseases is a progressive decrease in renal function, which ultimately results in ischemic nephropathy and end stage renal disease (ESRD).

3. **Clinical features.** Clinical features are outlined in Table 24.7.
4. **Screening tests for renovascular hypertension.** Rapid-sequence IV pyelogram, simple renogram, unstimulated plasma renin activity (PRA), IV digital subtraction angiogram, captopril–PRA test, and renal vein renins are not sufficiently accurate for routine use. Currently renal ultrasound with duplex Doppler velocimetry of the renal arteries is the preferred screening test. In the absence of renal cysts, a length difference >1.5 cm implies predominantly unilateral renal disease, and, in the context of hypertension, this is often RAS. The peak systolic blood flow velocity is measured in the aorta and along the renal arteries. A threefold step-up in velocity from the aorta to a renal artery suggests RAS.
5. **Diagnostic tests for renal artery stenosis.** Angiography is the gold standard for diagnosing RAS but is invasive and can cause contrast nephropathy. It is usually reserved until a plan for angioplasty has been agreed. To cause functionally significant renal ischemia, a stenosis must usually occlude >75% of the arterial lumen. The demonstration of an anatomic stenosis does not

TABLE 24.7	Clinical features suggestive of renovascular hypertension

Hypertension resistant to two or more drugs and a diuretic
Onset before age 20 y in women or after age 55 y
Accelerated or malignant hypertension
Arteriosclerotic disease elsewhere
Smoking history
Azotemia (especially with angiotensin-converting enzyme inhibitors or angiotensin receptor blockers)
Abdominal bruit (especially diastolic or flank)
Recurrent pulmonary edema
Kidney size difference >1.5 cm (in the absence of cysts)

prove that it is the cause of the hypertension. Where possible, a small catheter should be advanced past the stenosis to measure the pressure drop that, if >10 or 20 mm Hg implies a significant stenosis. Other imaging procedures are:

- **Spiral computed tomography.** This is noninvasive and accurate but requires >100 mL of contrast. Therefore, it is best avoided in those with renal insufficiency.
- **Magnetic resonance.** This is noninvasive and does not use nephrotoxic agents and is less expensive than angiography. The reported accuracy is quite high in experienced hands but can miss lesion of fibromuscular dysplasia within the kidney.

6. **Intervention.** The goal is to improve or cure hypertension or to delay the progression to ischemic nephropathy. Percutaneous transluminal renal angioplasty (PTRA) is combined with stenting (S) for osteal lesions. PTRAS can cause arterial rupture or dissection, atheroemboli to the kidney or lower limbs, acute renal failure from contrast-associated nephropathy, or bleeding at the puncture site. The technical success rate is >90%, and at 1 year, >75% of those arteries treated with stenting remain patent, but there is a progressive increase of restenosis with time. Within-stent stenosis cannot be assessed by magnetic resonance angiography but is assessed by ultrasound. It can be treated by repeated PTRA. Surgical revascularization is reserved for those who have failed PTRAS and for those with concomitant disease of the abdominal aorta requiring surgery.

7. **Management.** Controlled trials have failed to show a clear benefit of improvement in renal function over 6 to 12 months for patients with RAS randomized to PTRAS compared with medical therapy although some improvement in hypertension is often apparent. Therefore, the finding of RAS does not mandate intervention. Only those with renal artery narrowing of >75% should be considered for intervention. All patients with atherosclerotic RAS require cardiovascular risk factor management and careful control of hypertension. ACEIs or ARBs are excellent choices to reduce BP and counteract the adverse cardiovascular effect of angiotensin II. However, a few patients experience a significant (>20%) increase in serum creatinine. Such patients may benefit from PTRAS. Patients should be evaluated at weekly intervals until stable after ACEI or ARB therapy and at 3 to 4 months, then every 6 months to determine whether their condition is stable. Those with documented progression and no contraindications should be considered for intervention, whereas those who remain stable should normally be managed conservatively.

B. **Primary Hyperaldosteronism.**

1. **Pathophysiology and clinical features.** Hypertension is caused by excess aldosterone and is accompanied by suppression of renin. *Aldosterone-producing adenomas* (APAs) of the adrenal zona glomerulosa cells, also called Conn syndrome, previously accounted for most cases of primary hyperaldosteronism but currently bilateral adrenal hyperplasia, also called *idiopathic hyperaldosteronism* (IHA) is the most common cause. Multiple adenomas occur in <10% of patients. Rare causes include glucocorticoid-remediable hyperaldosteronism, also called *dexamethasone-suppressible hyperaldosteronism* that is caused by a chimeric mutation in the promoter for the aldosterone synthase gene that leads to its activation by the adrenocorticotrophic

hormone (ACTH). It is inherited as a dominant condition and is diagnosed by DNA analysis or from the reversal of hyperaldosteronism and hypertension after suppression of ACTH secretion with dexamethasone.

Excessive production of aldosterone results in renal salt retention, causing extracellular fluid volume expansion, hypertension, and enhanced secretion of K^+ and H^+ in the collecting ducts, leading to hypokalemic metabolic alkalosis. Aldosterone activates a mineralocorticosteroid receptor (MR) that is also activated by glucocorticosteroids, which are present in much higher concentrations than aldosterone. However, the MR normally is protected from glucocorticosteroids by coexpression of 11-beta-hydroxysteroid dehydrogenase (11-beta-HSD) that metabolizes glucocorticosteroids such as cortisol to inactive cortisone. The 11-beta-HSD can be inhibited by glycoyrrhinic acid present in licorice or chewing tobacco or may be defective due to a dominant mutation giving rise to pseudohyperaldosteronism.

Primary aldosteronism must be differentiated from secondary aldosteronism caused by excess renin secretion, as occurs in renovascular hypertension or edematous states, and from pseudohyperaldosteronism or Liddle syndrome that is caused by excessive reabsorption of Na^+ via the epithelial sodium channel in the collecting ducts. Patients with pseudohyperaldosteronism have the clinical and biochemical changes of primary hyperaldosteronism, but have suppressed levels of renin and aldosterone. The hallmarks of hyperaldosteronism are hypertension, hypokalemic metabolic alkalosis, and suppressed PRA, but elevated aldosterone.

2. **Screening tests.** Screening should be undertaken in selected patients. The features that should prompt screening are:

- unprovoked or diuretic-induced hypokalemia with alkalosis;
- hypertension resistant to therapy with two or more drugs; and
- suppression of PRA and/or elevation of SAC and of the SAC/PRA ratio.

Screening should follow the correction of potassium deficits because hypokalemia suppresses aldosterone secretion even from adenomas (Table 24.8). Blood for serum potassium must be taken without stasis or fist clenching.

3. **Diagnostic tests.** Primary hyperaldosteronism is diagnosed by failure to suppress 24-hour excretion of aldosterone or tetrahydroaldosterone after 3 days of high salt intake (10 g of salt daily).

Adrenal venous sampling is required to distinguish between an APA and IHA but is technically difficult. An SAC-to-cortisol ratio that is greater than fourfold higher on one side compared with the other suggests a unilateral source for aldosterone secretion that can be an adenoma or a microadenoma that will respond to adrenalectomy. Patients with IHA have elevated SAC in both adrenal veins.

TABLE 24.8	Screening test for primary hyperaldosteronism

24-h urine potassium >40 mEq despite hypokalemia
Low PRA
SAC >15 ng/dL; SAC to PRA ratio $\geq$25 ng·dL^{-1}/ng·m^{-1}·h^{-1}
PRA, plasma renin activity; SAC, serum aldosterone concentration.

4. **Treatment.** APAs should be removed laparoscopically. BP is normalized in 50% to 75% of patients, and the biochemical abnormalities are corrected in almost all. IHA is managed with a mineralocorticosteroid antagonist such as spironolactone or eplerenone. In those who develop adverse effects, high doses of amiloride (20 to 40 mg daily) usually control hypertension and hypokalemia.

V. **PHEOCHROMOCYTOMA.** Hypertension is caused by a tumor (pheochromocytoma) that secretes catecholamines. More than 90% are benign.

1. **Pathophysiology, associated conditions, and clinical features.** Some 90% of pheochromocytomas are in the adrenal medulla, but neural crest cells that can harbor a pheochromocytoma are found in autonomic ganglia, organs of Zuckerkandl (lying anterior to the aortic bifurcation), carotid bodies, and bladder. Tumors are bilateral in 10% to 20%.

   Pheochromocytomas may be inherited as an autosomal-dominant trait, either alone or as part of the syndromes of multiple endocrine neoplasia type 2 (medullary thyroid carcinoma, pheochromocytoma, and parathyroid hyperplasia), von Hippel–Lindau syndrome (retinal and cerebellar hemangioblastomas, renal cysts, and renal cell carcinomas), von Recklinghausen syndrome (neurofibromatosis and café-au-lait skin pigmentation), or tuberous sclerosis (mental deficiency, renal cysts, and tumors). Hypertension is sustained in approximately 60% but may be paroxysmal and cause severe hypertension, headache, sweating, and palpitations precipitated by exercise, urination, defecation, sexual intercourse, anesthesia, contrast agents, or certain drugs, including vasodilators. Other clinical features of weight loss, fever, anxiety, tremors, psychotic illness, and glucose intolerance are seen occasionally. Orthostatic hypotension is secondary to diminished plasma volume from pressure natriuresis and blunted sympathetic reflexes.

2. **Screening tests.** The features that suggest the need to screen for pheochromocytoma are:

   - hypertension accompanied by headache, palpitations, and sweating;
   - paroxysmal hypertension;
   - sustained, severe or resistant hypertension; and
   - hypertension and unexplained orthostatic hypotension.

   The most sensitive and specific screening test is plasma metanephrines. An increase of >three- to fivefold while the patient is hypertensive is highly suggestive of pheochromocytoma.

3. **Localization tests.** A CT scan, MRI, or selective adrenal venous sampling for catecholamines is used for localization. MRI is preferred because it is noninvasive, accurate, and can discriminate between pheochromocytomas and adrenal adenomas or cysts.

4. **Management.** Surgical excision is curative. Preoperative stabilization with alpha blockade and volume expansion is essential. Acute pheochromocytoma crisis responds to IV alpha blockade with phentolamine. Prolonged, predictable alpha blockade is achieved with phenoxybenzamine, which is a noncompetitive alpha antagonist. A shorter-acting combined alpha and beta blocker, such as labetalol or carvedilol, is useful for less severely hypertensive subjects.

VI. **OTHER CAUSES OF SECONDARY HYPERTENSION.** Additional causes of hypertension are presented in Table 24.9.

| TABLE 24.9 | Additional causes of secondary hypertension |

Cause	Clinical features
Preeclampsia	Third-trimester pregnancy, proteinuria, and edema
Cushing syndrome	Central obesity, hirsutism, glycosuria
Coarctation of the aorta	Delayed pulses in legs
Hyperparathyroidism	Increased calcium and parathyroid hormone levels
Congenital adrenal hyperplasia	
11-hydroxylase deficiency	Virilization
17-hydroxylase deficiency	Abnormal sexual development
Sleep apnea	Obesity, snoring, somnolence
Hypothyroidism	Bradycardia, hair loss, amenorrhea
Hyperthyroidism	Tachycardia
Acromegaly	Excessive growth, glycosuria

VII. SUGGESTED READINGS

Carey RM, Calhoun DA, Bakris GL, et al. Resistant hypertension: detection, evaluation, and management: a scientific statement from the American Heart Association. *Hypertension.* 2018;72(5):e53–e90.

Cooper SC, Murphy TP, Cutlip DE, et al. Stenting and medical therapy for atherosclerotic renal-artery stenosis. *New Engl J Med.* 2014;370(1):13–22.

Olin JW, Gornik HL, Bacharach JM, et al. Fibromuscular dysplasia: state of the science and critical unanswered questions: a scientific statement from the American Heart Association. *Circulation.* 2014;129(9):1048–1078.

Peixoto AJ. Acute severe hypertension. *New Engl J Med.* 2019;381(19):1843–1852.

Williams B, MacDonald TM, Morant S, et al. Spironolactone versus placebo, bisoprolol, and doxazosin to determine the optimal treatment for drug-resistant hypertension (PATHWAY-2): a randomised, double-blind, crossover trial. *Lancet.* 2015;386(10008):2059–2068.

25 Hypertension and Renal Disease in Pregnancy

Judit Gordon-Cappitelli

Both renal disease and hypertension present threats to the mother and fetus. Some causes of hypertension or renal failure are unique to pregnancy. Key questions for clinicians are whether pregnancy alters the course of the underlying renal disease or whether the kidney disease will alter the outcome of the pregnancy.

I. SPECIFIC RENAL PROBLEMS IN PREGNANCY

A. Urinary Tract Infection. Urinary tract infection (UTI) is the most common medical disorder occurring in pregnancy. The smooth muscle relaxation and ureteral dilation in pregnancy likely predispose to the greater risk of UTI that may lead to prematurity, fetal growth restriction, and pregnancy loss. Asymptomatic bacteriuria occurs in up to 7% of pregnant women, and, if untreated, a third develops into symptomatic UTI, and 1% to 2% into pyelonephritis. Routine practice includes screening urine culture by 16 weeks of gestation. Positive cultures, even without evidence of leukocyturia or symptoms, should be treated with oral antibiotics for 7 to 10 days. Several antibiotics present specific risks to the fetus (Table 25.1). Sulfonamides should be avoided for several weeks before delivery. Tetracyclines cause fetal dental abnormalities. Aminoglycosides entail a 2% to 3% risk of ototoxicity. Relapse of UTI requires an additional 2 to 3 weeks of antibiotics, followed by suppressive therapy until delivery. Pyelonephritis requires hospitalization, intravenous antibiotics, and fluids. While current practice often favors the use of the lowest recommended dose of a drug during pregnancy, this is inappropriate for antibiotics. Full doses of antibiotics should be prescribed. Several penicillins and cephalosporins are eliminated renally, and their clearance may be increased by >50% due to renal hyperfiltration.

B. Acute Kidney Injury. Since the glomerular filtration rate (GFR) is higher, and the serum creatinine (Scr) is lower in normal pregnancy, changes from baseline, or levels of Scr above 0.8 mg/dL should prompt evaluation. Prerenal acute kidney injury (AKI) may occur from severe hyperemesis gravidarum, or hemodynamic shifts from heart failure, pulmonary embolism, sepsis, or hemorrhage. AKI, during the first trimester, can be a consequence of septic abortion. Acute tubular necrosis in the third trimester can complicate concealed hemorrhage from placental abruption, that can occur in 1% to 2% of women with preeclampsia and in 7% of those with the *h*emolysis, *e*levated *l*iver function tests, *l*ow *p*latelets (HELLP) syndrome. Recognition of the normal gestational dilatation of the collecting system and ureters is key to avoiding misdiagnosis of obstructive uropathy.

C. Chronic Kidney Disease. Subtle renal insufficiency often goes unrecognized in pregnancy as the GFR is increased 30% to 50% even in women with advanced chronic kidney disease (CKD). Pregnancy outcome is affected adversely by renal dysfunction, hypertension, and proteinuria. CKD in women without advanced renal failure and absent or well-controlled hypertension, usually results in a live birth with little impact on renal disease progression. By contrast, about 20% of women with baseline Scr at or above 1.5 to 2.5 mg/dL and up to 45% of women with baseline Scr >2.5 mg/dL will suffer a precipitous or progressive loss of renal function during or following pregnancy. Even in the "low-risk" group with well-preserved GFR, preeclampsia occurs in 30% and worsened proteinuria in many. Lower preconception GFR, proteinuria of >1 g/day, and more severe hypertension predict severe maternal hypertension, prematurity, fetal growth restriction, and an increased chance of more rapid progression to renal failure.

D. Proteinuria. Although urinary protein excretion increases in normal pregnancy, more than 300 mg/24 hours is abnormal. A quantitative measure of 24-hour urine protein, or the ratio of urine protein/urine creatinine is required. Proteinuria occurring before 20 weeks of gestation usually indicates pre-existing renal disease or hypertension. Timing is critical as one-third of women who present with proteinuria after 20 weeks of gestation eventually have preeclampsia. Proteinuria that does not resolve after 3 months postpartum, should be assessed for underlying renal disease. The presence of nephrotic syndrome should prompt a search for the cause and selection of treatment that is safe during pregnancy. Renal biopsy should be thoughtfully reserved for cases where diagnosis will alter management such as de novo nephrotic range proteinuria during the first and second trimesters that is not explained by preeclampsia. The use of immunosuppressants is limited due to the teratogenicity (Table 25.1). If edema is

TABLE 25.1 Fetal risk with immunosuppressants and specific drugs

Risk level to fetus	Drug and comments	
Lowest risk/ recommended use	Hydroxychloroquine	Should use in SLE to reduce risk of flares
	Aspirin low dose	Use for all high-risk pregnancies to reduce risk of preeclampsia
	Low–molecular-weight heparin or heparin	If low risk of bleeding, can use for prophylaxis in hypercoagulable states or clotting. Avoid warfarin, and direct oral anticoagulants
	Methyldopa	Titrate to goal blood pressure <140/90
	Labetalol	
	Long-acting nifedipine	
	Hydralazine	
	Penicillin	Fosfomycin does not achieve therapeutic levels in the kidneys so should not be used if pyelonephritis is suspected.
	Cephalosporins	
	Amoxicillin-clavulanate	
	Fosfomycin	
	Aztreonam	
	Meropenem, ertapenem	

(*continued*)

TABLE 25.1   Fetal risk with immunosuppressants and specific drugs (*Continued*)

Risk level to fetus	Drug and comments	
Minimal risk/ acceptable use	Glucocorticoids	Use lowest possible dose
	Azathioprine	Maximum dose 2 mg/kg/day
	Tacrolimus and cyclosporine	Tacrolimus preferred over cyclosporine
	Intravenous immune globulin	Ideally before third trimester
	Nonsteroidal anti-inflammatory drugs	Acceptable up to 30 wks gestation but avoided in renal insufficiency completely
	Thiazide diuretics	Ideally avoided but use if
	Furosemide	needed for severe edema
Moderate risk/ selective use	Rituximab	Acceptable up to conception, afterward used in life-threatening case only
	Nitrofurantoin	Avoid use during the first
	Trimethoprim-sulfamethoxazole	trimester and at term
Highest risk/do not use	Renin–angiotensin–aldosterone system inhibitors	Discontinue before planned conception. If proteinuria is present can wait until pregnancy identified or by 8 weeks of gestation. Avoid after this time
	Mycophenolate mofetil	Avoid at least 6 wks before conception
	Sirolimus and enviroxime	Avoid 3 mo before conception
	Cyclophosphamide	Use only in life-threatening cases. The highest risk is during third trimester
	Methotrexate	Avoid 3 mo before conception and during pregnancy
	Tetracyclines	Avoid due to fetal
	Aminoglycosides	complications
	Fluoroquinolones	
	Imipenem	
	Statins	Discontinue before planned conception if possible

severe, compression stockings and low sodium diet (2 g per day) should be advised. Loop diuretics should be avoided if preeclampsia is present. In those with severe hypoalbuminemia (<2.5 to 3 g/dL) and low bleeding risk, and especially if the cause of nephrotic syndrome is membranous nephropathy, prophylactic anticoagulation should be considered. This should use low–molecular-weight heparin since warfarin is contraindicated. Novel oral anticoagulants should not be used.

E. Glomerulonephritis. Glomerulonephritis (GN) can flare during pregnancy. Prompt diagnosis is crucial to preserving kidney function. Kidney biopsy can be considered during the first two trimesters to establish the diagnosis of GN where serologies are insufficient. Preeclampsia does not require biopsy. Patients with systemic lupus erythematosus (SLE), IgA nephritis (IGAN), antineutrophil cytoplasmic antibody-associated (ANCA) vasculitis, focal segmental glomerulosclerosis, membranous nephropathy, and minimal change disease are at risk for renal flares.

SLE increases the risk of adverse maternal and fetal outcomes, while pregnancy can flare lupus nephritis (LN), which may be difficult to differentiate from preeclampsia. Systemic lupus flares can be decreased by continuing the use of hydroxychloroquine. Pregnant women with lupus anticoagulant or anticardiolipin antibodies should be treated with aspirin and low–molecular-weight heparin to prevent recurrent, usually mid-trimester, pregnancy loss. Flares of SLE are commonly treated with azathioprine and steroids, while cyclophosphamide is reserved for use in late in pregnancy when the severity of the pathology is justified by renal biopsy and early delivery is not practical. Mycophenolate is teratogenic and should be avoided. Patients should be taken off renin–angiotensin–aldosterone (RAAS) blockade and mycophenolate before pregnancy.

RAAS blockade is contraindicated in pregnancy, although most of their severe developmental toxicity occurs later in pregnancy. The benefit of RAAS blockade in women with diabetic nephropathy and significant proteinuria suggests that these women should continue their "renal protective" therapy until pregnancy is confirmed but by 8 weeks of gestation, they should be discontinued. Rituximab maybe used in the first trimester but there are concerns of neonatal B-cell depletion when used in later trimesters. Women with a history of lupus or GN should be counseled about the best timing of pregnancy, which is after 6 months of quiescent disease on medications that can be continued safely during pregnancy.

F. End-Stage Renal Disease. Pregnancy in end-stage renal disease (ESRD) is very rare due to extremely diminished fertility. There is a significant benefit of intensive and frequent hemodialysis (five to six times per week) with goals of providing near normal levels of serum urea nitrogen.

G. Transplantation. Although renal transplantation restores fertility, the first year after transplant carries the highest risk of rejection and maternal infection.

II. HYPERTENSIVE DISORDERS OF PREGNANCY. Systemic vasodilation decreases blood pressure (BP) in normal pregnancy by ~10 mm Hg (Table 25.2). Falls of 20 to 40 mm Hg are common in women with underlying hypertension. Hypertension increases the risk of maternal and neonatal morbidity and mortality.

A. Classification of Hypertension in Pregnancy. Hypertension in pregnancy is classified as chronic hypertension, gestational hypertension, preeclampsia, or preeclampsia superimposed on chronic hypertension. Vasodilation during pregnancy usually allows the discontinuation of antihypertensives in those with mild hypertension early in pregnancy. Gestational hypertension is new-onset hypertension without proteinuria or end-organ dysfunction on two separate occasions after 20 weeks of gestation. It can persist for more than 3 months postpartum. It often recurs in subsequent pregnancies and predicts essential hypertension later in life. Preeclampsia is defined as new-onset hypertension with proteinuria or other end-organ damage generally after 20 weeks of gestation and up to 6 weeks postpartum.

TABLE 25.2	Physiologic changes in normal pregnancy

Adaptations in pregnancy	Consequences
Increased renal perfusion and glomerular filtration rate (30–50%)	Serum creatinine >0.8 mg/dL or blood urea nitrogen >13 mg/dL is suspicious
Increased glomerular basement membrane permeability	Increased protein excretion up to 300 mg
Respiratory alkalosis with renal compensation	Normal $PCO_2 = 30$ mm Hg; normal $HCO^- = 19$–20 mmol/L
Retention of 8-L water; ~900 mEq Na+; plasma volume increased ~42%	Some edema is expected; volume sensed as normal
Reset of osmotic regulation, with osmolality decreased by 10 mOsm/L	Normal serum sodium ~135 mmol/L
Circulating renin, angiotensin, aldosterone increased, but angiotensin and aldosterone effects decreased	Difficult to diagnose secondary hypertension
Decreased blood pressure by ~10 mm Hg in healthy individuals and by 20–40 mm Hg in women with hypertension	Easy to miss underlying hypertension
Altered tubular function; increased urinary protein, glucose, uric acid, and amino acid excretion	Proteinuria worsens with underlying glomerular disease; normal uric acid 2.8–3.0 mg/dL
Increased progesterone levels in early pregnancy	Decreased peripheral vascular resistance; dilatation of the ureters and renal pelvis

B. **Blood Pressure Management in Pregnancy.** The goals of BP control are not well defined but most would initiate treatment if the systolic blood pressures (SBPs) ≥150 mmHg or diastolic blood pressures (DBPs) ≥100 mm Hg, and in many cases if SBP ≥140 mm Hg to or DBP ≥90 mm Hg. The BP should not be reduced below 120/80 mm Hg.

The most commonly used oral antihypertensives include methyldopa, labetalol, and nifedipine. Atenolol and propranolol are not recommended. There is less experience of amlodipine and nondihydropyridine calcium channel blockers. Clonidine is best avoided due to its side-effect profile. Hydralazine is a first-line agent for hypertensive emergencies. Diuretics are usually avoided due to the potential risk of intravascular volume depletion and fetal hypoperfusion. ACE inhibitors, ARBs, direct renin inhibitors and mineralocorticoid receptor antagonists are contraindicated after early pregnancy due to drug-induced fetopathy (oligohydramnios and patent ductus arteriosus) and potentially lethal fetal and neonatal acute renal failure. Salt restriction is not usually recommended.

Severe hypertension with SBP ≥160 mm Hg and/or DBP ≥110 mm Hg) persisting for ≥15 minutes, should be treated urgently and warrants hospitalization with parenteral hydralazine or labetalol. Postpartum hypertension should be evaluated to differentiate between transient new-onset postpartum hypertension and preeclampsia. Treatment choices will depend on whether the patient is breastfeeding or not. Hypertension beyond 6 months postpartum should be treated as chronic hypertension.

C. **Preeclampsia and Its Management.** Preeclampsia is a defined as new-onset hypertension with proteinuria (>300 mg/day) or other end-organ damage generally after 20 weeks of gestation and including up to 6 weeks postpartum. Other end-organ damage can consist of thrombocytopenia (<100,000/microL), renal insufficiency (doubling of Scr or Scr >1.1 mg/dL), pulmonary edema, new-onset headache, visual symptoms (blurry vision, flashing lights), and transaminitis (at least two times upper limit of normal). Preeclampsia superimposed on chronic hypertension can be identified if there is sudden increase in hypertension or proteinuria. Preeclampsia is the most common cause of nephrotic syndrome in pregnancy and must be differentiated from a flare in glomerulonephritis. Evaluation of serologic data and ultrasonographic evaluation of the placenta, uterine arteries and fetus are critical. Delivery is the definitive treatment for preeclampsia. This may be delayed in women with milder disease to gain added fetal maturation but should only be contemplated with close observation in the absence of ominous findings or disease progression and with careful BP control.

HELLP syndrome is a subtype of severe preeclampsia. Microangiopathy or the appearance of schistocytes on a blood smear should suggest the HELLP syndrome. Epigastric or right upper quadrant tenderness, especially with liver function test abnormalities suggests incipient hepatic hemorrhage or rupture. Also ominous are progressive renal dysfunction or neurologic findings (including headache or blurred vision), no matter how mild. Any of these ominous findings should prompt urgent delivery. HELLP syndrome must be differentiated from atypical hemolytic uremic syndrome (aHUS) and thrombotic thrombocytopenic purpura (TTP). AHUS can be triggered by pregnancy or postpartum. ADAMTS13 activity should be checked and plasmapheresis should be considered.

Eclampsia is grand mal seizures in a patient with preeclampsia. Eclamptic seizures may be prevented or treated with magnesium sulfate, but not with classic anticonvulsants. Dosing is decreased in women with renal insufficiency. Toxicity can manifest as areflexia or hypoventilation and is treated with calcium gluconate.

Preeclampsia and its subtypes are caused by an abnormal uteroplacental circulation, genetic and environmental factors, and compliment dysregulation. It is most common in nulliparas, at extremes of maternal age (<16 or >35), or with multifetal gestations. Risk is increased by maternal microvascular disease, diabetes mellitus, collagen vascular disease, underlying renal disease, and hypertension. Complement dysregulation and activation may also play a role. Systemic inflammation and infection such as UTI or periodontal disease can predispose to preeclampsia. Preeclampsia pathogenesis causes endothelial dysfunction, with hypertension (from disruption of endothelial control of vascular tone and angiotensin II hypersensitivity), proteinuria (from altered vascular permeability), coagulopathy (from enhanced endothelial expression of procoagulants), other end-organ manifestations such as headaches, seizures, visual symptoms, epigastric pain (from the endothelial dysfunction of each target organ), and fetal growth restriction (from the ischemic and hypoperfused placenta). Placenta formation requires extensive angiogenesis to create a sufficient vascular supply. Measurement of sFlt-1 (soluble FMS-like tyrosine kinase-1; an antiangiogenic factor), PIGF (placental growth factor; an angiogenic factor), and their ratio may be helpful in diagnosing preeclampsia versus pre-existing disease.

Patients at high risk of preeclampsia should be considered for aspirin 81 mg from 12 to 28 weeks of gestation in addition to prenatal vitamin, vitamin D and calcium. Women with preeclampsia have an increased risk of cardiovascular disease later in life, and thus should be monitored closely.

III. SUGGESTED READINGS

Blom K, Odutayo A, Bramham K, et al. Pregnancy and glomerular disease: a systematic review of the literature with management guidelines. *Clin J Am Soc Nephrol.* 2017;12(11):1862–1872.

Cerdeira AS, Agrawal S, Staff AC, et al. Angiogenic factors: potential to change clinical practice in pre-eclampsia? *Br J Obstet Gynecol.* 2018;125(11):1389.

Gonzalez Suarez ML, Kattah A, Grande JP, et al. Renal disorders in pregnancy: core curriculum 2019. *Am J Kidney Dis.* 2019;73(1):119–130.

Hui D, Hhladunewich MA. Chronic kidney disease and pregnancy. *Obstet Gynecol.* 2019;133:1182–1194.

Umans JG. Medications during pregnancy: antihypertensives and immunosuppressants. *Adv Chronic Kidney Dis.* 2007;14(2):191–198.

Zhang J-J, Ma X-X, Hao L, et al. A systematic review and meta-analysis of outcomes of pregnancy in CKD and CKD outcomes in pregnancy. *CJASN.* 2015;10(11):1964–1978.

Drug Use and the Kidney

26 Drug Dosing in Renal Insufficiency

Rupam Ruchi

The activity of a drug is related to the concentration of free drug in the tissue compartment in which the effect occurs (Fig. 26.1). The kidney is a major route of elimination for many drugs. Therefore, patients with renal disease, or with unsuspected chronic kidney disease, as in the elderly, are more susceptible to adverse drug reactions and toxicity. Uremia may alter drug pharmacokinetics, including absorption, volume of distribution (V_D), protein binding, and biotransformation. This can result in accumulation of the parent drug or its active metabolites to toxic levels (e.g., acyclovir, codeine, meperidine, and procainamide). The nephrotoxicity of commonly used drugs is discussed in Chapter 27.

I. **DRUG BIOAVAILABILITY AND ABSORPTION.** The bioavailability of a drug is the fraction of a dose absorbed into the circulation. It depends on the route of administration and on factors that could interfere with absorption, such as drug binding in the gut or first-pass biotransformation in the gut wall or liver. Gastrointestinal drug absorption can be impaired in uremia due to vomiting, delayed gastric emptying, diarrhea, or impaired gastric acidity. Phosphate binders may chelate drugs in the gut, preventing absorption.

II. **DRUG DISTRIBUTION.** Factors that affect the extent of drug distribution in the body include drug molecular size, plasma protein binding, and tissue binding. Edema and ascites can increase the V_D for hydrophilic and highly protein-bound agents. Decreased binding of acidic drugs to proteins in uremia increases the unbound drug levels and, consequently, their distribution and elimination. The alteration in protein binding may be caused by one of the following three mechanisms: (a) decreased serum albumin concentration; (b) accumulation of endogenous organic acids in uremic plasma that displace acidic drugs from albumin-binding sites; and (c) altered albumin drug-binding capacity. By contrast, binding of basic drugs to acidic glycoproteins can be increased in renal failure.

Reduced protein binding decreases the total plasma drug concentration while increasing the unbound fraction increases the total concentration. For example, because of decreased phenytoin binding to albumin in chronic kidney disease (CKD), total plasma drug concentrations underestimate free drug levels and therapeutic responses. There is a transient rise in free drug levels, but these later return to steady state as the total drug level decreases. The finding of a low total drug level may prompt the physician to increase drug dosage to reestablish therapeutic total plasma drug levels, with the danger of drug toxicity. Specific measurement of plasma free-drug concentrations avoids drug toxicity.

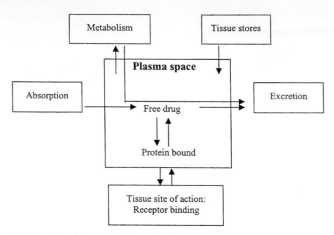

FIGURE 26.1: The relationships among absorption, distribution, protein binding, and excretion of a drug and its concentration at its site of action.

III. CLEARANCE. The total plasma clearance of a drug depends on renal elimination, hepatic metabolism, and conjugation. Renal elimination of drugs is determined by the glomerular filtration rate, tubular secretion, and tubular reabsorption. Glomerular filtration rate should be estimated from creatinine clearance or from a prediction formula such as the Cockcroft–Gault or eGFR creatinine CKD-EPI 2021 formula equations (see Chapter 1). Protein-bound drugs are poorly filtered, but they may be efficiently secreted by the proximal tubule. Unbound drugs are usually freely filtered through the glomerulus. Drugs with primarily hepatic elimination are preferred in patients with CKD. However, renal insufficiency may alter hepatic drug metabolism.

IV. PRESCRIBING FOR THE PATIENT WITH CKD

A. Calculation of Initial Loading Dosage. Because loading dose depends only on the V_D and not on drug clearance, patients with renal failure and normal extracellular volume are usually given a normal loading dose, whereas those with edema or ascites may require a larger loading dose. Similarly, those with volume depletion may need a small loading dose. Loading dose is calculated as

$$\text{Loading Dose} = \text{Desired plasma drug concentration} \times V_D$$

B. Calculation of Maintenance Dosage. The fraction of the normal dose for a patient with renal insufficiency can be calculated from the equation:

$$\text{Dose in renal failure} = \text{Dose in normal renal function} \times (t_{1/2} \text{ Normal}/t_{1/2} \text{ Renal failure})$$

Where $t_{1/2}$ is the half-life for elimination and is inversely proportional to clearance. Alternatively, the dose can often be kept constant and the dosing interval increased:

$$\text{Dose interval in renal failure} = \text{Normal dose interval}/(t_{1/2} \text{ Normal}/t_{1/2} \text{ Renal failure})$$

V. HEMODIALYSIS OF DRUGS. Drug removal by hemodialysis (HD) is directly proportional to the plasma concentration of free drug and to the clearance characteristics of the dialysis membrane. Large drug molecular size does not limit drug removal by HD with high-flux membranes (e.g., polysulfone, cellulose triacetate, polyacrylonitrile). It is only important with less "leaky" cellulosic (e.g., cuprophane or cellulose acetate) membranes. The most important variables limiting drug removal by HD are a large V_D and a high level of protein binding. Drug removal during HD can be substantial, for instance, this may require replacement of approximately 50% of total body stores of an aminoglycoside. As in the case of urea kinetic modeling, there can be substantial postdialysis redistribution of drug from tissue to the central (plasma-containing) compartment. This phenomenon can limit drug removal during HD and lead to overestimates of drug removal if plasma levels are measured immediately after dialysis before equilibration is complete.

Whenever possible, drug dosing in HD patients should be estimated using aids such as Table 26.1. Thereafter, the accuracy of these estimates should be confirmed by measurement of plasma drug levels. This strategy avoids the wide variation in drug levels that may result if drugs are only dosed when the plasma levels fall below the therapeutic target.

VI. DRUG DOSING DURING CONTINUOUS RENAL REPLACEMENT THERAPY. Drug removal by continuous renal replacement therapy (CRRT), either venovenous hemofiltration (CVVH) or venovenous hemodialysis (CVVHD), differs from that in intermittent HD because dialytic clearance by convection and diffusion is usually much higher, and intercompartmental redistribution during and after dialysis is relatively unimportant. The dialyzer membranes do not differ from those used in high-flux HD, offering an effective pore size that is larger than nearly all unbound drugs. Consequently, drug-dosing adjustments during CRRT are much more dependent on the relative contribution of CRRT to total body clearance of the drug than on the V_D of the drug. One simple approach to drug-dosing adjustment during CRRT is to estimate mean urea clearance from total dialysate or ultrafiltration volume (often in the range of 30 to 35 mL/min for CVVH and CVVHD), then to look up dose adjustments in Table 26.1 or similar published references for patients with CKD and residual function of 10 to 50 mL/min. More precise estimates can be made when protein-binding data and plasma drug levels are available. The ability of a drug to transit the dialyzer by convective clearance during continuous ultrafiltration is expressed as the *sieving coefficient(s)*:

$$S = \text{drug concentration in ultrafiltrate/drug concentration in plasma}$$

Because most unbound drugs are freely cleared by continuous hemofiltration, S can be approximated by:

$$\text{Free fraction of drug} = \text{fractional protein binding}$$

The drug clearance can be determined by:

$$\text{Drug clearance} = S \times \text{ultrafiltration rate}$$

Drug replacement is calculated as:

$$\text{Drug replacement} = \text{drug clearance} \times \text{drug concentration}$$

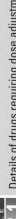

TABLE 26.1 Details of drugs requiring dose adjustments in patients with renal insufficiency and those receiving dialysis

Drug	Excreted unchanged (%)	Protein bound (%)	t₁/₂ Normal/renal failure (h)	Dose or frequency adjustment for GFR (mL/min)			Supplemental dose for dialysis		
				GFR >50	GFR 10–50	GFR <10	HD	PD	CRRT
Analgesics									
Narcotics									
Codeine	Hepatic	7	2.5–3.5/?	100%	75%	50%	?	?	Dose for GFR 10–50
Fentanyl	Hepatic	80–84	2–7/?	100%	75%	50%	Not applicable	Not applicable	Dose for GFR 10–50
Hydromorphone	Hepatic/renal	20	?/?	100%	100%	100%	100%	100%	100%
Meperidine[a]	Hepatic	70	2–7/7–32	100%	Avoid	Avoid	Avoid	Avoid	Avoid
Methadone	Hepatic	60–90	13–58/?	100%	75%	50–75%	None	None	Dose for GFR 10–50
Morphine[b]	Hepatic	20–30	1–4/unchanged	100%	75%	50%	None	?	Dose for GFR 10–50
Oxycodone	Hepatic/renal	45	3–4/lengthened	75%	75%	50%	50%	50%	Not applicable
Nonsteroidal anti-inflammatory drugs									
Acetaminophen	Hepatic	20–30	2/2	q4h	q6h	q8h	None	None	Dose for GFR 10–50
Aspirin	Hepatic/renal	80–90	2–3/unchanged	q4h	q4–6h	Avoid	Dose after HD	None	Dose for GFR 10–50
Ibuprofen	<1	99	2/unchanged	100%	100%	100%	None	None	Dose for GFR 10–50
Antimicrobials									
Aminoglycosides[c,d] (traditional multiple daily doses; see alternative once-daily dosing at the end of the table)									
Amikacin	95	<5	1.4–2.3/17–150	60–90% q12h or 100% q12–24h	30–70% q12–18h or 100% q24–48h	20–30% q24–48h or 100% q48–72h	½ full dose after HD	15–20 mg/L/day	Dose for GFR 10–50, monitor level

Gentamicin	95	<5	1.8/20–60	60–90% q8–12h OR 100% q12–24h	30–70% q12h OR 100% q24–48h, by level	20–30% q24–48h OR 100% q48–72h, by level	½ full dose after HD	3–4 mg/L/d	Dose for GFR 10–50, monitor level
Streptomycin	70	35	2.5/100	q24h	q24–72h	q27–96h	½ full dose	20–40 mg/L/day	Dose for GFR 10–50, monitor level
Tobramycin	95	<5	2.5/27–60	60–90% q8–12h	30–70% q12h	20–30% q24–48h	⅔ full dose	3–4 mg/L/day	Dose for GFR 10–50, monitor level
Carbapenems									
Imipenem[e]	20–70	13–21	1.0/4.0	100%	50%	25%	Dose after HD	Dose for GFR <10	500 mg q6h
Cephalosporins									
Cefaclor	70	25	1.0/3.0	100%	50–100%	50%	250–500 mg after HD	250–500 mg q8–12h	Not applicable
Cefazolin	75–95	80	2/40–70	100% q8h	100% q12h	50% q24–48h	15–20 mg/kg after HD	0.5 g q12h	Dose for GFR 10–50
Cefotaxime	60	37	1.0/15	q6h	q8–12h	q24h	1 g after HD	1 g/day	1 g q12h
Ceftazidime	60–85	17	1.2/13–25	q8–12h	q24–48h	q24h	1 g after HD	0.5 g/day	1 g q12h or 2 g load followed by 3 g/day continuous infusion
Ceftriaxone	30–65	90	7–9/12–24	100%	100%	100%	Dose after HD	750 mg q12h	Dose for GFR 10–50
Cephalexin	98	20	0.7/16	q8h	q12h	q24h	Dose after HD	Dose for GFR <10	Not applicable
Macrolides									
Azithromycin	6–12	8–50	10–60/?	100%	100%	100%	None	None	Dose for GFR 10–50

(continued)

TABLE 26.1 Details of drugs requiring dose adjustments in patients with renal insufficiency and those receiving dialysis (*Continued*)

Drug	Excreted unchanged (%)	Protein bound (%)	t₁/₂ Normal/renal failure (h)	Dose or frequency adjustment for GFR (mL/min)			Supplemental dose for dialysis		
				GFR >50	GFR 10–50	GFR <10	HD	PD	CRRT
Clarithromycin	15	70	2.3–6.0/?	100%	75%	50–70%	Dose after HD	None	Dose for GFR 10–50
Erythromycin	15	60–90	1.4/5–6	100%	100%	50–70%	None	None	Dose for GFR 10–50
Miscellaneous									
Clindamycin	10	60–95	2–4/3–5	100%	100%	100%	None	None	Dose for GFR 10–50
Linezolid	30	30	4.7–6.4/6.1–8.4	100%	100%	100%	No dose adjustment	No dose adjustment	600 mg q12h
Metronidazole	20	20	6–14/7–21	100%	100%	50%	Dose after HD	Dose for GFR <10	Dose for GFR 10–50
Sulfamethoxazole	70	50	10/20–50	q12h	q18h	q24h	1 g after HD	1 g/day	2.5–5 mg/kg q12h
Trimethoprim	40–70	30–70	9–13/20–49	q12h	q18h	q24h	Dose after HD	Dose for GFR <10	2.5–5 mg/kg q12h
Vancomycin	90–100	10–50	6–8/200	500 mg q12h	500 mg q24–48h	500 mg q48–96h	Dose for GFR <10	Dose for GFR <10	Dose for GFR 10–50
Penicillins									
Amoxicillin	50–70	15–25	2.3/5–20	q8h	q8–12h	q24h	Dose after HD	250 mg q12h	Not applicable
Ampicillin	30–70	20	1.5/7–20	q6h	q6–12h	q12–24h	Dose after HD	250 mg q12h	Dose for GFR 10–50
Aztreonam	75	45–60	2.9/6–8	100%	50–75%	25%	0.5 g after HD	Dose for GFR <10	Dose for GFR 10–50
Nafcillin	36	85	0.5/1.2	100%	100%	100%	None	None	Dose for GFR 10–50

(continued)

Penicillin G	60–85	<5	0.5/6–20	100%	75%	20–50%	Dose after HD	Dose for GFR <10	Dose for GFR 10–50
Piperacillin	75–90	30	0.8–2.0/3.0–5.1	q4–6h	q6–8h	q8h	2 g q8h plus 1 g after HD	Dose for GFR <10	Dose for GFR 10–50
Ticarcillin	85	45–60	1.2/11–16	1–2 g q4–6h	1–2 g q8h	1–2 g q12h	3 g after HD	3 g q12h	Dose for GFR 10–50
Quinolones[f]									
Ciprofloxacin	50–70	20–40	3–6/6–9	100%	50–75%	50%	250 mg q12h	250 mg q12h	400 mg q24h
Gatifloxacin	74–84	20	7–14/36	400 mg q24h	200 mg q24h	200 mg q24h	200 mg q24h after HD	200 mg q24h	Dose for GFR 30–50
Levofloxacin	67–87	24–38	4–8/76	100%	500 mg initially, then 250 mg q24–48h	500 mg initially, then 250 mg q48h	Dose for GFR <10	Dose for GFR <10	500 mg q48h
Ofloxacin	68–80	25	5–8/28–37	100%	50%	25–50%	100 mg q12h	Dose for GFR <10	300 mg q24h
Tetracyclines[g]									
Doxycycline	35–45	80–90	20/18–25	100%	100%	100%	None	None	Dose for GFR 10–50
Minocycline	6–10	70	16/12–18	100%	100%	100%	None	None	Not applicable
Antifungals									
Amphotericin B	5–10	90	24/unchanged	q24h	q24h	q24–36h	None	None	Dose for GFR 10–50
Amphotericin B lipid complex	<1	90	19–45/unchanged	q24h	q24h	q24h	None	None	Dose for GFR 10–50
Fluconazole	70	12	22/?	100%	50%	50%	200 mg after HD	Dose for GFR <10	200–400 mg q24h
Caspofungin	<2	97	9–11/?	100%	100%	100%	100% dose	100% dose	100% dose
Flucytosine	90	<10	3–6/75–200	q12h	q16h	q24h	Dose after HD	0.5–1.0 g q24h	Dose for GFR 10–50

TABLE 26.1 Details of drugs requiring dose adjustments in patients with renal insufficiency and those receiving dialysis (*Continued*)

Drug	Excreted unchanged (%)	Protein bound (%)	$t_{1/2}$ Norma/renal failure (h)	Dose or frequency adjustment for GFR (mL/min)				Supplemental dose for dialysis		
				GFR >50	GFR 10–50	GFR <10	HD	PD	CRRT
Itraconazole	35	99	21/25	100%	100%	50%	100 mg q12–24h	100 mg q12–24h	100% dose
Antiparasitics									
Chloroquine	40	50–65	4/5–50 days	100%	100%	50%	Dose for GFR <10	Dose for GFR <10	Dose for GFR 10–50
Pentamidine	20	69	2.8–12/118	q24h	q24–36h	q48h	Dose for GFR <10; 0.75 g after each HD	Dose for GFR <10	Dose for GFR 30–50
Dapsone	5–20	70–90	20–30/?	100%	?	?	None	Dose for GFR <10	?
Antituberculosis									
Ethambutol	75–90	10–30	4–7/15	q24h	q24–36h	q48h	Dose after HD	Dose for GFR <10	Dose for GFR 30–50
Isoniazid	5–30	4–30	0.7–4.0/8–17	100%	100%	50%	Dose after HD	Dose for GFR <10	Dose for GFR 30–50
Pyrazinamide	1–3	5	9/26	100%	100%	100%	40 mg/kg 24 h before 3×/wk dialysis	100%	Dose for GFR 10–50
Rifampin	15–30	60–90	1.5/1.8–11	100%	50–100%	50%	None	Dose for GFR <10	Dose for GFR 30–50
Antiviral^b									
Abacavir	Hepatic	50	1.5–2.7/none	100%	100%	100%	None	None	100% dose

Acyclovir (prodrug = valacyclovir)	40–70	15–30	2.1–3.5/19	5 mg/kg q8h	5 mg/kg q12h	5 mg/kg q24h	Dose after HD	Dose for GFR <10	5–10 mg/kg q24h
Amantadine	90	60	12/500	q24–48h	q48–72h	q7d	None	None	Dose for GFR 10–50
Cidofovir/probenecid	70–85%	<6%	2.6/not applicable	See note	Avoid	Avoid	Avoid	Avoid	Avoid; if needed, 2 mg/kg/wk
Didanosine	60	<5	1.3–1.6/4.5	q12h	q24h	q48h	25% of daily dose	Dose for GFR <10	Dose for GFR 10–50
Efavirenz	Hepatic	>99	40–76/?	?	?	?	?	?	Dose for GFR 10–50
Famciclovir	50–65	<25	1.6–2.9/10–22	q8h	250 mg q12h	250 mg q48h	250 mg after HD	?	Not applicable
Foscarnet	85	17	3/prolonged	28 mg/kg	15 mg/kg	6 mg/kg	Dose after HD	Dose for GFR <10	CMV induction 60 mg q24h, main, 60 mg q48h
Ganciclovir (prodrug = valganciclovir)	90–100	1–2%	3.6/30	q12h	q24–48h	q48–96h	Dose after HD	Dose for GFR <10	Induction: 2.5 mg/kg q24h; main: 1.25 mg q24h
Indinavir	Hepatic	60	1.8/?	?	?	?	No adjustment necessary	Dose for GFR <10	No data 100%
Lamivudine	68–71	36	5–7/15–35	150 mg q12h	100 mg q.d.	50 mg q.d.	Dose after HD	Dose for GFR <10	100 mg first day, then 50 mg/day
Lopinavir/ritonavir	Hepatic	98–99	5–6/?	400 mg q12h	400 mg q12h	400 mg q12h	No dose adjustment	?	100%
Nevirapine	<5	60%	20–45/?	100%	100%	100%	None	?	100%
Ribavirin	10–40	98–99	30–60/?	100%	Avoid	Avoid	Avoid	Avoid	100%

(continued)

Details of drugs requiring dose adjustments in patients with renal insufficiency and those receiving dialysis (*Continued*)

Drug	Excreted unchanged (%)	Protein bound (%)	$t_{1/2}$ Normal/renal failure (h)	Dose or frequency adjustment for GFR (mL/min)				Supplemental dose for dialysis		
				GFR >50	GFR 10–50	GFR <10	HD	PD	CRRT
Rimantadine	<25	10%	13–65/ prolonged	100 mg q12h	100 mg q.d.	100 mg q.d.	?	?	?
Ritonavir	Hepatic	98–99%	3–5/?	?	?	?	None	None	100%
Saquinavir	Hepatic	97%	1–2/?	?	?	?	?	?	100%
Stavudine	40	<1	1.0–1.4/5.5–8.0	100%	50%	50% q24h	Dose after HD	?	100%
Valacyclovir (prodrug of acyclovir)	<12%	13.5–18.0	2.5/3.3	1 g q8h	1 g q12–24h	0.5 g q24h	Dose after HD	Dose for GFR <10	Not applicable
Zalcitabine	75	<4	0.75 mg q12h	0.75 mg q8h	0.75 mg q12h	0.75 mg q24h	Dose after HD	?	0.75 mg q12h
Zidovudine	8–25	10–30	1.1–1.4/1.4–3.0	200 mg q8h	200 mg q8h	100 mg q12h	100 mg after HD	Dose for GFR <10	100%
Cardiovascular drugs									
Adenosine	<5	0	<10 s/ unchanged	100%	100%	100%	None	None	None
Amiodarone	<5	96	14–120 days/ unchanged	100%	100%	100%	None	None	None
Digoxin	76–85	20–30	36–44/80–120	100% q24h	25–75% q36h	10–25% q48h	None	None	Dose for GFR 10–50, monitor level
Dobutamine	<10	?	2 min/?	100%	100%	100%	?	?	?
Flecainide	25	52	12/19–26	100%	50%	50%	None	None	?
Lidocaine	10	60–66	2.2/3.0	100%	100%	100%	None	None	Dose for GFR 10–50

Drug			Half-life (normal/ESRD)	Dose for GFR >50	Dose for GFR 10–50	Dose for GFR <10	Supplement		
Mexiletine	10	70–75	8/13–16	100%	100%	50–75%	None	None	?
Propafenone	<1	>95	12/?	100%	100%	100%	None	None	Dose for GFR 10–50
Quinidine	20	70–95	6/4–14	100%	100%	75%	100–200 mg after HD	None	Dose for GFR 10–50, monitor level
Sotalol	60	<1	?	100%	30%	15–30%	Dose after HD	None	Dose for GFR 10–50
Tocainide	40	10–20	14/22–27	100%	100%	50%	200 mg	None	?
Angiotensin-converting enzyme inhibitors									
Benazepril	20	95	22/30	100%	75–100%	50%	25–30%	None	?
Captopril	30–40	25–30	1.9/21–32	100% q8–12h	75% q12–18h	50% q24h	25–30%	None	?
Enalapril	43	50–60	24/34–60	100% q8–12h	75–100%	50%	20–25%	None	?
Fosinopril	<1	95	11–12/12–20	100%	100%	75%	None	None	?
Lisinopril	80–90	0–10	12.6/40–50	100%	50–75%	25–50%	Dose after HD	None	?
Quinapril	30	97	1–2/6–15	100%	75–100%	50%	Dose for GFR <10	Dose for GFR <10	?
Ramipril	10–21	55–70	5.8/15.0	100%	50–75%	25–50%	Dose after HD	?	?
Angiotensin receptor blockers									
Candesartan	33	99	9/?	100%	100%	100%	No dose adjustment	No dose adjustment	?
Eprosartan	35–50	99	5–7/?	100%	100%	100%	100%	?	?
Irbesartan	20	90	13/No change	100%	100%	100%	No dose adjustment	?	?
Losartan	10	30	3/4	100%	100%	100%	None	None	?
Olmesartan	7	99	13/36	100%	100%	100%	?	?	?
Telmisartan	7	98	24/16	100%	100%	100%	?	?	?
Valsartan	13.2	85–99	6.1/?	100%	100%	?	None	?	?

(continued)

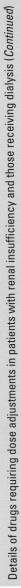

TABLE
26.1 Details of drugs requiring dose adjustments in patients with renal insufficiency and those receiving dialysis (*Continued*)

Drug	Excreted unchanged (%)	Protein bound (%)	t_{1/2} Normal/renal failure (h)	Dose or frequency adjustment for GFR (mL/min)			Supplemental dose for dialysis		
				GFR >50	GFR 10–50	GFR <10	HD	PD	CRRT
Beta-blockers									
Atenolol	>90	3	6.7/15–35	100% q24h	50% q48h	30–50% q96h	25–50 mg after HD	Dose for GFR <10	?
Carvedilol	<2	95	5–8/unchanged	100%	100%	100%	None	?	?
Labetalol	<5	50	3–9/unchanged	100%	100%	100%	None	None	?
Metoprolol	5	8	3.5/2.5–4.5	100%	100%	100%	None	None	?
Pindolol	40	50	2.5–4.0/3–4	100%	100%	100%	None	None	?
Propranolol	<5	93	2–6/1–6	100%	100%	100%	None	?	?
Calcium channel blockers									
Amlodipine	<10	>95	35–50/50	100%	100%	100%	None	None	?
Diltiazem	<10	98	2–8/3.5	100%	100%	100%	None	None	?
Nicardipine	<1	98–99	5/5–7	100%	100%	100%	None	None	?
Nifedipine	<10	97	5.5/5–7	100%	100%	100%	No dose adjustment	No dose adjustment	?
Verapamil	<10	83–93	3–7/2.4–4.0	100%	100%	100%	None	None	Dose for GFR 10–50
Centrally acting agents									
Clonidine	45	20–40	6–23/38–42	q12h	q12–24h	q24h	None	None	?
Methyldopa	25–40	<15	1.5–6.0/6–16	q8h	q8–12h	q12–24h	250 mg	None	?
Vasodilators									
Hydralazine	5–10	87	2.0–4.5/7–16	q8h	q8h	q8–16h	None	None	?
Minoxidil	15–20	0	2.8–2/unchanged	100%	100%	100%	None	None	?
Terazosin	20–30	90–94	9–12/8–12	100%	100%	100%	?	?	?

212

Antiulcer/proton pump inhibitors

Drug							Dose after HD	Dose for GFR <10	Dose for GFR 10-50
Cimetidine	50–70	20	1.5–2.0/5	100%	50%	25%	?	None	?
Esomeprazole	<1	97	1.0–1.5/unchanged	100%	100%	100%	None	?	Dose for GFR 10–50
Famotidine	65–80	15–22	2.5–4.0/12–19	50%	25%	10%	?	Dose for GFR <10	Dose for GFR 10–50
Lansoprazole	None	>98	1.3–2.9/unchanged	100%	100%	100%	?	?	?
Omeprazole	<1	95	0.5–1.0/unchanged	100%	100%	100%	?	?	?
Ranitidine	80	15	1.5–3.0/6–9	75%	50%	25%	50%	?	?
Anticonvulsants, antidepressants, antiparkinsonians, antipsychotics									
Amitriptyline	Hepatic	96	24–40/unchanged	100%	100%	100%	None	?	?
Carbamazepine	2–3	75	12–17/unchanged	100%	100%	75%	Dose for GFR <10, give after HD	Dose for GFR <10	100%
Carbidopa	30	?	2/?	100%	100%	100%	?	?	?
Clonazepam	Hepatic	47	18–50/?	?	?	?	?	?	?
Citalopram	12	80	35/?	100%	100%	?	None	?	?
Fluoxetine	Hepatic	94.5	24–72/unchanged	100%	100%	100%	?	?	?
Gabapentin	90	Unbound	5–7/132	400 mg t.i.d.	300 mg q12–24h	300 mg every other day	300 mg load, then 200–300 mg after HD	300 mg every other day	Dose for GFR 10–50
Haloperidol	Hepatic	90–92	10–19/?	100%	100%	100%	None	None	?
Lamotrigine	10	55	25–36/43–58	100%	75%	100 mg qod	100 mg after HD	Dose for GFR 10–50	Decrease dose by 50%

(continued)

T A B L E

26.1 Details of drugs requiring dose adjustments in patients with renal insufficiency and those receiving dialysis (*Continued*)

Drug	Excreted unchanged (%)	Protein bound (%)	$t_{1/2}$ Normal/renal failure (h)	Dose or frequency adjustment for GFR (mL/min)				Supplemental dose for dialysis		
				GFR >50	GFR 10–50	GFR <10		HD	PD	CRRT
Levetiracetam	65	<10	7/25	500–1,000 mg b.i.d.	250–750 mg b.i.d.	250–500 mg b.i.d.		500–1,000 mg q.d., then 250–500 mg after HD	?	?
Levodopa	None	5–8	0.8–1.6/?	100%	100%	100%		Dose after HD	?	?
Lithium	Renal	None	14–28/40	100%	50–75%	25–50%		Dose after HD	None	Dose for GFR 10–50
Nefazodone	Hepatic	99	2–4/unchanged	100%	100%	100%		?	?	?
Phenobarbital	Hepatic/renal	40–60	60–150/117–160	q8–12h	q8–12h	q12–16h		1/2 dose after HD	50%	Normal dose, monitor level
Paroxetine	2%	95	15–20/30	100%	50–75	50		?	?	?
Phenytoin	2	90	24/unchanged	100%	100%	100%		None	None	100%
Sertraline	Hepatic	97	24/?	100%	100%	100%		?	?	?
Topiramate	70–80	9–17	19–23/48–60	100%	50%	25%		Dose after HD	Dose for GFR 10–50	Dose for GFR 10–50
Valproic acid	3–7	90	5–16/ unchanged	100%	100%	100%		None	None	?
Venlafaxine	Hepatic	27	4/6–8	75%	50%	50%		None	?	?
Antidiabetics										
Chlorpropamide	47	91–99	24–48/50–200	50%	Avoid	Avoid		Avoid	Avoid	Not applicable
Glipizide	4.5–7.0	97	3–7/?	100%	100%	100%		?	?	Not applicable

Drug									
Glyburide	50	99	1.4–2.9/5	?	Avoid	Avoid	None	None	Not applicable
Metformin	90–100	Negligible	1–5/prolonged	50%	25%	Avoid	Not applicable	Avoid	Avoid
Antihyperlipidemics									
Pioglitazone	Hepatic	97	9/unchanged	100%	100%	100%	100%	?	?
Rosiglitazone	Hepatic	99	3–4/unchanged	100%	100%	100%	100%	?	?
Atorvastatin	<2	>98	14/?	?	?	?	?	?	?
Gemfibrozil	None	97–99	7.6/unchanged	100%	100%	100%	None	?	?
Lovastatin	None	>95	1.1–1.7/unchanged	100%	100%	100%	?	?	?
Niacin	None	?	0.5–1.0/?	100%	50%	25%	?	?	?
Pravastatin	<10	40–60	0.8–3.2/unchanged	100%	100%	100%	None	None	None
Simvastatin	<0.5	>95	?	100%	100%	100%	None	None	None

Creatinine clearance (ml/min)	>80	60–80	40–60	30–40	20–30	10–20	<10
Antibiotic dose	Dose q24h (mg/kg)				Dose q48h (mg/kg)		
Amikacin/kanamycin	15.0	12.0	7.5	4.0	7.5	4.0	3.0
Gentamicin/tobramycin	5.1	4.0	3.5	2.5	4.0	3.0	2.0

?, no data; CMV, cytomegalovirus; CRRT, continuous renal replacement therapy; GFR, glomerular filtration rate; HD, hemodialysis; Hepatic, predominantly eliminated by hepatic metabolism; PD, peritoneal dialysis.

[a] Active metabolite (normeperidine) lowers seizure threshold, accumulates in end-stage renal disease, and is poorly dialyzed.

[b] End-stage renal disease patients have increased sensitivity to morphine's effects.

[c] Aminoglycosides: see below for alternative once-daily dose.

[d] Measure serum levels; risk for nephrotoxicity and ototoxicity.

[e] Imipenem lowers seizure threshold in end-stage renal disease. Cilastatin decreases potential nephrotoxicity of metabolite.

[f] Quinolone malabsorption occurs in the presence of magnesium, calcium, aluminum, and iron-containing compounds.

[g] Tetracycline drugs: malabsorption occurs with magnesium, calcium, aluminum, and iron-containing compounds.

[h] See http://www.aidsinfo.nih.gov for updates.

Adapted from Aronoff GR, Berns JS, Brier ME, et al., eds. Drug prescribing in renal failure: dosing guidelines for adults, 4th ed. Philadelphia: American College of Physicians, 2007; Brater DC. Drug dosing in renal failure. In: Brady HR, Wilcox CS, eds. Therapy in nephrology and hypertension: companion to Brenner and Rector's The kidney, 3rd ed. Philadelphia: WB Saunders, 2008:939–954; Gilbert D, Moellering R, et al. The Sanford guide to antimicrobial therapy. Hyde Park: Jeb C. Sanford, 2008; Sandow N. Rx list: the Internet drug list. RxList LLC, 2008. Available at http://www.rxlist.com/.

More importantly, drug-dosing recommendations during CRRT should be based on clinical clearance data when available. Plasma drug-level monitoring may be needed for some drugs in critically ill patients.

VII. PERITONEAL DIALYSIS OF DRUGS. Like other solutes, most drugs may be transported bidirectionally across the peritoneal membrane during peritoneal dialysis. Intraperitoneally administered drugs enter the circulation rapidly. For example, antibiotics can achieve equivalent plasma levels after intravenous or intraperitoneal dosing. Although the peritoneal surface area is large, most dwell volumes are only approximately 2 L. Even if drug clearance were to approximate to peritoneal creatinine clearance, the net clearance would only be 6 to 8 mL/min. More importantly, because peritoneal volumes are much smaller than the V_D for most drugs, only a small fraction of drug in the body is present in the peritoneal cavity at any given time. This limits its contribution to drug clearance. This is especially true for drugs that bind strongly to plasma proteins. Both the modality of peritoneal dialysis and the degree of residual renal function can affect drug clearance. Importantly, the data on the peritoneal elimination of many drugs are inconsistent, increasing the need for drug-level monitoring.

VIII. DETAILS OF DRUG DOSING IN RENAL FAILURE. Table 26.1 provides details of commonly used or important drugs that require dose adjustments in patients with renal insufficiency and those receiving dialysis. When specific recommendations are unavailable, data on the usual importance of renal drug elimination, half-life, V_D, and protein binding allow an estimate of dose adjustments.

IX. SUGGESTED READINGS
Gilbert D, Moellering R, Eliopoulos G, et al. *The Sanford Guide to Antimicrobial Therapy*. Jeb C. Sanford; 2008.

Hirata S, Kadowaki D. Appropriate drug dosing in patients receiving peritoneal dialysis. *Contrib Nephrol*. 2012;177:30–37.

Ruchi R, Bozorgmehri S, Ozrazgat-Baslanti T, et al. Opioid safety and concomitant benzodiazepine use in end-stage renal disease patients. *Pain Res Manag*. 2019;3865924.

Sandow N. *Rx list: the Internet drug list*. RxList LLC. 2003. Accessed May 29, 2008. http://www.rxlist.com

27 Nephrotoxic Drugs, Contrast Nephropathy and Renal Protective Strategies

Afia Ashraf, Keiko I. Greenberg

Numerous medications have been associated with nephrotoxicity, including commonly used antibiotics, diuretics, antihypertensive agents, nonsteroidal anti-inflammatory medications (NSAIDs), and chemotherapeutic agents. Exposure to nephrotoxic medications is a common cause of acute kidney injury, particularly among hospitalized patients and the elderly, who may be at increased risk of developing drug-related nephrotoxicity due to intravascular volume depletion and comorbid conditions.

I. **MECHANISMS OF NEPHROTOXICITY.** Nephrotoxic medications cause kidney injury through a variety of pathogenic mechanisms that affect different segments of the nephron.

A. **Acute Tubular Injury.** Renal tubule cells, particularly those in the proximal tubule, are susceptible to drug-related toxicity because their apical surface is exposed to filtered nephrotoxins, or they take up nephrotoxins from the basolateral circulation. Once in the tubule cell, drugs cause injury by different mechanisms including mitochondrial injury and oxidative injury, that ultimately lead to cell death. Obstruction of tubules by apoptotic cells, tubular back leak of filtrate in obstructed tubules, and activation of tubuloglomerular feedback with afferent arteriole vasoconstriction are thought to contribute to the decline in glomerular filtration rate. Recovery of kidney function is seen in most patients but some may develop significant tubular atrophy and interstitial fibrosis.

Medications that enter proximal tubule cells from the apical surface include **aminoglycosides**. They bind to receptors on the apical membrane that leads to endocytosis and translocation into lysozymes to trigger an injury cascade. Cell injury and death may present as a proximal tubulopathy with hypokalemia, hypophosphatemia and Fanconi syndrome, and/or acute kidney injury. **Mannitol**, **sucrose and other sugars** contained in intravenous immunoglobulins preparations, and **hydroxyethyl starch and other starches** enter proximal tubule cells via pinocytosis. Accumulation of these substances within lysosomes leads to osmotic nephrosis, or the formation of large vacuoles and cell swelling. Swollen cells may cause significant narrowing or occlusion of the proximal tubular lumen.

Nephrotoxins can also enter the proximal tubule through the basolateral membrane via active transporters. These include the human organic anion transporters (hOAT) and human organic cation transporters (hOCT). **Tenofovir, cisplatin,** and **ifosfamide** are transported by hOAT or hOCT. Tubular injury can occur when these drugs accumulate intracellularly. Tenofovir causes mitochondrial dysfunction leading to cell apoptosis and necrosis, which can manifest clinically as Fanconi syndrome and/or acute kidney injury. Cisplatin causes formation of toxic compounds associated with oxidative stress, reactive oxygen, and nitrogen species and induction of pathways that lead to inflammation and apoptosis. The metabolism of ifosfamide within the tubule cell generates chloroacetaldehyde which inhibits the oxidative phosphorylation pathway. Like tenofovir, ifosfamide nephrotoxicity can manifest as a proximal tubulopathy and/or acute kidney injury.

Amphotericin B has direct toxic effects on tubular cell membranes, leading to apoptosis and cell death. It also causes renal vasoconstriction. Clinical manifestations of amphotericin B nephrotoxicity include acute kidney injury, hypokalemia, hypomagnesemia, distal renal tubular acidosis, and impaired urinary concentrating ability.

B. **Acute Interstitial Nephritis.** Many medications have been associated with acute interstitial nephritis (AIN), which is thought to be a delayed hypersensitivity reaction. Medications may induce AIN by binding to renal tissue, mimicking renal antigens, acting as haptens (substances that require binding to another molecule to elicit an immune response) or by other mechanisms. **Methicillin** was previously the commonest cause of AIN that is frequently accompanied by fever, rash, and arthralgias. Subsequently, a large number of medications have been linked to AIN but extrarenal manifestations are uncommon in AIN caused by drugs other than methicillin. These drugs include **allopurinol, beta-lactams, quinolones, rifampin, sulfonamides, vancomycin, acyclovir, indinavir, loop and thiazide diuretics, phenytoin, NSAIDs, proton pump inhibitors, and ranitidine**. In recent years, several anticancer agents have been associated with AIN. These include **PD-1 inhibitors, CTLA-4 inhibitors, ALK inhibitors (crizotinib), BRAF inhibitors (vemurafenib, dabrafenib), tyrosine kinase inhibitors (sunitinib, sorafenib, pazopanib)** as well as **immune checkpoint inhibitors (ipilimumab, nivolumab, pembrolizumab, atezolizumab).**

C. **Chronic Interstitial Nephritis.** Several medications have been associated with chronic interstitial nephritis, including **calcineurin inhibitors, carmustine, semustine, cisplatin, lithium, and aristolochic acid**. It can occur also with long-term use of analgesics, particularly **phenacetin**-containing combinations (phenacetin–aspirin–caffeine, phenacetin–acetaminophen). Each of these agents causes tubular injury (likely by different mechanisms) which leads to an inflammatory response occurring in the interstitium. Unlike AIN, chronic interstitial nephritis is insidious and is not usually accompanied by signs of hypersensitivity.

D. **Intratubular Obstruction.** When insoluble medications (or metabolites of medications) are excreted in the urine, they may form crystals within distal tubular lumens, causing "crystalline nephropathy." Such medications include **methotrexate, indinavir, acyclovir, foscarnet, ganciclovir, atazanavir, sulfadiazine, ciprofloxacin, ampicillin, sulfonamides, triamterene, oral sodium phosphate,** and **ethylene glycol** (which is metabolized to **oxalic acid**). Crystal formation obstructs flow in the distal tubule lumen and also triggers an inflammatory response in the interstitium. Risk factors for crystalline nephropathy include volume depletion causing slow urine flow rates, high medication dose, rapid infusion rates, and alterations in urinary pH.

E. **Cast Nephropathy.** The exact mechanism of vancomycin-associated acute kidney injury is unknown. Possible mechanisms that have been postulated include oxidative stress, complement activation, and mitochondrial damage causing acute tubular injury and necrosis. It has also been associated with AIN. Another potential mechanism described more recently in a series of patients with vancomycin-associated kidney injury is the formation of obstructive tubular casts. Immunohistologic staining demonstrated that these casts were composed of vancomycin aggregates and uromodulin. Casts were surrounded by reactive cells. Most patients had high vancomycin trough levels.

F. **Glomerulonephritis.** Some medications can cause autoimmune disease that, when the kidney is involved, manifests as glomerulonephritis. **Levamisole-adulterated cocaine, hydralazine, propylthiouracil, carbimazole,** and **methimazole** have been linked to ANCA-associated vasculitis. High MPO-ANCA titers are often seen in medication-related vasculitis. **Procainamide, hydralazine, quinidine**, and **TNF-alpha inhibitors** are among the medications that have been associated with lupus-like disease where antihistone antibodies are frequent. **Gold, penicillamine, mercury, captopril**, and **NSAIDs** have been associated with membranous nephropathy. Antiphospholipase A2 receptor antibodies should not be present in secondary membranous nephropathy.

G. **Thrombotic Microangiopathy.** Thrombotic microangiopathy is characterized by endothelial injury and platelet thrombi causing partial or complete obstruction of capillaries and arterioles. Potential mechanisms of medication-induced thrombotic microangiopathy include autoantibody formation, complement activation, and direct endothelial toxicity. Many anticancer agents have been linked to thrombotic microangiopathy, including **chemotherapeutic agents (gemcitabine, mitomycin C), proteasome inhibitors (bortezomib, carfilzomib, ixazomib), VEGF inhibitors (bevacizumab), tyrosine kinase inhibitors (sunitinib, sorafenib)**, and **immune checkpoint inhibitors (ipilimumab)**. Other medications associated with thrombotic microangiopathy include **quinine, cyclosporine, tacrolimus, clopidogrel, ticlopidine**, and **interferons**.

H. **Impaired Renal Perfusion/Altered Intraglomerular Hemodynamics.** Antihypertensive agents and diuretics can cause significant reduction in renal perfusion leading to prerenal acute kidney injury. Several medications can affect the kidney's ability to maintain intraglomerular pressure in the setting of renal hypoperfusion. **NSAIDs** impair afferent arteriolar vasodilation by blocking prostaglandin production. **Calcineurin inhibitors (cyclosporine, tacrolimus), contrast dye,** and **amphotericin-B** also cause afferent arteriolar vasoconstriction. **Angiotensin-converting enzyme inhibitors** and **angiotensin receptor blockers** impair vasoconstriction of efferent arterioles.

I. **Rhabdomyolysis.** Some medications can cause direct injury to muscle cells or create conditions that predispose muscle cells to injury (e.g., ischemia), leading to rhabdomyolysis. Rhabdomyolysis is characterized by muscle cell injury resulting in the release of myoglobin and other cell contents into the circulation. Myoglobin causes kidney injury via renal vasoconstriction, direct tubular injury, and distal tubular obstruction. Medications and toxins associated with rhabdomyolysis include **HMG-CoA reductase inhibitors (statins), alcohol, cocaine, heroin, ketamine, methadone,** and **methamphetamine.**

J. **Obstructive Uropathy.** Medications that cause urinary retention result in postrenal acute kidney injury. These include medications with anticholinergic activity

(antipsychotic agents, antihistamines, antidepressants), opioids, alpha adrenoceptor agonists, benzodiazepines, and detrusor relaxants.

II. **CONTRAST-ASSOCIATED NEPHROPATHY.** Acute kidney injury occurring within a few days after intravascular iodinated contrast administration was previously considered common and was called "contrast-induced nephropathy." In recent years, due to increased awareness of the potential nephrotoxic effects of iodinated contrast, use of strategies to prevent acute kidney injury, and development of newer contrast agents, rates of acute kidney injury following contrast administration are low and are overestimated by most practitioners. As many patients undergoing an imaging study or other procedure requiring iodinated contrast have other risk factors for acute kidney injury, such as hypotension or exposure to other nephrotoxic agents, it is often impossible to determine the exact role played by contrast in causing acute kidney injury. Therefore, the "contrast-associated acute kidney injury" is likely a more appropriate term to describe this condition.

Multiple mechanisms have been proposed for contrast-associated nephropathy. Contrast agents have direct cytotoxic effects on tubular cells, leading to injury, apoptosis, and necrosis. Apoptotic cells can cause tubular obstruction—contrast agents increase the viscosity of fluid in the tubules which may also contribute to obstruction of tubules. Activation of tubuloglomerular feedback leads to renal vasoconstriction. Contrast agents also induce renal vasoconstriction by changing nitric oxide, prostaglandin, and other substances. Increased viscosity of blood may lead to thrombosis of capillaries and small arterioles/venules.

Although slightly different definitions of contrast-associated nephropathy have been utilized over the years, current guidelines define it as acute kidney injury (by KDIGO criteria) occurring within 48 hours of contrast exposure. Severe reduction in kidney function and need for renal replacement therapy are quite uncommon. However, contrast-associated nephropathy has been associated with increased risk of mortality and progression of pre-existing chronic kidney disease.

Several risk factors associated with the development of contrast-associated nephropathy have been identified of which chronic kidney disease and diabetes are the strongest. The type of contrast agent used is a factor—high-osmolality contrast agents used in the past were associated with higher risk of contrast-associated nephropathy than the low-osmolality and iso-osmolality agents used today. Higher contrast volume has also been linked to an increased risk of contrast-associated nephropathy. Finally, intra-arterial administration of contrast is thought to be associated with higher risk of contrast-associated nephropathy than intravenous administration due to higher concentration of contrast in the renal arteries. A few models have been validated to estimate the risk of contrast-associated nephropathy for coronary intervention, for example, at https://qxmd.com/calculate/calculator_47/contrast-nephropathy-post-pci.

III. **RENAL PROTECTIVE STRATEGIES**
A. **Prevention of Contrast-Associated Nephropathy.** In general, low-osmolality or iso-osmolality contrast agents should be used and volume of contrast administered should be minimized. Repeated administration of contrast within 48 to 72 hours should be avoided.

In patients with significant chronic kidney disease or who are at high risk of developing contrast-associated nephropathy due to other factors, preventive measures should be considered. The only intervention that has been shown to prevent contrast-associated nephropathy is the administration of intravenous saline. The optimal fluid regimen is unknown—recommendations range from 1 to 1.5 mL/kg/h for 6 to 12 hours prior to a procedure and 6 to 24 hours after a procedure in hospitalized patients and 1 to 3 mL/kg/h from 1 to 3 hours prior to and 1 to 1.5 mL/kg/h for 4 to 6 hours after a procedure in the outpatient setting. Studies have not demonstrated any benefit to using intravenous sodium bicarbonate over saline. Acetylcysteine is frequently used for prevention of contrast-associated nephropathy but it was not shown to be protective in a large randomized controlled trial. Therefore, its use is not recommended.

There is little evidence of benefit from withholding certain medications, such as ACE inhibitors, ARBs, and diuretics, prior to contrast administration. It is reasonable to hold NSAIDs prior to contrast if possible. Holding metformin has been advocated due to concern for lactic acidosis should severe acute kidney injury occur, however, there is no evidence to support this recommendation. The removal of contrast with hemodialysis immediately after administration has not been shown to prevent contrast-associated nephropathy.

B. **Prevention of Drug-Induced Nephrotoxicity.** There are several measures that may be helpful for preventing acute kidney injury related with medications. Nonnephrotoxic medications should be used whenever possible and the use of multiple nephrotoxic medications should be avoided. Modifiable risk factors for acute kidney injury, such as volume depletion or hypotension, should be corrected prior to nephrotoxin administration. Renally cleared medications should be dose adjusted for baseline kidney function. Kidney function should be monitored in patients who are at higher risk for developing acute kidney injury, such as older patients and those with pre-existing chronic kidney disease, diabetes, heart failure, and liver disease. In some cases, there may be a safer form of a medication available (e.g., tenofovir alafenamide is preferable to tenofovir disoproxil fumarate and liposomal amphotericin to conventional amphotericin). Drug levels should be monitored for medications that cause dose-dependent toxicity such as vancomycin and lithium. Administration of intravenous saline should accompany intravenous acyclovir to prevent intratubular crystal formation.

IV. SUGGESTED READINGS

Goldstein SL. Medication-induced acute kidney injury. *Curr Opin Crit Care.* 2016;22(6):542–545.
Mehran R, Dangas GD, Weisbord SD. Contrast-associated acute kidney injury. *N Engl J Med.* 2019;380(22):2146–2155.
Naughton CA. Drug-induced nephrotoxicity. *Am Fam Physician.* 2008;78(6):743–750.
Perazella MA. Drug-induced acute kidney injury: diverse mechanisms of tubular injury. *Curr Opin Crit Care.* 2019;25(6):550–557.
Rosner MH, Perazella MA. Acute kidney injury in patients with cancer. *N Engl J Med.* 2017; 376(18):1770–1781.

28 Immunosuppressive Agents for Kidney Transplantation

Steven Gabardi, Winfred W. Williams

I. **INTRODUCTION.** Success following renal transplantation is highly dependent on an immunosuppressive (IS) regimen to prevent graft rejection and preserve renal function.

A "one-size-fits-all" approach is the dominant paradigm for IS medication (Table 28.1). The most frequent choice for IS is a calcineurin inhibitor (CNI), an antimetabolite, and corticosteroids. **CNIs** act by inhibiting T-cell (Tc) activation through downregulation of interleukin-2 (IL-2) synthesis thereby preventing clonal expansion of Tcs directed against the allograft. The **Antimetabolites** disrupt the synthesis of RNA, DNA, and cell division and thereby suppress B-cell and Tc replication and proliferation. **Corticosteroids** are lymphotoxic at high doses and suppress cytokine-driven clonal expansion and the inflammatory cascade associated with allograft rejection.

Tacrolimus (TAC) is the primary IS agent used in the United States. The next most effective are the antimetabolites Mycophenolic Acid (MPA) and Azathioprine (AZA). AZA has now been supplanted by mycophenolate mofetil (MMF) and enteric-coated MPA (EC-MPA). Methylprednisolone, prednisone, and prednisolone are the most common steroids used for organ transplant. Many U.S. transplant centers have incorporated IS regimens that withdraw corticosteroid therapy within the first 30 to 90 days following renal transplant to prevent their long-term adverse events.

The mammalian target of rapamycin (mTOR) inhibitors are used currently in patients intolerant of CNIs, those with basal or squamous cell carcinomas, or those with drug-resistant cytomegalovirus (CMV) disease. The newest IS agent is belatacept, that is a humanized fusion protein given intravenously to block the costimulatory pathway (Signal 2) and to induce Tc anergy (Fig. 28.1).

Tc activation requires three signals (Fig. 28.1). **Signal 1** represents antigen recognition by the Tc receptor at the Major Histocompatibility Complex (MHC) on Antigen Presenting Cells (APC) that activates nuclear transcription of the mRNA for cytokine IL-2. This, in turn, leads to autocrine IL-2 binding to CD25 (IL-2 receptor) and activation of the **Signal 3** pathway with Tc activation and proliferation. CNIs block Signal 1 by inhibiting calcineurin phosphatase. Activation of **Signal 2**, or the co-stimulatory pathway depends on Tc surface molecules that interact with ligands on the APC. Belatacept selectively blocks Tc activation via the co-stimulation pathway. **Signal 3** activates the pathway governing the cell cycle and thereby controls Tc proliferation and expansion.

	TABLE 28.1 Currently available immunosuppressive agents

Drug class	Induction or maintenance immunosuppression	Available agents—generic (trade) names
Antilymphocyte antibodies	Induction	Alemtuzumab (Campath)
		Antithymocyte globulin [equine] (ATGAM)
		Antithymocyte globulin [rabbit] (Thymoglobulin)
Antiproliferatives	Maintenance	Azathioprine (Imuran)
		Mycophenolate mofetil (CellCept)
		Mycophenolic acid (Myfortic)
Calcineurin inhibitors (CNIs)	Maintenance	Cyclosporine (Sandimmune)
		Cyclosporine modified (Gengraf, Neoral)
		Tacrolimus (Prograf)
		Tacrolimus extended release (Astagraf XL, Envarsus XR)
Corticosteroids	Maintenance	Methylprednisolone (Solumedrol)
		Prednisone (Deltasone)
Co-stimulation blocker	Maintenance	Belatacept (Nulojix)
Interleukin-2 receptor antagonist	Induction	Basiliximab (Simulect)
Mammalian target of rapamycin inhibitors (mTOR)	Maintenance	Everolimus (Zortress)
		Sirolimus (Rapamune)

mTOR is central to cell cycle activation and when inhibited by sirolimus (SRL) or everolimus (EVL), abrogates cell cycle activity.

II. IMMUNOSUPPRESSIVE AGENTS

A. Induction Therapy. Induction therapy is administered during the perioperative period to prevent Tc activation or induce Tc depletion. Current induction therapy is used for high- and low-risk transplant recipients. It allows for modifications in the maintenance regimen, including lowering TAC exposure, corticosteroid withdrawal regimens, and utilization of belatacept for maintenance.

Antibody induction agents include specific antilymphocyte depleting agents or IL-2 receptor antibodies (antagonists) that target Tc. Trials have reported that induction therapy with biologic antibodies plus conventional IS agents is superior to maintenance therapy alone in reducing kidney allograft rejection and allograft failure. These agents can delay initiation of CNIs in delayed graft function and accelerate corticosteroid withdrawal (see Table 28.2).

Infusion-related reactions include flu-like symptoms, GI distress, dizziness, and myalgias.

    1. Antilymphocyte antibodies. These agents deplete Tc to reverse or prevent acute rejection.

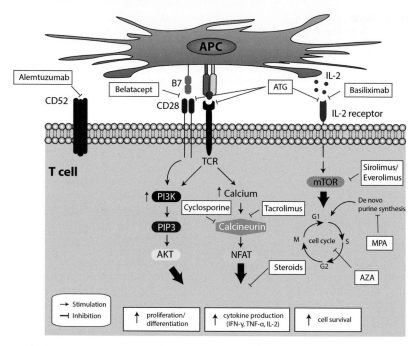

FIGURE 28.1: Illustration of the main mechanisms of action of induction and maintenance immunosuppressive drugs used in kidney transplantation. (From Riella LV, ed. Immunosuppression. In: *Kidney Transplant eBook.* 3rd ed. Apple; 2019:30–65.)

a. **Polyclonal antibodies.** Polyclonal preparations consist of antisera raised in animals. They contain a wide variety of antibodies directed against cluster determinant (CD) 2, CD3, CD4, CD8, CD18, and human leukocyte antigen (HLA) molecules. Two polyclonal lymphocyte-depleting antibodies are available currently: Antithymocyte globulin (rabbit) (rATG) is a polyclonal rabbit-derived antilymphocyte globulin used to treat cellular rejection and for induction. rATG causes Tc depletion, Fc receptor-mediated complement-dependent lysis, opsonization and phagocytosis by macrophages, and immunomodulation with apoptosis. Immune reconstitution may be prolonged over several months. A study reported benefit of giving the initial rATG dose IV at transplant.

b. **Monoclonal antibody.** The monoclonal antibody, alemtuzumab (Campath), is directed against the CD52 receptor. It causes profound lymphocyte depletion followed by immune reconstitution over months to a year.

c. **Anti–interleukin-2 receptor antibody.** The IL-2 receptor antibody, basiliximab, blocks the Signal 3 pathway (Fig. 28.1). Some centers use basiliximab with corticosteroids that may have less adverse effects and late complications than antilymphocyte antibodies, including posttransplant lymphoproliferative disease.

B. **Maintenance Immunosuppression**

1. **Calcineurin Inhibitors—Tacrolimus and Cyclosporine A.** CNIs reduce IL-2 production and receptor expression and thereby reduce Tc activation. The

T A B L E **28.2**	Induction immunosuppression		

Generic name	Depleting/ nondepleting protein	Common dosing	Common adverse events
Alemtuzumab	Depleting	30 mg IV/SC × 1 dose	Infusion-related reactions, myelosuppression
Antithymocyte globulin equine	Depleting	7.5–15 mg/kg/day IV × 3–14 days	Infusion-related reactions, myelosuppression
Antithymocyte globulin rabbit	Depleting	0.75–1.5 mg/kg/day IV × 3–6 days	Infusion-related reactions, myelosuppression
Basiliximab	Nondepleting	20 mg IV × 2 doses	None reported vs. placebo

CNIs block Signal 1. Cyclosporine A (CsA) binds to cyclophilin and TAC to FK-binding protein 12 (FKBP12). A complex is formed that inhibits the phosphatase activity of calcineurin thereby preventing dephosphorylation and subsequent gene transcription for IL-2 resulting in inhibition of T-lymphocyte activation. TAC is 10 to 100 times more potent than CsA. These two CNIs have variable effects and require therapeutic trough level monitoring (see Table 28.3).

a. **Tacrolimus.** The macrolide antibiotic TAC is the most common CNI in practice.

- Dose: This drug has significant variability. Starting doses are 0.1 mg/kg/day given in two divided doses with immediate release TAC, 0.15 to 0.2 mg/kg/day with Astagraf XL and 0.14 mg/kg/day with Envarsus XR. Maintenance doses are adjusted based on trough levels.
- Target trough levels: 0 to 6 months (8 to 10 ng/mL), 6 to 12 months (6 to 8 ng/mL), and after 12 months (4 to 6 ng/mL), if there are no rejection episodes or other complications.
- Metabolism: It is extensively metabolized via hepatic CYP3A4 and CYP3A5.

b. **Cyclosporine A.** This CNI is generally reserved for those who experienced adverse reactions to TAC. *Neoral*, *Gengraf*, and their generics are generally selected.

- Dose: This drug has significant variability. The microemulsion formulation has an oral bioavailability of 30% to 45%. Starting doses of CsA are 6 to 10 mg/kg, given in two divided doses. Maintenance doses are adjusted based on trough levels.
- Target trough level: 0 to 6 months (200 to 250 ng/mL), 6 to 12 months (150 to 200 ng/mL) and after 12 months (80 to 150 ng/mL), if there are no rejection episodes or other complications.
- Metabolism: It is extensively metabolized via hepatic CYP3A4 and CYP3A5. It is highly bound to plasma lipoproteins and to erythrocytes.

c. **Adverse effects of CNIs.** CNIs cause many side effects (see Table 28.3). There is a high incidence of renal allograft damage from interstitial fibrosis and vascular injury that affects >90% of renal transplant patients after 10 years but the frequency may be less with TAC. Kidneys show arteriolar

TABLE 28.3	Common side effects of cyclosporine and tacrolimus		
		Cyclosporine	Tacrolimus
Nephrotoxicity (acute and chronic)		++	++
Renal tubular toxicity ($\uparrow K^+$, $\downarrow Mg^{++}$, $\downarrow HCO_3^-$)		+	+
Hypertension and salt retention		++	+
Hyperuricemia and gout		+	−
Glucose intolerance and post-Tx diabetes		+	++
Hyperlipidemia		++	+
Hirsutism		++	−
Alopecia		−	+
Gingival hypertrophy		+	−
Neurotoxicity (tremor)		+	++
Neurotoxicity (posterior reversible encephalopathy syndrome; PRES)		+	+
Thrombotic microangiopathy		+	+
Liver toxicity (nonprogressive $\uparrow$ LFTs)		+	+/−
Gallstones		+	−
Diarrhea		−	+

mTOR inhibitors—Sirolimus (SRL) and Everolimus (EVL).

hyaline deposits, interstitial fibrosis and tubular atrophy, or "IFTA" (*interstitial fibrosis/tubular atrophy*). There is a progressive decline in GFR that ultimately contributes to graft failure.

Early nephrotoxicity can be related to toxic levels that cause intense afferent arteriolar vasoconstriction thereby reducing the GFR. Fortunately, this is reversible by reducing the dose of the CNI.

   2. mTOR Inhibitors
   a. Sirolimus and Everolimus. SRL is related to TAC. EVL is a metabolite of SRL with similar immunosuppression but a shorter half-life.
   - Mechanism: These also bind to FKBP12 that then irreversibly inhibits mTOR kinase activity that regulates cell growth and proliferation.
   - Dose: SRL single-dose loading is 6 to 12 mg/day followed after 24 hours by a once-daily dose of 1 to 4 mg. EVL is started 0.75 to 1.5 mg twice daily.
   - Target trough levels: Therapeutic drug monitoring is necessary. Both of the mTOR inhibitors can delay graft function, inhibit wound healing, and cause lymphocele formation, pneumonitis, and mucositis. If used early posttransplant a level of 8 to 12 ng/mL is appropriate for either agent. In patients greater than 6 months posttransplant, trough concentrations should range from 3 to 8 ng/mL.
   - Metabolism: Both mTOR inhibitors are absorbed in the upper GI tract, and undergo extensive GI metabolism by CYP3A5 and first-pass metabolism by the CYP3A4 enzyme. Importantly, SRL has a half-life of 60 hours, necessitating a loading dose, but allowing for once-daily dosing. EVL's half-life of approximately 30 hours necessitates twice-daily dosing.

TABLE 28.4	Other adverse effects of mTOR inhibitors
Skin	Skin rashes, acne flares, rash
Edema	Peripheral edema, which may be secondary to an increase urinary protein excretion
Hyperlipidemia	↑TG, ↑Chol; disproportionately high Chol
Thrombotic microangiopathy	Rare
Arthralgia	Unusual
Teratogenic	Avoid in pregnancy and breastfeeding
Interstitial pneumonitis	Occurs in 1–3% and can be life-threatening
Stomatitis, mouth ulcers	With SRL oral solution. Can be painful and debilitating, may respond to topical steroids and topical lidocaine, and lowering drug dose

Their major advantage is their antiproliferative properties that are beneficial in patients with basal cell or squamous cell carcinomas or those with renal cellular carcinoma. They have anti-CMV properties valuable in recurrent CMV disease.

Adverse effects of mTORi (see Table 28.4). The adverse effect profile of SRL and EVL limits their broad use.

i. **Nephrotoxicity.** Nephrotoxicity may entail delayed repair of tubular epithelial injury in patients who receive kidneys with prolonged cold-preservation ischemia times. Proteinuria and glomerulonephropathy have been reported following CNI conversion. Many do not use them in patients with a serum creatinine >2 mg/dL or those with proteinuria.

ii. **Impaired wound healing.** A major concern with mTOR inhibitor therapy is impaired wound healing, wound dehiscence, and infection. Thus, they are rarely used within the first 6 to 12 months following renal transplant.

3. **Antimetabolites**

a. **Azathioprine.** AZA was the initial agent used with steroids for kidney transplantation. Its use currently is reduced because of adverse effects including an increase in squamous cell skin cancers. It is reserved as an alternative MPA.

- Mechanism: AZA is rapidly converted to 6-mercaptopurine and subsequently to 6-thioguanine (6-TG) that is incorporated into replicating DNA to inhibit DNA synthesis and RNA transcription and thereby the replication of rapidly proliferating lymphocytes.
- Dose: Starting dose is 1 to 2 mg/kg once daily.
- Therapeutic monitoring: Clinical monitoring of complete blood counts is warranted.
- Metabolism: Extensively metabolized by xanthine oxidase (XO) and thiopurine methyltransferase (TPMT) that are subject to genetic variants. Slow metabolizers accumulate toxic metabolites causing myelosuppression that can be predicted by testing for TPMT activity. Allopurinol and febuxostat inhibit XO and cause accumulation of AZA metabolites with bone marrow suppression. This contraindicates their use with allopurinol or febuxostat.

- Adverse effects: Myelosuppression is common. It can also cause GI disturbances, pancreatitis, and skin cancer in the long term.
b. **Mycophenolic Acid.** MMF is a prodrug for MPA that is also available as an enteric-coated sodium formulation, EC-MPA.
  - Mechanism: MPA is a noncompetitive inhibitor of inosine monophosphate dehydrogenase (IMPDH) that is the rate-limiting step in the synthesis of purine nucleotides. The resulting depletion of guanine blocks DNA synthesis and lymphocyte proliferation. MPA decreases B-cell and Tc proliferation, suppresses Ab production, and limits monocyte recruitment.
  - Dose: Started at 1,000 mg twice daily. The equimolar dose of EC-MPA is 720 mg twice daily. The dose of MPA may be reduced after 6 to 12 months.
  - Therapeutic monitoring: MPA has significant variability due to variable plasma protein binding, enterohepatic recirculation, renal elimination, genetics, patient age, and drug–drug interactions.
  - Metabolism: MPA is metabolized in the liver to a metabolite that is hydrolyzed back to MPA by enteric flora in the GI tract and reabsorbed via enterohepatic recirculation causing a second peak of blood MPA concentration 4 to 6 hours after dosing that can lead to the prominent lower GI side effects. MPA is extensively protein bound to plasma albumin. Its metabolism is affected by renal function, acidosis, and changes in serum albumin concentration.
  - Adverse effects: Some 30% of patients experience nausea, bloating, crampy abdominal discomfort, or diarrhea and require dose reduction or discontinuation. EC-MPA may provide improved GI tolerability. Myelosuppression can occur.

  MPAs are teratogenic and cause severe developmental abnormalities in early gestation. Thus, they should be stopped well in advance of pregnancy and women of childbearing age should be appraised of their fetal risks. In general, patients can be converted to AZA but this is also teratogenic, but to a lesser extent and is considered the best alternative for pregnant renal transplant recipients.

4. **Corticosteroids.** Although effective, they are also notoriously problematic (see Table 28.5). The use of antilymphocyte antibodies can minimize or allow complete tapering of steroids. Most protocols utilize standard glucocorticoid dosing during the transplant operation and immediately postoperatively, followed by either gradual or rapid taper with complete withdrawal within 90 days.
  - Mechanism: At high doses, they are directly lymphocytic, but, at lower doses, they inhibit Tc and APC-derived cytokine expression and dendritic cell function. They downregulate IL-1, IL-2, IL-3, IL-6, TNF-α, and γ-IFN and adhesion molecules and inhibit monocyte migration to areas of inflammation.
  - Dose: Typically, a bolus of IV methylprednisolone of 100 to 500 mg is given with transplant and tapered over several days to a maintenance dose of approximately 20 mg/day of oral prednisone. Further dose reductions occur over subsequent weeks and months posttransplant, if an early steroid withdrawal protocol is not implemented. Doses of 2.5 to 5 mg/day are commonly used for long-term maintenance. Pulse dose corticosteroids are first-line therapy for the treatment of acute cellular or antibody-mediated rejection.
  - Metabolism: Metabolism occurs via hepatic microsomal enzymes. Levels are not monitored.

TABLE 28.5 Major adverse effects associated with systemic glucocorticoid therapy[a]

Dermatologic and appearance
Skin thinning, purpura, and/or ecchymoses
Weight gain
Cushingoid appearance
Acne
Hirsutism
Facial erythema
Striae

Ophthalmologic
Posterior subcapsular cataract
Elevated intraocular pressure/glaucoma
Exophthalmos

Cardiovascular
Fluid retention
Hypertension
Premature arteriosclerosis
Arrhythmias
Perturbations of serum lipoproteins

Gastrointestinal
Gastritis
Peptic ulcer disease
Steatohepatitis
Visceral perforation

Bone and muscle
Osteoporosis
Avascular necrosis
Myopathy

Neuropsychiatric
Euphoria
Dysphoria/depression
Insomnia
Akathisia
Mania/psychosis
Pseudotumor cerebri

Metabolic and endocrine
Hyperglycemia
Hypothalamic–pituitary–adrenal insufficiency

Immune system
Increased risk of infections[b]

Hematologic
Leukocytosis

The risk of adverse effects is generally dose- and duration-dependent.
[a]High-dose inhaled glucocorticoid therapy can rarely cause systemic adverse effects. Refer to UpToDate content for information on local adverse effects of inhaled glucocorticoids.
[b]Refer to UpToDate content on the effects of glucocorticoids on the immune system.

- Adverse Effects: Corticosteroids are associated with osteoporosis, hyperlipidemia, hypertension, insulin resistance, cataracts, poor wound healing, and growth retardation. Since the leading cause of death among renal transplant recipients is cardiovascular disease, their cardiovascular side effects must be balanced against long-term graft survival.

5. **Co-Stimulation Blockade.** Belatacept is the first IV biologic maintenance IS agent in transplant.
   - Mechanism: Belatacept blocks the CD80 and CD86 ligands on APCs that stimulate CD28 on inactive Tcs during costimulatory interaction (Signal 2; Fig. 28.1). Belatacept has been associated with lower rates of hypertension and dyslipidemia compared to CNIs. Although belatacept improves renal function and reduces donor-specific antibodies, there is an increase in acute rejection. Belatacept proved provide less problems with hypertension and dyslipidemia than CsA.

   Dosing: Dosing regimen is 10 mg/kg on the day of transplantation, followed by repeated doses of increased intervals of doses at 4 days, 2 weeks, and 4. 8 and 12 months posttransplant. After 16 weeks, it is dosed at 5 mg/kg every 4 weeks, requiring an infusion service. Monthly belatacept may have better adherence than daily CNIs. The lack of drug–drug interactions simplifies care of transplant recipients.

   Adverse Effects: The most common adverse effects are infection of the urinary tract and upper respiratory tracts and headache with the infusion. Belatacept may increase CMV and BK virus infection, causes peripheral edema, anemia, leukopenia, hypotension, arthralgia, and insomnia and carries a black-box warning for increased risk of posttransplant lymphoproliferative disorders. Thus, it is often restricted to patients who are immune to Epstein–Barr virus.

III. **CONCLUSION.** Modern IS protocols have achieved excellent success in reducing cellular rejection and improved short-term allograft survival but long-term allograft survival has not changed appreciably. Further understanding of the impact of pharmacogenetics on induction and maintenance immunosuppression should improve survival while research into nongenetic factors may improve precision.

IV. SUGGESTED READINGS

Gabardi S, Martin S, Roberts K, et al. Induction immunosuppressive strategies in renal transplantation. *Am J Health Syst Pharm*. 2011;68:211–218.

Halloran PF. Immunosuppressive drugs for kidney transplantation. *N Engl J Med*. 2004;351:2715–2729.

Kim M, Martin ST, Townsend K, et al. Antibody mediated rejection in kidney transplantation: a review of pathophysiology, diagnosis, and treatment options. *Pharmacotherapy*. 2014;34:733–744.

Lee RA, Gabardi S. Current trends in immunosuppressive therapies for renal transplant recipients. *Am J Health Syst Pharm*. 2012;69:1961–1975.

Oncology Drugs and the Kidney

Chintan V. Shah

INTRODUCTION

Recent advances in anticancer therapy have improved the care of patients with cancer dramatically. The 5-year relative survival rates have increased from 49% (1975–1977) to 69% (2008-2014). However, the improved prognosis combined with better surveillance techniques for the detection of cancer but the exposure to anticancer drugs and drug-related toxicity has increased. The kidneys are primarily at risk for drug toxicity from their role in the excretion of these drugs. We summarize key features of nephrotoxicity of oncology drugs based on site and type of renal injury (Table 29.1).

I. THROMBOTIC MICROANGIOPATHY

A. **Antiangiogenic Drugs.** Angiogenesis is vital for tumor growth. Vascular endothelial growth factor (VEGF) binds to vascular endothelial growth factor receptors (VEFRs) that activate the tyrosine kinase (TK) pathway to promote the growth of capillaries. This is the primary target for antiangiogenic drugs. Anti-VEGF antibodies (e.g., Bevacizumab) and VEGF-trap (decoy-soluble receptors, e.g., aflibercept) bind VEGF ligand whereas anti-VEGF receptor antibodies (e.g., ranibizumab, ramucirumab, axitinib) block VEGF receptors and TKIs (e.g., sunitinib, sorafenib) inhibit the intracellular signaling.

VEGF is released by renal podocytes to activate VEGF receptors on endothelial cells (ECs) that maintain the glomerular filtration barrier. Selective podocyte VEGF gene deletion in mice causes hypertension, proteinuria, and TMA. These are the features of drug toxicity in humans as well.

Hypertension is common and has been related to inhibition of nitric oxide and prostacyclin resulting in vasoconstriction. Hypertension is a mechanism-dependent toxicity reflecting effective inhibition of VEGF signaling and predicts a better tumor response. A retrospective analysis of more than 500 patients with metastatic renal cell carcinoma treated with sunitinib reported that the objective response rate was sixfold greater and median progression-free survival and overall survival more than fourfold longer for patients with sunitinib induced hypertension. Thus, hypertension can be a biomarker of response and should signal the continuation of therapy while implementing measures to control BP. Angiotensin-converting enzyme inhibition or calcium channel blockers are reasonable first-line options.

Proteinuria is the second commonest adverse event. It is a dose-dependent consequence of inhibition of VEGF in podocytes. Proteinuria occurs in 18% to 36% of patients. Mild proteinuria can be controlled with angiotensin-converting

| TABLE 29.1 | Classification of oncology drug-associated nephrotoxicity |

Thrombotic microangiopathy
- Antiangiogenic drugs
- Gemcitabine and mitomycin C

MCD/FSGS
- IFN
- Antiangiogenic drugs

Acute tubular necrosis
- Cisplatin, ifosfamide, pemetrexed
- Mithramycin

Fanconi syndrome
- Cisplatin, ifosfamide

Acute interstitial nephritis
- Immune checkpoint inhibitors
- Antiangiogenic drugs

Crystal nephropathy
- Methotrexate

Channelopathies

Magnesium wasting
- EGFR inhibitors (cetuximab, panitumumab)
- Cisplatin

Salt wasting
- Cisplatin, azacitadine

Nephrogenic diabetes insipidus
- Cisplatin, ifosphamide, pemetrexed

Syndrome of inappropriate diuretic hormone
- Cyclophosphamide, vincristine

MCD, minimal change disease; FSGS, focal segmental glomerulosclerosis; IFN, interferon; EGFR, endothelial growth factor receptors.

enzyme inhibitors or angiotensin receptor blockers while nephrotic syndrome warrants discontinuation of therapy.

Thrombotic microangiopathy (TMA) is the commonest lesion causing nephrotoxicity. The clinical findings include proteinuria worsening renal function and microangiopathic hemolytic anemia (MAHA).

B. Gemcitabine and Mitomycin C. Gemcitabine and mitomycin C can cause TMA. While mitomycin-associated toxicity is dose dependent, the cumulative dose of gemcitabine does not predict toxicity from hemolytic uremic syndrome (HUS). Plasmapheresis is ineffective in most patients with TTP-HUS from either of these drugs but rituximab and eculizumab may have some efficacy.

II. TUBULOPATHIES

A. Cisplatin. Cisplatin (cis-diamminedichloroplatinum II, CDDP) is widely used to treat carcinomas, sarcomas, and lymphomas. Nephrotoxicity is dose dependent and the dose-limiting adverse event observed in 30% to 40% of the patients. Tubular damage from CDDP can cause acute kidney injury (AKI), Fanconi syndrome, salt or magnesium wasting, or nephrogenic diabetes insipidus. Organic cation transporter 2 (OCT2) is required for transport of cisplatin into proximal tubular epithelial cells (PTECs) where it is concentrated fivefold. Thus, serum levels considered to be nontoxic can cause renal toxicity. Magnesium replacement downregulates the expression of OCT2 in PTECs and the risk of nephrotoxicity by fourfold. Magnesium supplementation (2 to 4 g magnesium sulfate) with low-volume hydration (1 to 2 L NS) is used to prevent cisplatin nephrotoxicity.

B. **Ifosfamide.** Ifosfamide is an alkylating agent resembling cyclophosphamide but its major metabolite is far more nephrotoxic. It can cause tubulopathies including proximal tubular injury or Fanconi syndrome, nephrogenic diabetes insipidus or AKI which is usually reversible. Fanconi syndrome is characterized by proximal tubular dysfunction with variable degrees of glucosuria in the setting of normoglycemia, renal phosphate and potassium wasting, proximal renal tubular acidosis, hypouricemia, and aminoaciduria. Nephrotoxicity occurs in about 5% of patients.

C. **Pemetrexed.** Pemetrexed is an antifolate agent resembling methotrexate. While methotrexate causes tubular injury via crystal deposition, pemetrexed directly damages tubules since most of the drug is excreted unchanged in the urine. Pemetrexed is concentrated in proximal tubular cells by apical uptake via folate receptors and/or basolateral uptake via folate carriers. Intracellular accumulation inhibits folate metabolic enzymes and impairs cellular RNA/DNA synthesis, thereby causing tubular injury with ATN, acute interstitial nephritis or nephrogenic diabetes insipidus.

III. **CHANNELOPATHIES. Magnesium wasting** with epithelial growth factor receptor (EGFR) inhibitors (cetuximab, panitumumab).

Magnesium is primarily reabsorbed in the distal nephron. Binding of EGR to EGFR on the basolateral membrane of the distal convoluted tubule (DCT) leads to insertion of TRPM6 channels into the apical membrane that facilitates the reabsorption of magnesium from the urinary space into the cell. The EGFR is overexpressed in several tumors of epithelial origin (e.g., colorectal, head/neck, breast, and lung cancers). Cetuximab is a chimeric monoclonal antibody directed against EGFR and is used in combination with chemotherapy and thereby inhibits magnesium reabsorption. More than one-half of patients develop hypomagnesemia while serum magnesium concentrations decline in almost all. Daily infusions of up to 6 to 10 g of magnesium sulfate are required on occasion to correct the deficit. Hypomagnesemia usually resolves within 4 weeks of discontinuation of cetuximab. Patients developing significant hypomagnesemia often develop hyperkalemia or hypocalcemia due to parathyroid hormone resistance.

IV. **ACUTE INTERSTITIAL NEPHRITIS**

A. **Immune Checkpoint Inhibitors.** Immune checkpoint inhibitors (ICPIs) for targeted immune therapy have revolutionized anticancer treatment. Immune check points maintain the balance between activation and suppression of T-cells. The tumor microenvironment provides a sanctuary for tumor cells by preventing their destruction by T-cells. ICPIs "remove the brakes" and allow the T-cells to attack the cancer cells. These check points include cytotoxic T lymphocyte–associated protein 4 (CTLA-4), programmed cell death protein 1 (PD-1), and PD-ligand 1 (PD-L1). One CTLA-4 inhibitor (ipilimumab), three PD-1 inhibitors (nivolumab, pembrolizumab, cemiplimab), and three PD-L1 inhibitors (atezolizumab, avelumab, durvalumab) have been approved by the Food and Drug Administration.

These drugs cause immune-related adverse events (IrAEs) that include pneumonitis, thyroiditis, and hepatitis but rash and colitis are the most frequent. While extrarenal IrAEs occur in >50% of the patients, the involvement of kidneys occurs in ~2%. AKI, from acute interstitial nephritis (AIN) is the most common renal toxicity. Occasional patients develop acute tubular injury or glomerular lesions.

While ICPI can be continued in patients with stage 1 AKI, it should be discontinued in patients with worse AKI. Glucocorticoids are the mainstay of treatment for AKI from ICPI. Therapy with intravenous pulse-dose corticosteroids (e.g., methylprednisolone 250 to 500 mg daily for 3 days) that is followed by oral prednisone treatment (1 mg/kg per day) may be required for severe AKI. Oral prednisone alone is used for less severe AKI. A slow taper of steroids over 3 to 6 months is required because of the long half-life of ICPIs.

V. CRYSTAL NEPHROPATHY

A. Methotrexate. Methotrexate is a classical antifolate used in a variety of cancers, including acute lymphoblastic leukemia, lymphoma, osteosarcoma. Lethal doses of methotrexate (1,000 to 33,000 mg/m^2) can be used with pharmacokinetically guided leucovorin (LV) rescue. Over 90% of methotrexate is cleared via the kidneys. However, methotrexate and its metabolites are poorly soluble at acidic pH and precipitate as crystals leading to renal damage. Methotrexate-induced renal dysfunction results in sustained, elevated plasma methotrexate concentrations that can cause significant systemic toxicities, including myelosuppression, mucositis, hepatitis, and dermatitis.

An increase in urine pH from 5.0 to 7.0 results in a 10-fold increase in the solubility of methotrexate and its metabolites. Thus, hydration and alkalinization with intravenous D5W with 100 to 150 mEq of sodium bicarbonate per liter should be administered by continuous infusion at 125 to 150 mL/h to maintain urine pH >7, starting 12 hours prior to the initiation of the methotrexate infusion and maintained until plasma levels are below 0.1 microM/L. Even with aggressive hydration and alkalinization, renal dysfunction following high-dose methotrexate occurs occasionally. The recombinant bacterial enzyme carboxypeptidase G2 can decrease plasma methotrexate levels rapidly but its availability is limited. Renal failure is typically nonoliguric and is reversible in almost all cases. Plasma creatinine levels usually peak within the first week and return toward baseline within 1 to 3 weeks.

VI. SUGGESTED READINGS

Eremina V, Jefferson JA, Kowalewska J, et al. VEGF inhibition and renal thrombotic microangiopathy. *N Engl J Med.* 2008;358(11):1129–1136.

Lameire N. Nephrotoxicity of recent anti-cancer agents. *Clin Kidney J.* 2014;7(1):11–22.

Perazella MA. Onco-nephrology: renal toxicities of chemotherapeutic agents. *Clin J Am Soc Nephrol.* 2012;7(10):1713–1721.

Perazella MA, Shirali AC. Immune checkpoint inhibitor nephrotoxicity: what do we know and what should we do? *Kidney Int.* 2020;97(1):62–74.

Volarevic V, Djokovic B, Jankovic MG, et al. Molecular mechanisms of cisplatin-induced nephrotoxicity: a balance on the knife edge between renoprotection and tumor toxicity. *J Biomed Sci.* 2019;26(1):25.

Drug Use in Hypertension and Volume Overload

30 Diuretic Drugs and Resistance

Mohammed A. Alshehri, Christopher S. Wilcox

Thiazide diuretics retain their position as excellent, inexpensive first-line therapy for all categories of mild-to-moderate edema. They are also preferred drugs for hypertension with the established benefit of reducing cardiovascular mortality and lowering stroke events in randomized controlled clinical trials. The eighth report of the Joint National Committee on Prevention, Detection, Evaluation, and Treatment of High Blood Pressure (JNC8) recommends a thiazide, a calcium channel blocker (CCB), an angiotensin-converting enzyme inhibitor (ACEI), or an angiotensin receptor blocker (ARB) as first-line treatment for uncomplicated hypertension. The report recommends thiazides over ACEIs and ARB in Black patients without proteinuria. The 2018 guidelines issued jointly by the European Society of Hypertension and the European Society of Cardiology recommend a combination of ACE inhibitors or ARBs with a thiazide diuretic or CCB as first-line treatment in most patients (see Chapter 23). When compared with an ACE inhibitor (lisinopril) or a CCB (amlodipine) in the ALLHAT study, thiazides had a better outcome in heart failure (vs. amlodipine) and in stroke (vs. lisinopril).

Diuretic therapy for hypertensive patients with normal renal function is usually based on thiazides. Loop diuretics are not effective as antihypertensives because of their short duration of action and postdiuretic renal salt retention, unless given two or three times daily with restriction of dietary salt intake. However, loop diuretics are used to control fluid retention and hypertension in patients with renal failure who become refractory to thiazides.

I. CLASSES OF DIURETICS AND THEIR USES

A. Proximal Tubule Diuretics (See Fig. 30.1)

1. **Carbonic anhydrase inhibitors**. As in all tubular segments, the energy for transport of Na^+ from the lumen into the cell is provided indirectly by the basolateral sodium-potassium adenosine triphosphatase (Na^+/K^+ ATPase). This maintains a low intracellular $[Na^+]$ and a high intracellular $[K^+]$ that establishes a steep negative intracellular potential difference (PD). Luminal exchange of Na^+ for H^+ by the sodium hydrogen exchanger 1 (NHE1) in the proximal tubule (PT) accounts for the reabsorption of >65% of Na^+, bicarbonate, and water. Therefore, carbonic anhydrase inhibitors (CAIs) that prevent Na^+/H^+ exchange impair Na^+, HCO_3^-, and water reabsorption from the PT (Fig. 30.1). Cellular bicarbonate, formed by the action of carbonic anhydrase (CA), exits the cell via the electrogenic basolateral sodium bicarbonate transporter (NBCI). The cellular H^+ that is also formed by the action of CA exits the cell via NHE3 into the tubular lumen where it reacts with filtered HCO_3^- to generate carbonic acid (H_2CO_3). This is metabolized by CA on the luminal brush border membrane to H_2O and CO_2. Thus, the

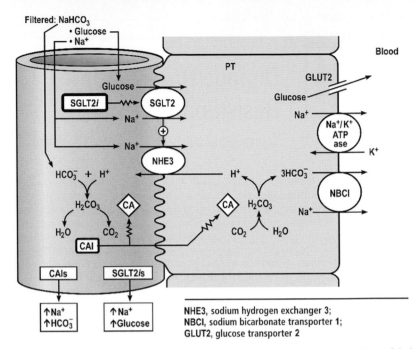

Filtered: NaHCO₃

FIGURE 30.1: Proximal tubule diuretics: Carbonic anhydrase inhibitors (CAIs) and sodium glucose-linked transport inhibitors (SGLT2*is*).

net effect of the combined actions of CA and NHE3 is to reabsorb $NaHCO_3$ from the tubular fluid of the PT to the blood. However, although CAIs cause a brisk diuresis, tolerance develops over a few days because the ensuing loss of HCO_3^- reduces the plasma HCO_3^- concentration below the threshold (about 17 to 19 mmol/L) at which the distal nephron can reabsorb the reduced load of HCO_3^- presented to it from the PT and thereby curtails the diuresis. CAIs are especially effective in patients with high serum levels of HCO_3^- due, for example, to metabolic alkalosis. Escalating doses of loop diuretics induce a metabolic alkalosis that can cause hypoventilation, CO_2 retention, and cardiac arrhythmia. Therefore, CAIs are a rational choice to add to loop diuretics in these circumstances but require careful monitoring.

CAIs are used to treat glaucoma because they reduce the formation of aqueous humor where methazolamide is the preferred agent. CAIs are used prophylactically to prevent high-altitude sickness. Side effects include hypovolemia, metabolic acidosis, or, uncommonly, allergic reactions, hepatitis, blood dyscrasias, and erectile dysfunction. Acetazolamide is the CAI that is used most commonly. It is prescribed as 250 to 500 mg twice daily.

2. **Sodium glucose cotransport 2 inhibitors.** Sodium glucose-linked transporter (SGLT2) is located in the PT where it reabsorbs much of the filtered glucose accompanied by Na^+ (Fig. 30.1). SGLT2 is linked to NHE3. Therefore, sodium glucose transport 2 inhibitors (SGLT2is) inhibit Na^+ reabsorption by SGLT2 and NHE3 and are quite potent diuretics even in patients who are not diabetic and do not have increased glucose concentrations in the

Agent	Dose range (mg)	Dose frequency
Empagliflozin	10–25	q.d.
Canagliflozin	100–300	q.d.
Dapagliflozin	5–10	q.d.

PT fluid. Empagliflozin, canagliflozin, and dapagliflozin are SGLT2is that have been in use for type 2 diabetes (Table 30.1). These drugs reduce blood pressure (BP) and body weight and enhance sodium and water excretion and cause a synergistic diuresis with loop or thiazide diuretics. Therefore, they can be considered PT diuretics. Recent clinical trials have reported not only renal and cardiac protection with SGLT2is but also prevention of recurrent heart failure both in diabetic and nondiabetic patients. Adverse effects include genital infection and normoglycemic ketoacidosis. The three SGLT2is that are available have broadly similar actions (Table 30.1).

B. Loop Diuretics (See Fig. 30.2)

1. **Mechanism of action.** Loop diuretics inhibit the coupled transport of Na^+/K^+/$2Cl^-$ via the sodium-potassium-2-chloride channel (NKCC2) that is expressed on the luminal membrane of the thick ascending limb (TAL) of the loop of Henle (LH) where 20% to 25% of filtered sodium is reabsorbed. Therefore, they are the most powerful diuretics. Again, the energy for the uptake of

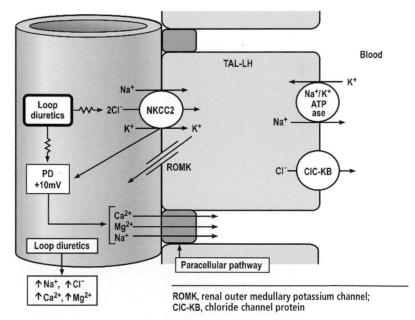

FIGURE 30.2: Loop diuretics: Inhibition of the sodium potassium two chloride transporter 2 (NKCC2) and the lumen-positive potential difference (PD).

luminal Na^+ into the cell derives from the basolateral Na/K ATPase that maintains a low intracellular $[Na^+]$ (Fig. 30.2). The Cl^- transported by NKCC2 exits the basolateral membrane by the chloride channel protein (CLC-KB). The K^+ transported by NKCC2 is secreted via the renal outer medullary potassium channel (ROMK) back into the tubular fluid, thereby setting up a futile cycle for K^+ without net transport across the cell. The outcome is the reabsorption of one Na^+ and two Cl^-. This is therefore effectively electrogenic transport and creates a lumen-positive PD that drives the paracellular transport of Na^+, Ca^{2+}, and Mg^{2+}. Therefore, loop diuretics that inhibit NKCC2 reduce the reabsorption of Na^+, Cl^-, and also of Ca^{2+} and Mg^{2+}. Accordingly, they can be used to treat acute hypercalcemia, and can cause hypomagnesemia. Loop diuretics, when administered acutely, can increase prostaglandin secretion. This can cause venodilation that reduces preload in patients with left ventricular failure, but leads to renin secretion.

2. **Pharmacokinetics.** Loop diuretics are bound strongly to albumin and therefore are not filtered. They are transported into the tubular lumen via an organic anion transporter (OAT) located on the basolateral membrane of PT cells. Other organic anions, that include nonsteroidal anti-inflammatory agents; antiviral agents such as adefovir, methotrexate; and a number of endogenous organic anions such as urate, compete with diuretics for transport by OAT. During renal insufficiency, a reduction in renal blood flow reduces the delivery of loop diuretics to the kidney while an increase in organic acids such as urate impairs their secretion via OAT. These together account for the requirement for increased doses of loop diuretics in patients with chronic kidney disease (CKD). Moreover, protein binding is required for secretion by OAT. Therefore, hypoalbuminemia is a cause of diuretic resistance (see Diuretic Resistance).

3. **Clinical use.** Loop diuretics increase the renal excretion of Na^+, free water, K^+, Ca^{++}, Mg^{++}, and H^+. They are the diuretics of choice for severe edema and for refractory hypertension in patients with a GFR <35 mL/min. They are useful to correct hyperkalemia in CKD. Most patients suffering from congestive heart failure (CHF) require treatment with a loop diuretic to control fluid overload.

Randomized placebo-controlled trials in patients with acute renal injury (AKI) have reported that loop diuretics can sometimes increase urine output but do not affect renal recovery, death, or the need for dialysis. Therefore, loop diuretics for patients with AKI should be reserved for those with volume overload.

4. **Individual agents.** The five available loop diuretics differ in oral bioavailability, half-life, and metabolism (Table 30.2). Bumetanide and torsemide are preferred in renal failure because they are metabolized mainly by the liver and are more predictable in their action than furosemide. Moreover, torsemide has a less variable bioavailability than furosemide and is less likely to cause hypokalemia. Therefore, many consider torsemide to be the loop diuretic of choice for patients with heart failure. Soaanz is an extended release formulation of torsemide with a more gradual, less abrupt diuresis useful in patients with overactive bladder (OAB). Ethacrynic acid lacks a sulfhydryl moiety and therefore it is used for patients who become allergic to loop or thiazide diuretics. Ceiling doses shown in Table 30.2 are the maximal effective once daily dose for subjects without azotemia and should not normally be exceeded, although the dose can be given twice daily for refractory patients. Oral or intravenous ceiling doses can be increased up to twofold for patients with GFR <30 mL/min or severe heart failure.

TABLE 30.2	Loop diuretics				
Agent	Duration (h)	Equivalent oral dose (mg)	Metabolism	Ceiling dose (mg)	Infusion dose (mg/h)
Bumetanide	2–4	1	L > K	4	0.5–1.0
Ethacrynic acid	3–6	25	L > K	100	5–20
Furosemide	3–6	20	K > L	80	5–40
Soaanz	8–12	10	L > K	40	N/A
Torsemide	5–8	10	L > K	40	5–20

Note: Equivalent doses are compared with 1 mg of oral bumetanide. Ceiling doses are maximally effective doses in subjects without azotemia or severe heart failure.
>; is greater than, K; kidney, L; liver, N/A; not applicable.

5. **Adverse effects.** Prerenal azotemia is more common when loop diuretics are used in combination with thiazides (Table 30.3). Hypokalemia and alkalosis can be prevented or treated by prescribing KCl or a potassium-sparing diuretic or mineralocorticosteroid receptor antagonist (MRA). Ototoxicity is a risk in patients with CKD given high doses of intravenous loop diuretics.

C. **Thiazides and Distal Convoluted Tubule Diuretics (See Fig. 30.3).** Thiazide diuretics, and the thiazide-like distal convoluted tubule (DCT) diuretics such as chlorthalidone, act in the early DCT by blocking the coupled Na^+/Cl^- cotransporter via sodium chloride cotransporter (NCC) that is expressed at the luminal membrane, where 3% to 5% of filtered Na^+ and a significant fraction of free water are reabsorbed (Fig. 30.3). Again, the energy for this uptake of Na^+ from the tubular lumen derives from the basolateral Na^+/K^+ ATPase that maintains a low intracellular $[Na^+]$. The K^+ pumped into the cell via Na^+/K^+ ATP provides a lumen-negative PD. This drives the reabsorption of Ca^{2+} via the transient receptor potential V5 (TRPV5) and of Mg^{2+} via the TRPM6. Ca^{2+} exits the cell at the basolateral membrane in exchange for Na^+ via the sodium calcium exchanger

TABLE 30.3	Adverse effects of loop diuretics	
Adverse effect	**Prevention or treatment**
Hypokalemia	KCl, potassium-sparing diuretic, or MRA
Hypomagnesemia	MgO_2
Metabolic alkalosis	KCl, potassium-sparing diuretic, MRA, or carbonic anhydrase inhibitor
Hyperuricemia	Allopurinol
Impotence	Sildenafil
Ototoxicity	Reduce dose, change to oral route
Prerenal azotemia	Hold diuretic, volume repletion
Hyperglycemia	Potassium-sparing diuretic or MRA
Hyperlipidemia	Statins
Allergy	Switch to ethacrynic acid
Hyponatremia	Restrict free water intake

MRA; mineralocorticosteroid receptor antagonist.

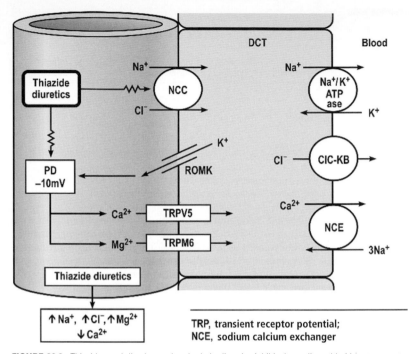

FIGURE 30.3: Thiazides and distal convoluted tubule diuretics inhibit the sodium chloride cotransporter (NCC) and the reabsorption of magnesium but enhance the reabsorption of calcium.

(NCE). The pathway for cellular exit of Mg^{2+} is not established. Blockade of NCC by thiazides reduces the intracellular $[Na^+]$ and the activity of Na^+/K^+ ATPase. The outcome is a reduced K^+ secretion via ROMK and a reduced lumen-negative PD that reduces the driving force for the reabsorption of Mg^{2+}. However, the reduced intracellular $[Na^+]$ during thiazide therapy increases the basolateral $3Na^+/Ca^{2+}$ exchange via the NCE and thereby increases net Ca^{2+} reabsorption. Thiazide diuretics impair urinary dilution because they impair solute removal from dilute tubular fluid, but they do not affect urinary concentrating capacity. Thus, they are prone to cause hyponatremia. They may also cause hypokalemia, metabolic alkalosis, and hypomagnesemia, but, in contrast to loop diuretics, thiazides reduce renal Ca^{2+} excretion and are used to reduce the reoccurrence of nephrolithiasis.

Thiazides are among the drugs of first choice for uncomplicated essential hypertension. They are useful for the treatment of mild edema and as additions to loop diuretics for refractory edema (see Diuretic Resistance). Thiazide diuretics have a greater antihypertensive effect than loop diuretics in patients with preserved renal function because of their longer duration of action. Higher doses of thiazides are needed in renal insufficiency. Thiazides usually have to be changed to loop diuretics at a GFR <35 mL/min. Commonly used thiazides are shown in Table 30.4.

Adverse effects of thiazides include glucose intolerance, hypokalemic metabolic alkalosis, and hyperuricemia. Hypokalemia and alkalosis with

| | Thiazide diuretics | | |

TABLE 30.4

Agent	Dose range (mg)	Dose interval	Duration of action (h)
Bendrofluazide	2.5–10	q.d.	Long
Chlorothiazide	250–1,000	b.i.d.	6–12
Chlorthalidone	25–100	q.d.	Up to 72
Cyclopenthiazide	25–100	q.d.	Long
Hydrochlorothiazide	12.5–100	q.d.	6–12
Hydroflumethiazide	50–100	q.d.	36
Indapamide	1.25–5	q.d.	24
Metolazone	1–10	q.d.	Up to 24
Mefruside	25	q.d.	Long
Polythiazide	0.5–4	q.d.	36

loop diuretics or thiazides are caused by increased delivery and reabsorption of Na^+ to the collecting ducts and by stimulation of the renin–angiotensin–aldosterone system (RAAS). Both of these actions enhance K^+ and H^+ secretion by the collecting ducts. Hyperuricemia is secondary to competition of urate with diuretics for proximal secretion by OAT. Glucose intolerance is largely due to impaired insulin release and impaired glucose uptake from hypokalemia. The combination of a thiazide with an ACE inhibitor, an ARB, a distal K^+-sparing diuretic, or an MRA reduces the risk of hypokalemia and carbohydrate intolerance. Treatment of mild asymptomatic hyperuricemia probably is not necessary, but gout requires specific therapy and, where possible, discontinuation of diuretic therapy. Thiazides inhibit free water excretion and can cause serious hyponatremia, which is most commonly observed in elderly women. Hyponatremia entails decreased free water excretion because of thiazide-induced failure to dilute the urine during maintained free water intake. However, some subjects develop recurrent thiazide-dependent hyponatremia from a genetic polymorphism of a prostaglandin transporter that causes the accumulation of prostaglandin E_2 (PGE_2) in the lumen of the distal nephron. PGE_2 enhances the action of arginine vasopressin (AVP) to increase free water reabsorption. Hyponatremia is less common with loop diuretics because they block both the urinary diluting and the urinary concentrating mechanisms. In fact, loop diuretics can be used to treat hyponatremia, when combined with hypertonic saline, for the syndrome of inappropriate antidiuretic hormone.

D. **Potassium-Sparing Diuretics and Mineralocorticosteroid Receptor Antagonists (See Fig. 30.4).** The aldosterone-sensitive distal nephron, comprising the late DCT, the connecting tubule (CNT), and the cortical collecting duct (CCD), reabsorbs only 1% to 3% of filtered Na^+, but it is the primary site for the secretion of the positively charged ions K^+ and H^+. Their secretion is driven by a steep lumen-negative electrical gradient caused by the reabsorption of the positively charged Na^+ via the epithelial sodium channel ($E_{Na}C$) without an accompanying anion (Fig. 30.4). Again, the energy for cellular Na^+ uptake from the tubular fluid derives from the basolateral Na^+/K^+ ATPase that maintains a low intracellular $[Na^+]$. The cellular K^+ transported by Na^+/K^+ ATPase is secreted into the tubular fluid by ROMK while the cellular H^+ is secreted by a luminal H^+ ATPase or H^+/K^+ ATPase. The activities of both transporters are enhanced by the lumen-negative PD.

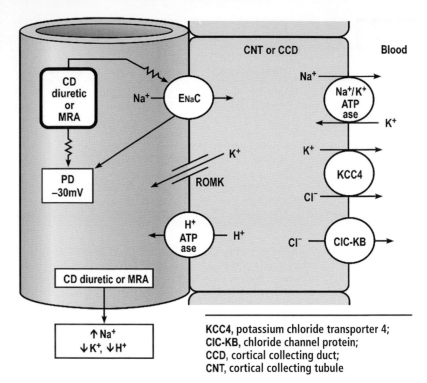

FIGURE 30.4: Collecting duct (CD) or potassium-sparing diuretics and mineralocorticosteroid receptor antagonists (MRAs) inhibit sodium reabsorption by the epithelial sodium channel (ENaC) and thereby the lumen-negative potential difference (PD) that drives the secretion of potassium and hydrogen ions.

Therefore, diuretics that block $E_{Na}C$ reduce the lumen-negative PD and thereby reduce the tubular secretion of K^+ and H^+. Two groups of diuretics act predominantly at this site. Amiloride and triamterene block $E_{Na}C$ directly whereas spironolactone, eplerenone and finerenone are MRAs that reduce the expression and activity of $E_{Na}C$. Potassium-sparing diuretics are most often used to prevent or treat hypokalemic metabolic alkalosis that has been provoked by loop or thiazide diuretics. MRAs also are used for the treatment of primary hyperaldosteronism, cirrhosis with ascites, or nephrotic syndrome. An important additional use for MRAs is to reduce mortality in patients with heart failure with reduced ejection fraction even in those receiving ACE inhibitors or ARBs. MRAs are recommended as fourth-line therapy for patients with drug-resistant hypertension. They reduce the severity of obstructive sleep apnea.

Amiloride is excreted by the kidney in active form, whereas triamterene is partly metabolized by the liver and accumulates in patients with cirrhosis. Spironolactone is metabolized to canrenoate that is active over 72 hours. Side effects of all these distal agents include hyperkalemia and metabolic acidosis. This is a special risk in patients with CKD or when used with ACE inhibitors, ARBs, or NSAIDs that predispose to these conditions. Spironolactone has antiandrogenic and proprogestogenic actions that, when used in high doses or for prolonged periods of time may cause impotence, loss of libido, and painful

TABLE 30.5	Distal potassium-sparing diuretics and mineralocorticosteroid receptor antagonists (MCAs)				
Agent	**Dose range (mg)**	**Dose interval**	**Duration of action (h)**	**Other info**
Amiloride	5–20	q.d.	Up to 24	—
Triamterene	50–100	b.i.d.	7–9	—
Spironolactone	12.5–100	q.d.	24–72	MRA
Eplerenone	50–100	q.d.	12–24	MRA

gynecomastia in men and irregular menses or postmenopausal bleeding in women. These effects often limit the use of spironolactone to doses >25 mg daily. Eplerenone and finerenone lacks these off-target effects.

Available agents are listed in Table 30.5.

E. Osmotic Diuretics. Mannitol is an osmotic diuretic that is freely filtered by the glomerulus but is not reabsorbed. Therefore, it provides an osmotic gradient that prevents fluid reabsorption and causes a rapid increase in the excretion of fluid, Na^+, K^+, and other ions. Mannitol is used to treat cerebral edema because it does not penetrate the blood–brain barrier. Trials in patients with acute kidney injury generally report that mannitol is no more effective than hydration alone in preserving renal function (see Chapter 27). Side effects include hypernatremia, hyperkalemia, acidosis, and intravascular volume expansion that occur in patients with renal failure who cannot eliminate it.

F. Other Newer Diuretics

1. **Natriuretic peptides and neutral endopeptidase inhibitors.** Atrial or brain natriuretic peptides enhance Na^+ and fluid excretion, promote vasodilation, and increase the glomerular filtration rate (GFR). They act primarily in the glomerulus and the medullary collecting tubule. Nesiritide is a recombinant brain-type natriuretic peptide that was approved for use in patients with decompensated CHF. However, the ASCEND-HF trial failed to document benefits from nesiritide and it led to a higher incidence of hypotension. Since natriuretic peptides are degraded by neutral endopeptidase inhibitors increase their plasma levels and cause natriuresis. Vasopeptidase inhibitors block neutral endopepidase, ACE, and bradykinin. Entresto is a combination tablet of valsartan with a vasopeptidase inhibitor, sacubitril. Entresto causes marked vasodilation and reduction in BP. It is licensed for the treatment of heart failure with reduced ejection fraction (HFrEF). Currently, renal actions have not been studied extensively. Its inhibition of bradykinin breakdown predisposes to angioedema with ACE inhibitors that are therefore contraindicated in conjunction with Entresto.

2. **Aquaretics.** Arginine vasopressin (AVP) type 2 (V2) receptor antagonists such as tolvaptan are therapeutic agents for euvolemic and hypervolemic hyponatremia (see Chapter 17). They block the binding of AVP to the V2 receptor on the basolateral membrane of collecting duct cells and are therefore aquaretics rather than diuretics. The vasopressin V2 receptor activates guanyl cyclase that is implicated in renal cyst growth, thereby providing a rationale for the use of tolvaptan in patients with autosomal dominant polycystic kidney disease (ADPKD). Recent trials report that the progression of renal cyst growth and renal dysfunction in patients with ADPKD can be slowed by tolvaptan (see Chapter 14). Adverse effects include volume depletion and hepatotoxicity.

APPROACH TO DIURETIC THERAPY

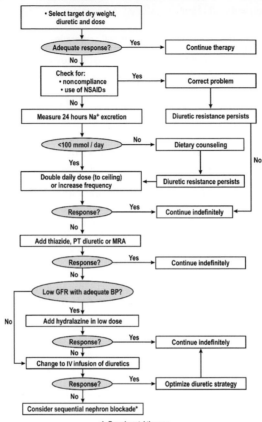

FIGURE 30.5: Algorithm for the management of diuretic resistance. GFR; glomerular filtration rate, NSAIDs; nonsteroidal anti-inflammatory drugs.

II. DIURETIC RESISTANCE AND ITS MANAGEMENT (SEE FIG. 30.5). Diuretic resistance implies persistent edema or congestion requiring treatment in a patient receiving a ceiling dose of a loop diuretic. The approach is outlined in Fig. 30.5.

The evaluation starts by the differentiation of renal edema from lymphatic or venous obstruction, idiopathic edema, or a complication of therapy, such as with a CCB or an NSAID. The first step is to establish a target dry weight and select a diuretic. There can be many components to diuretic resistance as follows:

1. *Nonadherence.* Therapy with a loop or thiazide diuretic almost invariably reduces the serum potassium and increases the plasma bicarbonate and urate concentrations. Therefore, failure to detect these changes suggests nonadherence. Resistance to diuretics can be a consequence of a failure to adhere to a restriction of sodium intake (<2 to 3 g or 80 to 120 mmol/day). Sodium and potassium intakes can be quantified from a 24-hour urine (corrected for incomplete collection by creatinine excretion), even in

patients receiving regular diuretic therapy. Non-adherence is a special problem for patients with overactive bladder (OAB) who may benefit from the equally effective but gentler diuresis with Soaanz that is an extended formulation of torsemide.

2. *Pharmacokinetic or pharmacodynamic limitations.* Diuretic absorption may be incomplete in uncompensated edema because of poor intestinal blood flow. These patients may respond better to intravenous administration of a loop diuretic.

3. *"Braking phenomenon."* After a few days (depending on the degree of edema), a brake develops on the progressive loss of NaCl and fluid and a new steady state is achieved when losses match intake and body weight stabilizes. The first step in treating edema or congestion in a patient who is not responding to a daily dose of furosemide is to use more frequent dosing or a continuous intravenous infusion.

4. *Tachyphylaxis.* During prolonged use of loop diuretics for resistant edema, the cells of the distal nephron become hypertrophic. This enhances their capacity to reabsorb Na^+ and Cl^- and thereby prevents the loop diuretic from increasing Na^+ and fluid excretion. This is best treated by the addition of a thiazide or a potassium-sparing diuretic that block the enhanced reabsorption at these sites.

5. *Hypoalbuminemia.* Severe hypoalbuminemia causes diuretic resistance by increasing the volume of distribution of the diuretic (decreased plasma protein binding) and thereby reducing its delivery to the kidney, inhibiting the secretion of the diuretic by the OAT transporter in the PT, promoting the metabolism of furosemide within the tubular cells, and enhancing NaCl reabsorption in the collecting ducts. However, diuretic resistance rarely responds to albumin infusions and this can cause hypertension, heart failure, and nephropathy. Nephrotic patients should receive an ACE inhibitor or an ARB to minimize proteinuria.

6. *Segmental nephron blockade.* The upregulation of renal transporters at other sites underlies much of diuretic resistance and the development of hypokalemia and alkalosis. Therefore, segmental nephron blockade with multiple diuretics used together is being explored to manage severe diuretic resistance. Recently, a combination of loop diuretics plus PT and DT diuretics, an MRA, an aquaretic (tolvaptan), and KCl given to patients with CHF and severe diuretic resistance have been reported to induce a remarkable daily fluid and Na^+ loss with no significant changes in serum electrolytes or creatinine. This therapy is experimental presently.

7. *Ultrafiltration.* Patients who are resistant to these approaches may require plasma ultrafiltration ("aquapheresis") to remove excessive extracellular fluid, but the expense combined with a failure to demonstrate superior outcomes to intensive diuretic therapy have limited enthusiasm presently.

III. SUGGESTED READINGS

Hoorn EJ, Wilcox CS, Ellison DH. Diuretics. In: Brenner BM, ed. *Brenner & Rector's The kidney*. 11th ed. Saunders; 2020:1708–1740.

Roush GC, Sica DD. Diuretics for hypertension: a review and update. *Am J Hypertens*. 2016; 29(10):1130–1137.

Wilcox CS. Antihypertensive and renal mechanisms of SGLT2 (sodium-glucose linked transporter 2) inhibitors. *Hypertension*. 2020;75(4):894–901.

Wilcox CS, Testani JM, Pitt, B. Pathophysiology of diuretic resistance and its implications for the management of chronic heart failure. *Hypertension*. 2020;76(4):1045–1054.

31 Alpha- and Beta-Blockers and Sympatholytics

Christopher S. Wilcox

Beta-blockers and diuretics once were considered equivalent in reducing cardiovascular mortality in patients with hypertension (primary prevention). However, the role of beta-blockers as first-line therapy has been questioned because of adverse metabolic effects (such as glucose intolerance), a spectrum of other adverse effects, and apparent inferiority, at least for the cardioselective agent atenolol, in the prevention of stroke. Newer beta-blockers might address these concerns. However, beta-blockers retain certain specific and important roles. For example, many trials have reported that they reduce the probability of reinfarctions in patients with a myocardial infarction (MI) and have benefit in treatment of patients with heart failure (HF) and reduced ejection fraction (HFrEF) (secondary prevention). Alpha-blockers inhibit peripheral vasoconstriction. Although effective in reducing blood pressure (BP), they frequently require coadministration of another agent (beta-blocker and diuretic) for sustained efficacy and have not been successful as in single-drug therapy in preventing HF or progression of CKD in the Antihypertensive and Lipid Lowering Treatment to Prevent Heart Attack (ALLHAT) trial. Thus, they are considered presently as fourth-line antihypertensive agents. However, combined alpha- and beta-blockers such as carvedilol or labetalol are very effective in lowering BP and are useful especially in resistant hypertension or hypertensive emergencies (see Chapter 24). Central sympatholytics are agonists of the alpha2-receptor. They are among the oldest antihypertensives, and are very effective in reducing BP, but patients often suffer from adverse effects especially at high dosage. Alpha-methyldopa is well studied for the treatment of hypertension in pregnancy (see Chapter 25).

I. BETA-BLOCKERS

A. Mechanism of Action. Beta-blockers antagonize the effects of the sympathetic nervous system by competing with epinephrine and norepinephrine for beta-receptors on target organs. Beta1-receptors predominate in the heart and in the renin-containing cells of the renal afferent arteriole, whereas beta2-receptors are located primarily in the bronchioles and vascular smooth muscle cells. Beta-blockers are nonselective when they block both subtypes and selective when they block only beta1-receptors. Both classes of beta-blockers lower BP by decreasing cardiac output, decreasing sympathetic outflow from the brain, and inhibiting renin release from the juxtaglomerular apparatus in the kidney. Selective beta-blockers are less prone to induce bronchospasm. Beta-blockers with intrinsic sympathomimetic activity (ISA) cause less bradycardia, or metabolic disturbances. Table 31.1 provides details of individual agents. Table 31.2 lists the adverse effects commonly associated with their use. Carvedilol and labetalol are two nonselective beta-blockers that also have alpha1-receptor–blocking

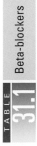

TABLE
31.1 Beta-blockers

Agent	ISA	Half-life (h)	Elimination	Maximal daily dose (mg)	Usual dosage (mg) GFR >50	GFR 10–50	GFR <10
Nonselective							
Nadolol		20–24	K	320	40–240	50%	25%
Penbutolol	+	17–24	K	80	20–40	50%	25%
Pindolol	+	3–11	L	60	10–40 b.i.d.	No change	50%
Proparanolol[a]		3–4	L	640	40–120 b.i.d.	No change	No change
Timolol		3–4	L	60	20–40 b.i.d.	No change	No change
Beta-1-selective							
Acebutolol	+	10	L	1,200	400–800	50%	30–50%
Atenolol		14–16	K	200	50–100	50%	30–50%
Betaxolol		14–22	L	40	10–40	No change	50%
Bisoprolol		9–12	K = L	20	5–20 q.d.	75%	50%
Esmolol		9 min	Red blood cells	7.2 mg/kg		No change	No change
Metoprolol[a]		3–7	K	400	100–200	No change	50%
Beta/alpha							
Carvedilol[a]		7–10	L	50	6.25–25 b.i.d.	No change	No change
Labetalol		3–4	L	2,400	100–600 t.i.d.	No change	No change

Dose for GFR indicates percentage of usual dose for patients with these levels of GFR (mL/min).

[a]Sustained-release formulation is available for once-daily dosing.

GFR, glomerular filtration rate; K, kidney; L, liver; ISA, intrinsic sympathomimetic activity.

TABLE 31.2	More frequent adverse effects of beta-blockers

Bradycardia
Depression
Malaise
Decreased exercise capacity
Bronchospasm
Hyperkalemia
Sexual dysfunction
Increase risk of diabetes
Increased triglycerides
Claudication
Raynaud's phenomenon
Sleep disturbance

properties and vasodilator actions (Table 31.1). Carvedilol has significant antioxidant effects. Both are often effective in the elderly, African Americans, and in patients with low- renin hypertension in whom beta-blockers often have little antihypertensive effect. Combined alpha- and beta-blockers are also useful in treating hypertension associated with catecholamine excess such as cocaine intoxication or pheochromocytoma. Nebivolol and celiprolol (not available in the United States) have vasodilator properties related to vascular nitric oxide generation (Table 31.3).

B. **Pharmacokinetics.** The various beta-blockers differ widely in oral bioavailability, hepatic first-pass metabolism, and route of elimination. Agents that have significant renal elimination require a dose reduction in renal failure. Beta-blockers that are hydrophilic may have less blood–brain barrier penetrance and, therefore, fewer central nervous system side effects. See Tables 31.1 and 31.3 for dosage suggestions for individual agents.

C. **Indications and Contraindications.** Beta-blockers are indicated for the treatment of hypertension in patients with coronary artery disease or those that have had an MI or those with HFrEF. A comprehensive meta-analysis published in *Lancet* in 2005 concluded that beta-blockers, compared with other antihypertensive

TABLE 31.3	Beta-blockers with vasodilator properties

Agent	α activity	β blocking	Elimination	Maximum daily dosage (mg)	Usual dose (mg) GFR >50	10–50	NO generation
Celiprolol	α2 agonist	β1	K	200	200	100	+
Nebivolol		β1	L	20	5 b.i.d.	2.5 b.i.d.	++

Labetalol and carvedilol are alpha–beta blockers with significant vasodilator properties (Table 31.1).
NO, nitric oxide; K, kidney; L, liver.

TABLE 31.4	Coincident diseases that may benefit from treatment with beta-blockers

Migraine (prophylaxis)
Supraventricular tachycardia
Angina
Essential tremor
Preoperative cardiovascular protection
Congestive heart failure with reduced ejection fraction
Thyrotoxicosis
Vasovagal syncope
Palpitations

agents, are associated with an increased risk of stroke of 16%. This relates especially to the cardioselective agent atenolol, whose use in the Losartan Intervention for Endpoint (LIFE) study of patients with left ventricular hypertrophy was associated with a greater cardiovascular mortality and a greater rate of stroke than those randomized to the angiotensin receptor blocker (ARB), losartan. Accordingly, some national advisory committees, including the JNC8, no longer recommend beta-blockers as first-line therapy for uncomplicated hypertension. However, other trials have shown that beta-blockers decrease perioperative MI and mortality in patients at risk for coronary artery disease, and reinfarction in those with a prior myocardial infarction. To date, three beta-blocking drugs—carvedilol, bisoprolol, and metoprolol—have been shown to improve mortality in patients with moderate heart failure with reduced ejection fraction (HFrEF). The protective mechanism is most likely due to a decrease in ventricular arrhythmias, improved diastolic relaxation, and protection from cardiac remodeling.

For concomitant diseases that may be treated with beta-blockers, see Table 31.4. Nonselective beta-blockers are contraindicated in patients with asthma. Relative contraindications to the use of beta-blockers include mild cardiac conduction abnormalities, asymptomatic bradycardia, and severe peripheral vascular disease.

II. **ALPHA-BLOCKERS.** Alpha-blockers antagonize the effects of the sympathetic nervous system by competing with epinephrine and norepinephrine for postsynaptic alpha1-receptors on resistance vessels. The net effect is a decrease in peripheral vascular resistance. Selective alpha1-blockers have no affinity for presynaptic alpha2-receptors, and thereby cause little reflex tachycardia or increase cardiac output. Moderately selective alpha-blockers retain some affinity for the presynaptic alpha2-receptors, which results in an increase in local norepinephrine release by sympathetic nerve endings and an increase in heart rate and cardiac output. Table 31.5 lists the various agents.

The selective alpha-blockers are considered fourth-line agents for the treatment of hypertension but are widely used to improve the obstructive symptoms of benign prostatic hypertrophy. Selective alpha-blockers are associated with a profound hypotensive effect when the first dose is taken. Administration of a low initial dose at nighttime while lying and a gradual uptitration of dosage are recommended. All of the selective alpha-blockers are associated with a decrease in triglycerides, total cholesterol, and low-density lipoprotein,

Alpha-blockers

Agent	Half-life	Metabolism	Initial dosage (mg)	Daily dose range (mg)
Selective				
Doxazosin	9–22 h	Liver	1 q.d.	1–16
Prazosin	2–4 h	Liver	1 b.i.d.	2–20
Terazosin	12 h	Liver	1 q.d.	1–20
Moderately selective				
Phenoxybenzamine	24 h	Liver	10 b.i.d.	20–120
Phentolamine	19 min	Liver	5 IV PRN	—

with a concomitant increase in high-density lipoprotein. Moderately selective alpha-blockers are used mainly for the treatment or perioperative management of pheochromocytoma, in which alpha-blockade should precede beta-blockade to prevent paradoxical hypertension.

III. CENTRAL SYMPATHOLYTIC AGENTS

A. Central Sympatholytic Agents. Alpha2-agonists reduce sympathetic outflow from the brain by binding to pre- and postsynaptic alpha-2 receptors in the midbrain and medulla. Consequently, they reduce plasma catecholamines, peripheral vascular resistance, and heart rate. Table 31.6 lists the various agents.

Common side effects of these agents include sedation, dry mouth, and depression. Alpha-methyldopa can cause hypersensitivity reactions, hepatitis, and Coombs-positive hemolytic anemia. Abrupt withdrawal from clonidine can cause severe rebound hypertension that is accentuated by beta-blockers. Clonidine is available as a skin patch (Catapres-TTS) that provides a steady drug delivery over 1 week. The patch is useful in noncompliant patients and in those who cannot take medication orally. Alpha-methyldopa has been the most widely studied agent in pregnancy. It is considered a first-line agent for pregnancy-associated hypertensive disorders. Both alpha-methyldopa and guanfacine carry a pregnancy category B rating from the U.S. Food and Drug

Central sympatholytic agents

Agent	Half-life (h)	Metabolism	Initial dosage (mg)	Daily dose range (mg)
Catapres-TTS		L = K	TTS-1 is equivalent to 0.1 mg t.i.d.	1–3 qwk
Clonidine	6–23	L = K	0.1 t.i.d.	0.2–1.2
Guanabenz	7–10	L	4 b.i.d.	8–64
Guanfacine	12–24	L = K	1 q.d.	1–3
a-Methyldopa	6–23	L	250 b.i.d.	500–3,000

K, kidney; L, liver, TTS transdermal patch.

Administration, whereas all other antihypertensives are considered category C or D (see Chapter 25).

IV. SUGGESTED READINGS

ALLHAT Officers and Coordinators for the ALLHAT Collaborative Research Group. The Antihypertensive and Lipid-Lowering Treatment to Prevent Heart Attack Trial. Major outcomes in high-risk hypertensive patients randomized to angiotensin-converting enzyme inhibitor or calcium channel blocker vs diuretic: the Antihypertensive and Lipid-Lowering Treatment to Prevent Heart Attack Trial (ALLHAT). *JAMA*. 2002;288(23):2981–2997.

Chang TI, Beddu S, Chertow GM. Antihypertensive therapy. In: Brenner BM, ed. *The Kidney*. 11th ed. WB Saunders; 2020:1654–1707.

Khan N, McAlister FA. Re-examining the efficacy of beta blockers for the treatment of hypertension: a meta analysis. *CMAJ*. 2006;174(12):1737–1742.

Lindholm LH, Carlberg B, Samuelsson O. Should beta blockers remain first choice in the treatment of primary hypertension? A meta-analysis. *Lancet*. 2005;366(9496):1545–1553.

Wiysonge C, Bradley H, Mayosi B, et al. Beta-blockers for hypertension. *Cochrane Database Syst Rev*. 2007;24(1):CD002003.

32

Angiotensin-Converting Enzyme Inhibitors, Angiotensin Receptor Blockers, Renin Antagonists and Mineralocorticosteroid Receptor Antagonists

Christopher S. Wilcox

I. **RENIN–ANGIOTENSIN–ALDOSTERONE SYSTEM.** The renin–angiotensin–aldosterone system (RAAS) has a unique role in hypertension and renal disease because angiotensin II (Ang II), acting on its type I receptors (AT1Rs), not only contracts blood vessels but also enhances renal salt retention. Ang II increases renal vascular resistance and the filtration fraction and increases NaCl reabsorption in the proximal tubule, loop segment, and distal nephron. Moreover, Ang II stimulates aldosterone, whose actions in the collection ducts further enhance Na^+ reabsorption. Ang II coordinates the body's response to salt depletion and hypotension. Renin secretion is enhanced by salt restriction, activation of the sympathetic nervous system, diuretic therapy, or a decrease in blood pressure (BP) during antihypertensive therapy. Exceptions are beta-blockers, that lower BP and inhibit renin secretion. Ang II itself inhibits renin secretion (Fig. 32.1).

Prolonged action of Ang II on AT1Rs causes oxidative stress and inflammation that lead to hypertrophy of the left ventricle, remodeling of blood vessels, sclerosis of glomeruli, and fibrosis of the renal interstitium. Ang II type 2 receptors (AT2Rs) enhance bradykinin (Bk) release that activates its type 2 receptors to generate nitric oxide and cyclic guanosine monophosphate. The actions of AT2Rs generally offset those of AT1Rs (Fig. 32.1). Angiotensin receptor blockers (ARBs) stimulate renin secretion and Ang II generation, and thereby activate AT2Rs.

Renin cleaves angiotensinogen (A0) to produce angiotensin I (Ang I) that is itself inactive. Renin inhibitors or antagonists (RAs) are competitive antagonists of this reaction. Angiotensin-converting enzyme (ACE) is a carboxypeptidase that not only cleaves two amino acids from the inert Ang I to form the active Ang II, but also inactivates Bk. Therefore, angiotensin-converting enzyme inhibitors (ACEIs) diminish Ang II and enhance Bk. It is presently unclear whether

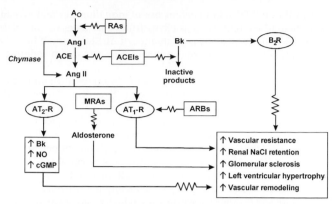

FIGURE 32.1: Diagrammatic representation of the renin–angiotensin–aldosterone system and the sites of action of renin antagonists (RAs), angiotensin-converting enzyme inhibitors (ACEIs), angiotensin receptor blockers (ARBs), and mineralocorticosteroid receptor antagonists (MRAs). Ang, angiotensin; A0, angiotensinogen; AT1R, angiotensin II type 1 receptor; AT2R, angiotensin II type 2 receptor; Bk, bradykinin; B2R, bradykinin type 2 receptor; cGMP, cyclic guanosine monophosphate; NO, nitric oxide.

there are special clinical benefits of ACEIs mediated via Bk, of ARBs mediated via AT2R, or of renin inhibitors mediated by blockade of the entire system. ACEIs, ARBs, and RAs are equally effective antihypertensive agents.

The circulating RAAS is complemented by a tissue RAAS expressed in the heart, kidney, blood vessels, brain, and adrenal glands, where Ang II acts as a locally produced autocoid.

II. ANGIOTENSIN-CONVERTING ENZYME INHIBITORS

A. Mechanism of Action. ACEIs reduce BP by peripheral vasodilation and natriuresis. Unlike some other vasodilators such as minoxidil, they reset the baroreflex and therefore do not cause tachycardia or stimulate the sympathetic nervous system. Their natriuretic actions prevent compensatory renal fluid retention. Peripheral vasodilation involves a reduction in vascular smooth muscle contraction, sympathetic tone, and aldosterone secretion. ACEIs also are venodilators, which may benefit patients with congestive heart failure (CHF).

B. Adverse Effects. ACEIs can induce functional renal insufficiency in some patients with renal artery stenosis that is bilateral or affects a single-functioning kidney, or in some patients with CHF, especially those receiving excessive diuretic therapy or those whose mean BP (MBP) is below the lower limit for renal autoregulation (about 85 mm Hg, equivalent to a BP of about 100/70 mm Hg). In these circumstances, there is a compromised glomerular ultrafiltration pressure because ACEIs lower the MBP and prevent the effects of Ang II to constrict the efferent arterioles. The glomerular filtration rate (GFR) normally returns promptly after withdrawal of ACEIs. ACEIs do not affect the GFR of normal subjects or those with essential hypertension. The kidneys of patients with chronic renal disease (CKD) generally have lost the ability to autoregulate. Therefore, any abrupt decrease in BP can reduce the GFR in the short term.

ACEIs can cause hyperkalemia in predisposed patients. CKD is not a contraindication to the use of ACEIs, but the serum potassium concentration (S_k) must be monitored before and within 1 week of initiation of therapy and after an increase in ACEI dose since the frequency of hyperkalemia with ACEIs increases as the GFR falls. Concurrent use of loop diuretics and avoidance of foods with high K^+ content (such as citrus fruits and juices or chocolate) may obviate hyperkalemia and allow continuance of ACEI therapy. If hyperkalemia persists, a potassium binding drug (patiromer or zirconium sodium) can be administered.

A dry cough during ACEI therapy occurs in up to 20% and angioedema in <1%. These adverse effects likely represent Bk action. Therefore, they are not normally encountered with ARBs, RAs, or mineralocorticosteroid receptor antagonists (MRAs), which, therefore, are alternative therapies for those who cough with ACEIs. ACEIs are contraindicated in pregnancy, where they can affect fetal survival during the third trimester. ACEIs do not perturb lipids and may improve carbohydrate tolerance. They do not normally provoke erectile dysfunction or depression and are generally well tolerated.

C. **Differences Between Agents.** ACEIs are structurally heterogeneous. All ACEIs, except captopril and lisinopril, are prodrugs, which prolongs their action. Some agents are highly lipophilic and provide superior ACE inhibition in tissues, but the clinical consequences of this are not yet clear (Table 32.1). Benazepril, fosinopril, quinapril, and trandolapril are relatively lipid-soluble agents with a balanced hepatic and renal excretion that are preferred in patients with CKD and those on dialysis since their high degree of plasma protein binding limits loss of the drug during hemodialysis. In contrast, the relatively low plasma protein binding of captopril and lisinopril render them readily dialyzable.

D. **Patient Selection and Drug Interactions.** Patient groups with low-renin hypertension are less responsive to monotherapy with ACEIs. These include African Americans, the elderly, individuals with diabetes, obese patients, and those consuming a high-salt diet. The addition of a diuretic stimulates the RAAS, thereby potentiating the antihypertensive effect of ACEIs. Thiazide diuretics counteract ACEI-induced hyperkalemia, whereas ACEIs counteract diuretic-induced glucose intolerance. Thus, ACEIs and thiazide diuretics make an ideal, and even synergistic, combination.

Nonsteroidal anti-inflammatory drugs blunt the effects of ACEIs. Close biochemical monitoring is required when ACEIs are used with other drugs that cause hyperkalemia, such as KC1 supplements, MRAs, distal diuretics, trimethoprim-sulfamethoxazole, pentamidine, or heparin. Certain ACEIs should not be taken with food (Table 32.1).

E. **Clinical Trials.** The results of comprehensive meta-analyses of ACEIs in patients with hypertension generally concur in showing similar overall benefit among ACEIs, diuretics, and calcium channel blockers (CCBs) for the prevention of cardiovascular mortality, with ACEIs and diuretics being more effective in preventing heart failure, and CCBs often more effective in preventing stroke. This conclusion was confirmed in the huge Antihypertensive and Lipid Lowering Treatment to Prevent Heart Attack (ALLHAT) Trial.

However, ACEIs were superior in some trials such as in the Heart Outcomes Prevention Evaluation (HOPE) study. ACEIs reduced stroke incidence and recurrence, even in normotensives, in the Perindopril Protection Against Recurrent Stroke Study, and were as effective as other antihypertensives in preventing complications in patients with diabetes mellitus in the U.K. Prospective Diabetes Study—Hypertension in Diabetic Study (UK PD). ACEIs were more effective than equivalent antihypertensive therapy in preventing progression of renal disease in patients with proteinuria >1 g/day in the effects of ACEIs in diabetic nephropathy, ramipril efficacy in nephropathy, but not in those

TABLE
32.1

Angiotensin-converting enzyme inhibitors

Agent	Serum half-life (h)	Initial dose (mg/day)	Dosing frequency (per day)	Usual dose (mg/day)	Principal elimination	Affected by food	Protein binding (%)	Dialysis (%)
Benazepril (Lotensin)	22	10	Once or twice	20–40	L	No	>95	N
Captopril (Capoten)[a]	2	25	Three times	12.5–50	K	Yes	25	50
Enalapril (Vasotec)	11	5	Once or twice	10–40	L	—	50	50
Fosinopril (Monopril)	12	5	Once	5–40	L	—	95	—
Lisinopril (Zestril, Prinivil)	12	10	Once	20–40	K	—	10	50
Moexipril (Univasc)	5	7.5	Twice	7.5–30	L	Yes	50	—
Quinapril (Accupril)	25	10	Once	20–80	L	Yes	97	—
Ramipril (Altace)	15	2.5	Once	2.5–20	L	Yes	73	—
Trandolapril (Mavik)	20	1	Once	2–4	L	No	85	—

The dosage of all, except fosinopril, should be reduced 50% at an eGFR of 10–15 mL/min.
[a]Contains a sulfhydryl group; N, not significantly affected.
K, kidney; L, liver.

with nephrosclerosis and low-grade proteinuria in the African American Study of Kidney Disease and Hypertension (AASK) Trial. ACEIs are of established benefit in preventing recurrent MI and prolonging life expectancy in moderate or severe CHF, even in the absence of hypertension. Therefore, ACEIs or ARBs are preferred agents for patients with CKD and proteinuria >1 g/day, including those with diabetic nephropathy, and for those with a myocardial infarction or CHF. They are also an excellent choice for patients with essential hypertension, especially those with associated cardiovascular risk factors.

III. **ANGIOTENSIN RECEPTOR BLOCKERS.** ARBs bind selectively to the AT1R, where they are competitive or insurmountable antagonists. They block all the primary action of Ang II to raise BP since the AT2R has effects that generally counter those of the AT1Rs.

A. **Actions, Uses, Interactions, and Adverse Effects.** The major effects and uses of ARBs are similar to those of ACEIs. However, ARBs do not stimulate Bk and therefore do not cause a dry cough or angioedema. Consequently, they have an even lower profile of adverse effects. Some ARBs are prodrugs. They have variable bioavailability (Table 32.2). Losartan is the only uricosuric ARB. Eprosartan is a purely competitive antagonist of the AT1R, whereas the active metabolite of losartan (EXP 3174) and all other ARBs are insurmountable antagonists because they bind very tightly to the receptor. The outcome is that these drugs have a more prolonged duration of action than is predicted by their plasma half-life because of their prolonged sojourn on the receptor.

B. **Clinical Trials.** Results of controlled clinical trials have reported that ARBs were superior to beta-blockers for the prevention of stroke in hypertensive patients in the Losartan Intervention for Endpoint Reduction in Hypertension (LIFE) Trial, and superior to equivalent antihypertensive therapy in reducing proteinuria and progression of nephropathy due to diabetes mellitus type 2 in the Irbesartan Diabetic Nephropathy Trial, Irbesartan in Type 2 Diabetes and Microalbuminuria Study, and the Reduction of Endpoint in NIDDM with Angiotensin II Antagonist Losartan (RENAAL) Trial. Therefore, they are excellent choices in those conditions.

| TABLE 32.2 | Angiotensin receptor blockers | | | |

Agent	Initial daily dose (mg)	Dose range (mg/day)	Active metabolites	Interaction with food
Azilsartan (Edarbi)	40	40–80	No	No
Candesartan (Atacand)	8–16	8–32	No	No
Eprosartan (Teveten)	200	400–800	No	No
Irbesartan (Avapro)	150	150–300	No	No
Losartan (Cozaar)[a]	25–50	50–100	Yes	No
Olmesartan (Benicar)	20	20–40	Yes	No
Telmisartan (Micardis)	20–40	40–80	No	Yes
Valsartan (Diovan)	80	80–160	No	Yes

Note: All agents are >90% protein bound, are eliminated predominantly by the liver, have a duration of action of <24 hours, can be given once daily and are not significantly dialyzable.
[a]Uricosuric action.

TABLE 32.3	Major renal protective mechanisms of ACEIs and ARBs

Normalize pressure natriuresis
Inhibit renal tubular sodium reabsorption
Decrease blood pressure
Decrease aldosterone production
Decrease proteinuria
Decrease glomerular capillary pressure
Reduce renal oxidative stress and fibrosis

IV. RENAL PROTECTION MECHANISMS OF ACEIs AND ARBs. These are reviewed in Table 32.3 and Chapters 5 and 36.

V. RENIN ANTAGONISTS. Aliskiren (Tekturna) is the first approved RA. Although it has a very low bioavailability of 2% to 3%, this is offset somewhat by its profound affinity for binding to prorenin at the renin receptor. Prorenin, which circulates in higher concentration than renin, is activated to renin by binding to the renin receptor. Presently, it is not clear whether aliskiren also blocks the signaling from an activated renin receptor that, if proven, would extend its spectrum of action.

Aliskiren has a long half-life of about 40 hours, which predicts that it will be cumulative with once-daily dosing. At its recommended doses of 150 or 300 mg daily, it is well tolerated, but higher doses cause diarrhea. Early studies suggest that, although its antihypertensive effect is similar to that of ACEIs or ARBs, it may have more potent renal effects. However, clinical trials to date have not shown superiority to ACEIs or ARBs.

VI. MINERALOCORTICOSTEROID RECEPTOR ANTAGONISTS. Aldosterone binds to the mineralocoticosteroid receptor (MR) in the collecting ducts that activates the epithelial Na^+ entry channels. The ensuing increase in cellular Na^+ uptake increases Na^+ absorption and enhances the negative charge across the luminal cell membrane, thereby increasing tubular secretion of the positively charged K^+ and H^+ ions. Aldosterone secretion is enhanced by the activation of the AT1R. Therefore, it is increased in patients with salt restriction, renovascular hypertension, CHF, and advanced cirrhosis with ascites and in those taking diuretics, and is inhibited by ACEIs and ARBs. Aldosterone secretion also is enhanced by hyperkalemia and metabolic acidosis independent of Ang II. This accounts for its elevated levels in patients with renal failure. The highest aldosterone levels are found in patients with primary hyperaldosteronism (see Chapter 24).

MRAs enhance renal Na^+ loss, but the effect may take some days to become apparent. The blockade of distal K^+ and H^+ secretion increases S_k and combats metabolic alkalosis. These effects are used to advantage when MRAs are combined with loop or thiazide diuretics to prevent hypokalemic metabolic alkalosis and the associated magnesium depletion while enhancing net NaCl depletion. Aldosterone also contributes to vasoconstriction, vascular inflammation, endothelial dysfunction, myocardial and renal fibrosis, and left ventricular hypertrophy.

MRAs added to conventional therapy, including ACEIs, reduce hospitalization and prolong life in patients with CHF from heart failure with reduced ejection fraction (HFrEF) studied in the Randomized Aldactone Evaluation (RAALS) Study and the Eplerenone Post-AMI Heart Failure Efficacy and Survival (EPHASUS) Study. Therefore, they should be added to ACEIs in patients with CHF, unless there is a contraindication.

Spironolactone (Aldactone) and eplerenone (Inspra) block the nuclear (genomic) MR. They are the preferred drugs for the medical management of primary hyperaldosteronism (see Chapter 24). They are particularly useful in patients with uncompensated edema due to advanced cirrhosis and ascites, or those with CHF, in whom hypokalemia and alkalosis often complicate diuretic therapy. They are also effective in essential hypertension and have been shown in the PATHWAY trial to be preferred drugs for patients with resistant hypertension. However, the use of spironolactone is limited by adverse effects and the use of eplerenone by high costs.

Spironolactone is well absorbed. It is metabolized to canrenoate that is fully active and has long half-life of 17 hours. It should be given only once daily.

Some side effects of MRAs are predictable, for example, hyperkalemia and metabolic acidosis, which preclude its use in any patients with even a borderline elevation of S_k. Additionally, spironolactone has pronounced, dose-dependent antiandrogenic and proprogestogenic effects that cause loss of libido, impotence, and painful gynecomastia in men, and menstrual irregularities and postmenopausal bleeding in women. Wherever possible, the dose should be limited to 12.5 to 25 mg daily to obviate these adverse effects.

Eplerenone (Inspra) is an MRA without antiandrogenic or proprogestogenic actions. It is better tolerated than spironolactone. It is cleared by hepatic metabolism, with a limited half-life of 4 to 6 hours. The effective daily dose range is 50–100 mg.

VII. SUGGESTED READINGS

Azizi M, Webb R, Nussberger J, et al. Renin inhibition with aliskiren: where are we now, and where are we going? *J Hypertens.* 2006;24(2):243–256.

Brenner BM, Cooper ME, DeZeeuw D, et al. Effects of losartan on renal and cardiovascular outcomes in patients with type 2 diabetes and nephropathy. *N Engl J Med.* 2001;345(12):861–869.

Casas JP, Chua W, Loukageorgakis S, et al. Effect of inhibitors of the renin-angiotensin system and other antihypertensive drugs on renal outcomes. Systematic review and meta-analysis. *Lancet.* 2005;366(9502):2026–2033.

Chang TI, Beddu S, Chertow GM. Antihypertensive therapy. In: Alan Yu, Glenn MC, Valérie AL, et al., eds. *Brenner and Rector's The Kidney.* 11th ed. Elsevier; 2020:1654–1707.

Whelton PK, Carey RM, Aronow WS, et al. ACC/AHA/AAPA/ABC/ACPM/AGS/APhA/ASH/ASPC/NMA/PCNA guideline for the prevention, detection, evaluation, and management of high blood pressure in adults: a report of the American College of Cardiology/American Heart Association Task Force on Clinical Practice Guidelines. *Circulation.* 2018;138(17):e484–e594.

33 Calcium Channel Blockers and Other Vasodilators

Mohammed A. Alshehri, Christopher S. Wilcox

I. CALCIUM CHANNEL BLOCKERS

A. Mechanism of Action. Calcium channel blockers (CCBs) antagonize the influx of Ca^{2+} into vascular smooth muscle cells (VSMCs) via voltage-operated, L-type calcium channels. The ensuing fall in intracellular $[Ca^{2+}]$ relaxes blood vessels and coronary arteries and decreases the peripheral vascular resistance and vascular reactivity. They are weak inhibitors of distal NaCl reabsorption in the kidneys, but are powerful dilators of the afferent arteriole. The efferent arteriole does not contain L-type Ca^{2+} channels and is unresponsive to CCBs. Therefore, unlike renin–angiotensin system inhibitors (RASi), CCBs do not reduce, and may increase the glomerular capillary pressure. This may account for lesser renal protection provided by CCBs than RASis.

B. Classification and Differences Between Calcium Channel Blockers. CCBs can be divided into *nondihydropyridines* (verapamil and diltiazem) and *dihydropyridines* (the remainder). Dihydropyridines block L-type Ca^{2+} channels on VSMCs quite selectively, whereas nondihydropyridines also block L-type Ca^{2+} channels in the gastrointestinal tract and in cardiac tissue and therefore are prone to cause constipation and to depress conduction through the atrioventricular node and reduce cardiac rate and contractility. All agents lower blood pressure (BP) and most of them are available in formulations that permit once-daily dosing (Table 33.1).

C. Metabolism and Elimination. CCBs undergo oxidative biotransformation. The nondihydropyridines are metabolized by hepatic cytochrome P450 CYP 3A. The absence of significant renal clearance prevents accumulation, or the need for major dosage modifications, in renal insufficiency.

D. Drug Interactions. Verapamil and diltiazem inhibit the metabolic clearance of other drugs that are substrates for hepatic cytochrome P450 CYP 3A, whereas dihydropyridines generally do not (Table 33.2). Both verapamil and diltiazem delay the metabolic clearance of tacrolimus and cyclosporine, necessitating a reduction in the dosage. Cimetidine, sulfinpyrazone, rifampin, phenytoin, and ketoconazole reduce the metabolic clearance of nondihydropyridine CCBs. They can thereby cause bradyarrhythmias when administered with verapamil or diltiazem. Additionally, verapamil and diltiazem inhibit P-glycoprotein–mediated drug transport. This may delay the intestinal absorption of drugs and their distribution into the central nervous system.

E. Use for Hypertension, Renal Disease, and Cardiovascular Protection. Long-acting CCBs are especially effective antihypertensives in low-renin hypertension that is

TABLE 33.1   Calcium channel blockers

Drug	Daily dose (mg)	Dosing frequency (per day)	Elimination [half-life (h)]	Special features
Amlodipine	2.5–10.0	Daily	30–50	Combinations with benazepril (Lotrel) or atorvastatin (Caduet) available
Barnidipine	120–360	Daily	24	Not available in the United States
Diltiazem[a,b]	180–480	Daily	2–8	Can cause bradycardia and impair LV function
Felodipine	5–10.0	Daily	10–14	Combination with enalapril (Lexxel)
Isradipine[a]	2.5–10.0	Twice daily	2–5	
Nicardipine[a,b]	60–120	Daily	5–8	Intravenous form for emergent hypertension
Nifedipine[a]	30–90	Daily	4–6	
Nimodipine	60	Each 4 h	1–3	Used for cerebral artery spasm in subarachnoid hemorrhage
Nisoldipine[a]	10–60	Daily	6–8	
Verapamil[a,b]	180–480	Daily	3–7	Can cause bradycardia, LV dysfunction, and constipation

[a]Available in long-acting, once-daily form.
[b]Also available for intravenous use.

TABLE 33.2   Interactions between nondihydropyridine CCBs and other drugs

Drug affected	Clinical effect
Digoxin	Digoxin toxicity
Carbamazepine	Neurotoxicity
Astemizole	Prolonged QT interval
Terfenadine	Torsade de pointes
Cisapride	Torsade de pointes
Quinidine	Torsade de pointes
Atorvastatin, lovastatin, simvastatin	Myopathy, rhabdomyolysis
Cyclosporine, tacrolimus	Nephrotoxicity
Beta-blockers	Bradyarrhythmias

common in African Americans, the elderly, obese patients, diabetics, and those with renal insufficiency.

CCB therapy has been reported to be superior to placebo in preventing stroke and coronary artery disease but inferior to therapy with a diuretic, beta-blocker, or angiotensin-converting enzyme inhibitor (ACEI) for preventing heart failure. In the Antihypertensive and Lipid Lowering Treatment to Prevent Heart Attack Trial (ALLHAT), patients were randomized to amlodipine, a diuretic, or an ACEI. The primary end points of fatal coronary disease or nonfatal myocardial infarction were similar between groups, but patients randomized to amlodipine were significantly more likely to experience heart failure than those randomized to diuretics but had a reduced number of strokes. The Anglo-Scandinavian Cardiac Outcome Trial (ASCOT) randomized patients to amlodipine, with the subsequent addition of an ACEI, or a thiazide diuretic. Those randomized to the CCB/ACEI arm had lower rates of cardiovascular morbidity and all-cause mortality. The Avoiding Cardiovascular Events through Combination Therapy in Patients Living with Systolic Hypertension (ACCOMPLISH) trial, compared the combination of benazepril/amlodipine to benazepril/hydrochlorothiazide. The patient in the former arm had lower rates of cardiovascular events. These data support the use of CCB/ACEI combinations for hypertension.

A meta-analysis of 16 trials for the prevention of diabetic nephropathy (defined as new development of microalbuminuria) reported a 42% reduced risk of nephropathy in those randomized to ACEI compared with CCBs. The African American Study of Kidney Disease and Hypertension (AASK) trial randomized 1,094 African Americans with CKD, hypertension, and presumed nephrosclerosis to a usual (102 to 107 mm Hg) or low (92 mm Hg) mean BP goal and to one of three primary treatments: beta-blocker (metoprolol), ACEI (ramipril), or CCB (amlodipine). The primary end point was the rate of decline of GFR. In this group of patients with a low rate of proteinuria, the end point was not changed in those with the lower BP goal but was more frequent in those randomized to amlodipine, which prompted the premature discontinuation of this arm. There was no significant difference in the primary end point between those randomized to the beta-blocker or the ACEI.

A recurring finding of meta-analysis in hypertension is that there is little difference between classes of drugs in the prevention of cardiovascular disease, but that a greater reduction in BP is associated with a greater reduction in cardiovascular risk. Subgroup analysis shows that CCBs may be somewhat less effective in preventing heart failure and progression of chronic kidney disease (CKD), but somewhat more effective in preventing stroke.

Proteinuria is little changed by dihydropyridines but is reduced by nondihydropyridines. An ACEI given with a nondihydropyridine CCB reduces proteinuria more than either agent alone.

A recent meta-analysis from 2019 for 71 RCTs of hypertensive renal transplant patients concluded that CCBs improve graft function and reduce graft loss. However, current practice guidelines do not yet recommend one particular class of antihypertensive for the treatment of hypertension in transplant recipients. CCBs might improve the allograft function by alleviating the renal afferent arteriolar vasoconstriction caused by calcineurin inhibitors.

CCBs are indicated specifically in hypertensives with angina pectoris or Raynaud's phenomenon. Nondihydropyridines slow the ventricular rate in patients with atrial fibrillation. CCBs are effective as part of a multidrug antihypertensive regimen in patients with CKD and in those with end-stage renal disease. They are not removed by dialysis. CCBs are very helpful as third-line antihypertensives in patients receiving a diuretic and an ACEI or an angiotensin receptor blocker (ARB) to achieve the low BP goal recommended by the JNC8 Guidelines (see Chapter 23).

F. Adverse Effects. CCBs are generally well tolerated. Nondihydropyridines can cause bradyarrhythmias and may worsen congestive heart failure. Nondihydropyridines can cause constipation and headache. Dihydropyridines cause dose-dependent edema by redistribution of plasma fluid into the interstitium because of arteriolar vasodilatation. The edema is relatively resistant to diuretics but is reduced by dose reduction. Dihydropyridines can activate the sympathetic nervous system. Therefore, they are best used in combination with beta-blockers to treat patients with myocardial ischemia and angina.

II. OTHER VASODILATORS. Hydralazine and minoxidil are direct-acting arteriolar vasodilators. Minoxidil opens potassium channels on VSMCs and on the nephron. The ensuing hyperpolarization closes voltage-gated Ca^{2+} channels, thereby reducing intracellular $[Ca^{2+}]$ and causing vasorelaxation but, in the kidney, leads to salt retention and edema.

These agents are effective antihypertensives. However, long-term therapy is limited by tachyphylaxis and a spectrum of adverse effects. Minoxidil leads to the reflex activation of the sympathetic nervous system, most notable in younger patients, that can worsen angina pectoris and myocardial ischemia and cause tachyarrhythmias. It also causes renal salt and fluid retention, leading to edema or worsening of congestive heart failure. Minoxidil can cause carbohydrate intolerance, hirsutism, and pericardial effusions that occasionally cause cardiac tamponade. Headache is frequent. Tachycardia and edema can develop with hydralazine if it causes a marked drop in the BP. Hydralazine also can cause a lupus-like syndrome with higher doses. Hydralazine increases sodium excretion when it is dosed appropriately.

Hydralazine is used in patients who are resistant to alpha-methyldopa to control pregnancy-associated hypertension (see Chapter 25). Minoxidil is used as a short-term treatment in severe, drug-resistant hypertension, especially in those with renal insufficiency (see Chapter 24). It requires coadministration of a beta-blocker to prevent reflex tachycardia and a diuretic to prevent fluid retention. Minoxidil should not be used for long-term therapy.

III. SUGGESTED READINGS

Dahlof B, Sever PS, Poulter NR, et al. Prevention of cardiovascular events with an antihypertensive regimen of amlodipine adding perindopril as required versus atenolol adding bendroflumethiazide as required, in the Anglo-Scandinavian Cardiac Outcomes Trial—Blood Pressure Lowering Arm (ASCOT-BPLA): a multicenter randomised conrolled trial. *Lancet.* 2005;366(9489):895–906.

Jamerson K, Weber MA, Bakris GL, et al. Benazepril plus amlodipine or hydrochlorothiazide for hypertension in high-risk patients. *N Engl J Med.* 2008;359(23):2417–2428.

Pisano A, Bolignano D, Mallamaci F, et al. Comparative effectiveness of different antihypertensive agents in kidney transplantation: a systematic review and meta-analysis. *Nephrol Dial Transplant.* 2020;35(5):878–887. doi:10.1093/ndt/gfz092

Sica DA, Prisant LM. Pharmacologic and therapeutic considerations in hypertension therapy with calcium channel blockers: focus on verapamil. *J Clin Hypertens*. 2007;9(Suppl 2):1–22.

Whelton PK, Carey RM, Aronow WS, et al. 2017ACC/AHA/AAPA/ABC/ACPM/AGS/APhA/ASH/ ASPC/NMA/PCNA guideline for the prevention, detection, evaluation, and management of high blood pressure in adults: a report of the american college of cardiology/american heart association task force on clinical practice guidelines. *J Am Coll Cardiol*. 2018;71(19): e127–e248.

Pressor Agents

Chanigan Nilubol

I. **INTRODUCTION.** Acute kidney injury (AKI) is a common condition that is independently associated with increased risk of mortality, morbidity, and cost of hospitalization. More than 90% of AKI in the intensive care unit (ICU) is due to acute tubular necrosis (ATN), often caused by ischemia or nephrotoxins. Mortality of those requiring renal replacement therapy is approximately 50%. AKI can be precipitated by microcirculatory imbalance between vasodilators and vasoconstrictors in several forms of AKI, including sepsis. While experimental ischemia–reperfusion injury responds to agents that improve renal perfusion pressure and blood flow, those benefits have not been confirmed in clinical trials. This chapter reviews prevention or treatment of AKI. The anticipated actions of individual agents are summarized in Table 34.1.

II. **PREVENTION AND TREATMENT OF ACUTE KIDNEY INJURY**

A. **Dopamine.** The increase in renal blood flow provided by dopamine in normal human subjects is often lacking in patients with hypovolemia, shock, hypoperfusion, ATN, or other disease states. Dopamine was used previously to prevent AKI complicating many conditions but results of clinical trials have not been encouraging. Thus, two randomized controlled trials in AKI in the ICU both reported that dopamine was not effective in preventing AKI and increased the risk of new-onset atrial fibrillation. Numerous controlled trials have failed to confirm benefits from dopamine in the prevention of contrast nephropathy and many have reported adverse arrhythmias. Current evidence does not support the use of dopamine in the prevention of AKI, as confirmed in the 2012 KDIGO Guideline for Acute Kidney Injury that also does not recommend dopamine or fenoldopam or atrial natriuretic peptide, to prevent ischemic ATN.

B. **Fenoldopam.** While fenoldopam has been reported to improve the serum creatinine in patients undergoing liver transplantation, it has not been successful in preserving kidney function during cardiovascular surgery or contrast-induced nephropathy. The largest randomized controlled trial of the use of fenoldopam in critically ill patients with AKI reported no effect on renal replacement therapy, length of ICU stay, or mortality but an increased risk of hypotension. On the other hand, in septic or critically ill patients with AKI, those randomized to fenoldopam had a decreased time of stay in the ICU, but no mortality benefit. A meta-analysis of 16 controlled trials reported that fenoldopam reduced the incidence of AKI, the need for renal replacement therapy, and reduced the time of stay in ICU. Current evidence is insufficient to recommend fenoldopam for routine use in patients with AKI.

C. **Norepinephrine.** Norepinephrine is used in patients with septic shock to raise their blood pressure. While norepinephrine can cause renal vasoconstriction,

TABLE
34.1

Pharmacology and principal effects of pressor agents

Agents	Origins	Receptors	Effects
Dopamine	• Proximal tubular cells • Sympathetic nervous system	Dopamine type I (DA-1) on blood vessels or proximal tubules (0.5–3 µg/kg/min) Adrenergic (>5 µg/kg/min)	• Interlobular artery vasodilatation • Afferent and efferent vasodilation • Net increase in renal blood flow and natriuresis Raises blood pressure by vasoconstriction
Fenoldopam	Synthetic	Selective DA-1	• Low dose (0.03–0.1 µg/kg/min): increases renal blood flow • High dose (>1 µg/kg/min): reduces blood pressure Lacks some of the adverse effects of dopamine
Norepinephrine	Sympathetic nervous system	Alpha adrenergic	Increases systemic vascular resistance and perfusion pressure during distributive or septic shock
Epinephrine	Sympathetic nervous system	Combined alpha and beta adrenergic	Effects depend on prior restored volume status Increases renal blood flow Raises blood pressure
Phenylephrine	Synthetic	Alpha adrenergic	Raises blood pressure
Arginine vasopressin	Posterior pituitary gland	Vasopressin type I (vascular smooth muscles) Vasopressin type II (distal tubules)	Vasoconstriction Reabsorption of free water (antidiuretic)

trials of norepinephrine in patients with hypotensive septic shock generally report an improvement in blood pressure, creatinine clearance, and urine output. Phenylephrine has a similar mechanism of action, whereas epinephrine has additional actions to stimulate the heart but can increase serum lactate. Norepinephrine infused at 0.5 to 3.0 mg/h in combination with albumin is effective in increasing arterial pressure and improving kidney function in patients with hepatorenal syndrome, although this is not as effective as vasopressin analogs (see Chapter 38).

D. Arginine Vasopressin. The addition of arginine vasopressin to norepinephrine may improve creatinine clearance and urine output but one randomized trial reported that the early use of vasopressin in patients with septic shock was no more effective than norepinephrine alone. Present evidence suggests that vasopressin should not be used in place of norepinephrine.

Vasopressin analogs infused with albumin have been reported to improve renal function in the hepatorenal syndrome but can cause severe vasoconstriction leading to myocardial infarction or intestinal ischemia (Also see Chapter 38).

E. Summary. Presently, there is insufficient evidence to recommend dopamine for prophylaxis or treatment of AKI. Fenoldopam has some promise and lacks the adverse arrhythmogenic effects of dopamine but its use is not yet supported by adequately powered controlled clinical trials. Norepinephrine is the recommended agent for seriously ill, hypotensive patients with septic shock, and some data suggests that it may be beneficially combined with arginine vasopressin. Trials of dopamine or fenoldopam in patients with impending or established AKI are summarized in Ford et al. (see Suggested Readings).

III. SUGGESTED READINGS

Bellomo R, Chapman M, Finfer S, et al. Low-dose dopamine in patients with early renal dysfunction: a placebo-controlled randomised trial. Australian and New Zealand Intensive Care Society (ANZICS) clinical trials group. *Lancet.* 2000;356(9248):2139–2143.

Ford D, Cullis B, Denton M. Dopaminergic and pressor therapy. In: Wilcox CS, ed. *Therapy in Nephrology and Hypertension.* 3rd ed. WB Saunders; 2008.

Francoz C, Durand F, Kahn JA, et al. Hepatorenal syndrome. *Clin J Am Soc Nephrol.* 2019;14(5): 774–778.

KDIGO. Clinical practice guideline for acute kidney injury. *Kidney Int Suppl.* 2012;2(Suppl 1):8.

Landoni G, Biondi-Zoccai GGL, Tumlin JA, et al. Beneficial impact of fenoldopam in critically ill patients with or at risk of acute renal failure: a meta-analysis of randomized clinical trials. *Am J Kidney Dis.* 2007;49(1):56–68.

Lauschke A, Teichgräber UKM, Frei U, et al. 'Low-dose' dopamine worsens renal perfusion in patients with acute renal failure. *Kidney Int.* 2006;69(9):1669–1674.

Diagnosis and Management of Renal Failure

Acute Kidney Injury

Saraswathi Gopal, Azra Bihorac

Acute kidney injury (AKI) has replaced the traditional term acute renal failure and refers to a sudden decrease in glomerular filtration rate (GFR), with a rise in blood urea nitrogen (BUN), creatinine (Cr), and/or decrease in urine output. A doubling in serum Cr (S_{Cr}) in acutely ill patients increases mortality to 30%, and another doubling in S_{Cr} increases this mortality to 60%. There are several different staging criteria for AKI but the Kidney Disease Improving Global Outcomes (KDIGO) staging system for AKI is preferred (Table 35.1).

S_{Cr} usually lags behind GFR during the onset or recovery of AKI. S_{Cr} reflects GFR, Cr production by muscle, its dilution in the plasma, and its proximal tubular secretion. BUN reflects GFR and protein intake or catabolism. Thus, S_{Cr} and BUN are not faithful indices of AKI.

The first step is to distinguish AKI from chronic kidney disease (CKD) or an acute decrement in GFR superimposed on long-standing stable CKD. Evidence of an acute rise in S_{Cr} or change in urinalysis is very helpful. Evidence of chronicity includes prior laboratory data like previous S_{Cr} levels, laboratory or radiographic evidence of CKD bone mineral disorder, bilaterally small (<10-cm length) and echogenic kidneys on renal ultrasound, and broad polymorphonuclear white blood cell casts on urinalysis that denote tubular dilatation in the setting of nephron loss or normocytic anemia.

I. **CLASSIFICATION OF ACUTE KIDNEY INJURY.** AKI is classified as prerenal (renal hypoperfusion), intrinsic (damage to kidney parenchyma), or postrenal (obstruction). Oliguria is a daily urine output of <500 mL and anuria as <100 mL.

A. **Prerenal Acute Kidney Injury.** This occurs when actual or functional hypovolemia results in insufficient blood flow to the kidneys. Definitive diagnosis depends on improving GFR with volume repletion. Specific etiologies are discussed in Table 35.2.

Decreased renal perfusion leads to prostaglandin-dependent afferent arteriolar dilatation and angiotensin-dependent efferent arteriolar constriction. Maintenance of GFR in this setting depends on these two systems. Thus, nonsteroidal anti-inflammatory drugs, angiotensin-converting enzyme inhibitors, and angiotensin receptor blockers can exacerbate AKI. Renal hypoperfusion is apparent from a reduced urinary Na (U_{Na}) and urea nitrogen concentration and concentrated urine with a high specific gravity, urine osmolality, or urine Cr concentration. Increased urea production and reabsorption, out of proportion to the decrement in GFR, is detected by a rise in the serum BUN to Cr ratio. If hypovolemia is not corrected, prerenal AKI may progress to acute tubular necrosis (ATN). Common clues in the presentation of prerenal AKI are summarized in Table 35.3.

TABLE 35.1	AKI staging KDIGO criteria	
Stage	**Serum creatinine**	**Urine output**
1	1.5–1.9 times baseline or ≥0.3 mg/dL increase	<0.5 mL/kg/h for 6 h
2	2–2.9 times baseline	<0.5 mL/kg/h for 12 h
3	3 times baseline or increase in serum creatinine to ≥4 mg/dL or initiation of renal replacement therapy	<0.3 mL/kg/h for 24 h or anuria for ≥12 h

Volume resuscitation is essential in the management of prerenal AKI. Crystalloids (e.g., buffered crystalloids) are used first, with colloids or blood as required later. It is difficult to restore effective renal perfusion in patients with redistribution of volume from the intravascular space (e.g., capillary leak, low serum albumin, congestive heart failure) without precipitating symptomatic volume overload or pulmonary edema. In these cases, addressing the underlying precipitating cause along volume management is needed.

1. **Hepatorenal syndrome.** Hepatorenal syndrome (HRS) is a severe and volume unresponsive form of prerenal AKI in the setting of advanced liver disease (usually cirrhosis) without other identifiable causes. Oliguria results from

TABLE 35.2	Etiologies of prerenal acute kidney injury

Intravascular volume depletion (effective)
  Cirrhosis
  Excessive use of diuretics
  Gastrointestinal fluid losses
  Hemorrhage
  Inadequate fluid replacement
  Nephrotic syndrome
  Renal fluid losses
  Third spacing of fluid
  Cardiogenic shock
  Congestive heart failure
  Massive pulmonary embolism
  Pericardial tamponade

Systemic vasodilation
  Anaphylaxis
  Sepsis
  Vasodilator drugs

Renal vasoconstriction
  Acute hypercalcemia
  Drugs that block renal responses to volume depletion
  Early sepsis
  Hepatorenal syndrome
  Infused vasopressor drugs

T A B L E 35.3	Clinical presentation of prerenal acute kidney injury		

History and symptoms	Signs	Laboratory tests
• History of fluid loss (vomiting, diarrhea, burns) • Use of non-steroidal anti-inflammatory drugs, angiotensin converting enzyme inhibitors, angiotensin receptor blockers or calcineurin inhibitors especially in the setting of effective volume depletion • Negative fluid balance; output greater than input • Preexisting congestive heart failure or cirrhosis • Thirst	• Orthostatic hypotension or tachycardia • Dry axillae • Flat neck veins in supine position • Dry skin and mucus membranes • Loss of tissue turgor	• Serum blood urea nitrogen to Cr ratio >20:1 (also seen with increased protein catabolism) • Urine specific gravity >1.03 • Urine osmolality >500 mOsm/Kg H_2O • U_{Na} <20 mEQ/L • FE_{Na} <1% [$FE_{Na} = (U_{Na} \times S_{Cr})/(S_{Na} \times U_{Cr}) \times 100$] • FE_{Un} <35% [$FE_{Un} = (U_{Un} \times S_{Cr})/(S_{Un} \times U_{Cr}) \times 100$] • Bland urine sediment, may have hyaline or granular cast • Renal sonogram; normal renal size and echogenicity

Cr, creatinine; FE_{Na}, fractional excretion of sodium; FE_{Un}, fractional excretion of urea nitrogen; S_{Cr}, serum creatine; S_{Na}, serum sodium; S_{Un}, serum urea nitrogen; U_{Cr}, urine creatinine; U_{Na}, urinary sodium concentration; U_{Un}, urine urea nitrogen.

intense renal vasoconstriction and systemic vasodilatation. The U_{Na} is usually <10 mEq/L, and the fractional excretion of sodium (FE_{Na}) is <1%, even after a volume challenge with albumin. HRS may be precipitated by infection or gastrointestinal bleeding or diuretic use. Mortality remains significantly high (see Chapter 38).

B. Intrinsic Acute Kidney Injury. Primary glomerular disease (glomerulonephritis [GN] or vasculitis) or tubular damage (ATN or acute interstitial nephritis [AIN]) can lead to intrinsic renal failure.

 1. **Acute tubular necrosis.** Decreased renal perfusion leading to ischemia accounts for ~50% of ATN, whereas nephrotoxins, such as aminoglycosides and radiocontrast agents, account for 30% (Table 35.4). Renal dysfunction from ATN appears within hours to days and lasts typically for 1 to 3 weeks, but occasionally for much longer. ATN causes irreversible cellular injury. Therefore, normalization of hemodynamics or removal of the toxic insult does not restore normal function immediately. However, restoration of normal renal perfusion is critical in ATN, because autoregulation is impaired in the injured kidney, rendering it more susceptible to recurrent injury from even mild hypotension.

 ATN is characterized by early damage to the proximal tubule and thick ascending limb of the loop of Henle. Shedding of brush borders and cell cytoplasm leads to tubular obstruction from solid casts, whereas leak of glomerular filtrate through damaged tubules reduces the effective glomerular filtration further. Remaining tubules function poorly, thereby impairing tubular reabsorption of electrolytes and excretion of potassium and hydrogen ions. Laboratory abnormalities include hyperkalemia, anion-gap metabolic acidosis, hyponatremia, hyperphosphatemia, hypermagnesemia, hypocalcemia, and hyperuricemia. A diagnostic urine sediment may reveal free tubular epithelial cells (large cells)

TABLE 35.4 Some toxic causes of acute tubular necrosis

Exogenous
    Antibiotics (e.g., aminoglycosides, amphotericin B, pentamidine)
    Radiographic contrast
    Chemotherapeutic agents (e.g., cisplatin)
    Immunosuppressive agents (e.g., cyclosporin)
    Organic solvents (e.g., ethylene glycol)
    Heavy metals (e.g., mercury, lead, arsenic, bismuth)
Endogenous
    Myoglobin (from rhabdomyolysis)
    Hemoglobin

with tubular epithelial cell casts. Many coarsely granular, pigmented, or muddy brown casts are suggestive of ATN. A U_{Na} >40 mEq/L and an FE_{Na} >1% in the setting of oliguria suggest ATN. However, FE_{Na} <1% may be observed early in nonoliguric ATN, especially that secondary to radiocontrast agents, rhabdomyolysis, or severe renal hypoperfusion due to hepatic failure, sepsis, burns, or congestive heart failure (Table 35.5).

  2. **Aminoglycoside-induced acute tubular necrosis.** This is usually nonoliguric and not evident until 7 to 10 days of treatment. Advanced age, pre-existing renal insufficiency, volume depletion, higher dosage, and exposure to other nephrotoxins increase the risk. All aminoglycosides are nephrotoxic, but once-daily aminoglycoside administration may decrease the risk. Monitoring peak and trough levels is prudent but does not eliminate the risk.

  3. **Contrast (radiocontrast)-induced nephropathy.** Contrast-induced nephropathy (CIN) occurs in up to 50% of high-risk patients who have volume depletion, pre-existing renal insufficiency, and diabetes mellitus. The BUN and S_{Cr} rise 24 to 48 hours after contrast administration, peak at 3 to 5 days, and may return to normal in 5 to 7 days. A low FE_{Na} and a high urine specific gravity (due to urine contrast) suggest contrast injury. Provided there are no

TABLE 35.5 Clinical presentation of acute tubular necrosis

History and symptoms	Laboratory tests
• Recent hypotension, shock, especially in the setting of anesthesia or sepsis • Recent nephrotoxin exposure	• Serum blood urea nitrogen to Cr ratio ~8–10:1 • Urine specific gravity 1.010–1.012 • Urine osmolality <350 mOsm/kg H_2O • U_{Na} >40 mEq/L • FE_{Na} >2% • FE_{Un} >35% • Urine sediment with renal tubular cells, tubular cell casts, pigmented granular casts

Cr, creatinine; FE_{Na}, fractional excretion of sodium; FE_{Un}, fractional excretion of urea nitrogen; S_{Cr}, serum creatine; S_{Na}, serum sodium; S_{Un}, serum urea nitrogen; U_{Cr}, urine creatinine; U_{Na}, urinary sodium concentration; U_{Un}, urine urea nitrogen.

contraindications to volume expansion, an infusion of 0.9% saline should be given to replace any defects and to maintain urine output at 1 to 2 mL/min before and for 12 hours after contrast exposure in high-risk groups. There is no additional benefit of using sodium bicarbonate solution over normal saline to prevent CIN. Meta-analyses looking at N-acetylcysteine use to decrease the risk of contrast nephropathy have shown conflicting results. Using lower doses of contrast agent is safer. Low-osmolal or iso-osmolal, nonionic contrast agents are preferred. Dopamine, fenoldopam, or diuretics are of no benefit in preventing CIN.

4. **Amphotericin B-induced acute tubular necrosis.** The risk of nephrotoxicity increases with the dose and duration of treatment. Patients with chronic renal insufficiency and those receiving diuretics are at an increased risk. Distal nephron damage is manifested as polyuria secondary to nephrogenic diabetes insipidus, hypokalemia, hypomagnesemia, and renal tubular acidosis. Lipid-complex formulations are less nephrotoxic.

5. **Rhabdomyolysis-induced acute tubular necrosis.** Rhabdomyolysis sufficient to cause ATN can be caused by muscle damage (trauma, pressure, crush, burns, or ischemia),increased muscle metabolism (seizures, exercise, heat stroke, myopathy), metabolic disorders (ketoacidosis, hypokalemia, hypophosphatemia), toxins (e.g., alcohol, carbon monoxide, statin drugs), severe infections, or drugs (statins).

The clinical features include muscle pain, dark brown urine, urine dipstick positive for blood (heme) in the absence of free hemoglobin, and urinary red blood cells. Hyperkalemia, hyperphosphatemia, hyperuricemia, early hypocalcemia with later hypercalcemia are also seen. Elevated levels of S_{Cr} kinase, myoglobin, and urine myoglobin support the diagnosis.

ATN can be prevented by aggressive volume replacement with isotonic saline from 200 to 1,500 cc/h. The goal of therapy is to increase urine output to >100 cc/h, but this must be terminated if the patient is anuric. Alkalinization of the urine has not shown to be of clinical benefit. Mannitol and diuretic therapy have no benefit over aggressive fluid resuscitation. Complications of rhabdomyolysis include acute renal failure, acidosis, compartment syndrome, hepatic dysfunction, disseminated intravascular coagulation, arrhythmias, and cardiac arrest.

6. **Multiple myeloma.** Multiple myeloma may cause AKI even before diagnosis of the underlying condition. The AKI is accompanied by anemia, hypercalcemia, and elevated serum globulins (see Chapter 11). Hypercalcemia can cause volume depletion and intrarenal vasoconstriction, leading to prerenal AKI, whereas ATN, cast nephropathy, primary amyloidosis, and light-chain deposition disease may cause intrinsic AKI. Monoclonal immunoglobulin light chains are not detected by standard dipstick tests, whereas sulfosalicylic acid detects all urinary proteins. Sulfosalicylic acid, urine and serum electrophoresis, and immunofixation are indicated if multiple myeloma is suspected.

7. **Glomerulonephritis, vasculitis, acute renovascular disease, or interstitial nephritis.** GN or vasculitis should be suspected as a cause of AKI in the setting of a multisystem illness with proteinuria and/or hematuria (see Chapters 8 and 9). There may be a history of autoimmune disease, recent infection, or hepatitis. Signs and symptoms include fever, skin rash, arthralgia, hemoptysis, hypertension, and volume overload. Laboratory tests reveal an elevated erythrocyte sedimentation rate, hypocomplementemia, and autoantibodies

T A B L E 35.6	Clinical presentation of obstructive uropathy

History and symptoms	Signs	Laboratory tests
• Elderly male (with presumed prostatism) • Previous history of urinary tract obstruction • History of bilateral nephrolithiasis • Symptom of bladder outflow obstruction (e.g., dysuria, nocturia, frequency, or hesitation) • Urinary incontinence • Use of anticholinergic medications • Predisposition to papillary necrosis (e.g., diabetes mellitus, sickle cell disease, analgesic abuse) • Pelvic or retroperitoneal disease or surgery	• Complete anuria or wide fluctuations in urine output; however, urine output can also be normal • Distended bladder on physical exam • Large postvoid residual urine on bladder catheterization	• Serum blood urea nitrogen to Cr ratio maybe normal or elevated • Urine specific gravity >1.02 acutely but lower with chronic obstruction • Urine osmolality >400 mOsm/kg H_2O acutely but ~300 chronically • U_{Na} <20 mEq/L acutely, >40 mEq/L chronically • FE_{Na} <1% acutely but >1% chronically • Bland urine sediment • Renal sonogram; dilated collecting system above the level of obstruction but may falsely not show obstruction early or with volume depletion or advanced renal failure

Cr; creatinine, FE_{Na}; fractional excretion of sodium, U_{Na}; urinary sodium concentration.

(like anti–double-stranded DNA or antineutrophil cytoplasmic antibodies or antiglomerular basement membrane antibodies). Careful urinalysis is key. Final diagnosis often depends on renal biopsy (see Chapters 8, 9, and 10).

AIN is often precipitated by drugs or infections and accompanied by eosinophilia, eosinophiluria, fever, and rash. Tubular function abnormalities may exceed the decrement in GFR. Pyuria or white blood cell casts in the absence of urinary tract infection or GN are suggestive of AIN (see Chapter 12).

Acute renovascular causes of ischemic ATN include thrombosis, dissection of aortic aneurysms, or renal arteries that often complicate trauma or a vascular intervention. Cholesterol renal atheroembolic disease usually follows an intravascular procedure. It is often associated with other signs of systemic emboli in the skin or nail beds, with fever, elevated erythrocyte sedimentation rate, hypocomplementemia, and eosinophilia. Renal vein thrombosis can complicate severe nephrotic syndrome or genetic thrombophilias. It may present as decreased renal function with flank pain and hematuria. Thrombotic microangiopathy should be suspected when AKI is accompanied by thrombocytopenia, intravascular hemolysis, fever, and neurologic abnormalities (see Chapter 10).

C. **Postrenal (Obstructive) Acute Kidney Injury.** Obstruction of urine flow at any point from the tubules to the urethral outlet may result in postrenal AKI. Even partial obstruction with preserved urine output may decrease GFR. It is crucial to diagnose functional obstruction because bladder catheterization, urethral dilation and stenting, or percutaneous nephrostomy may restore and preserve renal function. Obstructive symptoms or the use of anticholinergic medications should raise suspicion. To cause clinically apparent AKI, obstruction must be bilateral or affect a single functioning kidney (Table 35.6). Urine chemistries early in the course of obstructive uropathy may resemble those in prerenal AKI due to solute reabsorption from relatively stagnant tubular fluid. Unequivocal diagnosis may depend on a furosemide renogram (see Chapter 2), retrograde pyelography, or response to urinary drainage.

1. **Crystal-induced acute kidney injury.** Obstructive AKI may result from intratubular deposition of uric acid crystals during chemotherapy for malignancies with high cell turnover such as leukemia, aggressive lymphomas, or sarcomas. The collecting system is not dilated. Therefore, imaging strategies are not useful. Aggressive hydration, alkaline diuresis, and allopurinol may prevent kidney injury. Allopurinol should be started several days before chemotherapy and maintained during induction. The benefits of alkaline diuresis may be limited because it may precipitate calcium phosphate. Recombinant urate oxidase may be preferable. Crystal-induced intratubular obstruction also may complicate therapy with high-dose acyclovir or indinavir.

II. **MAKING THE DIAGNOSIS OF ACUTE KIDNEY INJURY.** The focus in diagnosing AKI should be on the time course of kidney injury, its relationship to possible inciting factors, and the assessment of volume status and relevant comorbidities. Changes in S_{Cr} lag behind changes in GFR. Urinalysis requires a fresh urine specimen. It is often more sensitive when the sediment is stained with drops of methylene blue. Bladder catheterization is required when urine output is uncertain or obstruction is possible. The kidneys of most AKI patients should be imaged by ultrasound. Subsequent evaluation often includes calculation of urinary diagnostic indices, followed by other laboratory tests or therapeutic trials focused on specific diagnoses.

Urinalysis should always include dipstick measures of urinary concentration, blood, protein, and pH. Suspected proteinuria should be confirmed by a quantitative assay indexed to urine Cr. The urine sediment may provide unequivocal diagnosis of ATN or GN. Hospital laboratories often fail to identify cellular casts, perhaps because they disintegrate before examination. Urinary eosinophils are best detected using Hansel stain. Their presence is consistent with, but not diagnostic of, AIN and not particularly sensitive (see Chapter 4).

Estimates of GFR by 24-hour Cr clearance or by formulas (see Chapter 1) usually underestimate the severity of AKI because Cr is not in a steady state after an abrupt decrease in GFR.

The FE_{Na} can often distinguish ATN from prerenal AKI but may fail to distinguish obstructive AKI. It is falsely elevated after diuretics, when the fractional excretion of urea may be preferable.

III. **MANAGEMENT.** The clinical course of AKI can be divided into the following phases (Fig. 35.1):

■ *Acute Kidney Injury:* The period between the exposure to an insult and a fall in renal function, this can last up to 7 days.

■ *Acute Kidney Disease (AKD):* Last from greater than 7 days to 90 days, during which renal damage might not be completely reversed. Patients may be anuric, oliguric, or nonoliguric.

■ *Recovery:* Marked by a decreasing serum BUN and Cr toward normal and/ or increasing urine output. Patients may enter a polyuric phase that can cause fluid and electrolyte abnormalities. Recovery of renal function may be complete or incomplete.

■ *Chronic Kidney Disease:* Any abnormalities in kidney structure or function that persists for >90 days is termed CKD.

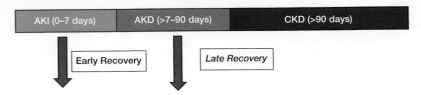

FIGURE 35.1: The spectrum of acute kidney injury (AKI), acute kidney disease (AKD), recovery and chronic kidney disease (CKD).

Reversible causes of renal dysfunction must be sought and treated expeditiously. It is essential to maintain hemodynamics, as the ATN kidney is particularly susceptible to recurrent injury.

After intravascular volume is normalized, fluids should be matched to urine output plus insensible losses. Hyperkalemia should be treated with glucose and insulin, sodium bicarbonate (if the serum bicarbonate is low), sodium polystyrene sulfonate resin, intravenous calcium gluconate for cardiac instability, or dialysis (see Chapter 18). Serum pH should be maintained >7.20 and symptomatic hypocalcemia should be treated (see Chapter 20).

AKI is a hypercatabolic state, but nutritional support has not been shown to be beneficial. Enteral nutrition is preferred to parenteral support but should not include more than 1.5 g of protein/kg/day. Drug doses should be adjusted (see Chapter 26). Magnesium- and phosphorous-containing medications should be avoided. Indications for dialysis are given in Chapter 42. Hemodialysis, continuous renal replacement therapy, and peritoneal dialysis are effective in treating metabolic abnormalities and fluid overload. Intermittent or continuous renal replacement therapy, there is no evidence to support mortality benefit in one group over the other.

IV. PROGNOSIS. Patients who recover from AKI may or may not return to their baseline kidney function. Incomplete recovery is more common in patients over age 65 years, those with pre-existing CKD and other comorbid conditions (like heart failure). Hospital-acquired AKI is associated with higher in-hospital and long-term mortality. Those who experience significant AKI (stage 2 and above) during hospitalization and discharged alive should have follow-up evaluation to monitor for resolution of AKI and/or worsening or new-onset CKD.

V. SUGGESTED READINGS

Bellomo R, Kellum JA, Ronco C. Defining acute renal failure: physiological principles. *Intensive Care Med.* 2004;30(1):33–37.

Carvounis CP, Niser S, Guro-Razuman S. Significance of the fractional excretion of urea in the differential diagnosis of acute renal failure. *Kidney Int.* 2002;62(6):2223–2229.

Chawla LS, Bellomo R, Bihorac A, et al. Acute kidney disease and renal recovery: consensus report of the Acute Disease Quality Initiative (ADQI) 16 workgroup. *Nat Rev Nephrol.* 2017;13(4):241–257.

Esson ML, Schrier RW. Diagnosis and treatment of acute tubular necrosis. *Ann Intern Med.* 2002;137(9):744–752.

Prowle JR, Echeverri JE, Ligabo EV, et al. Fluid balance and acute kidney injury. *Nat Rev Nephrol.* 2010;6(2):107–115.

Singbartl K, Kellum JA. AKI in the ICU: definition, epidemiology, risk stratification, and outcomes. *Kidney Int.* 2012;81(9):819–825.

Wilcox CS, ed. *Therapy in Nephrology and Hypertension.* 3rd ed. WB Saunders; 2008.

36 Chronic Kidney Disease

Amir Kazory, Limeng Chen

I. **BACKGROUND**. Chronic kidney disease (CKD) refers to irreversible loss of renal function, and is defined by a decrease in glomerular filtration rate (GFR) to less than 60 mL/min/1.73 m² of body surface area, or presence of at least one marker of kidney damage (e.g., albuminuria, structural abnormalities detected by imaging, abnormal histologic examination) for 3 or more months. According to the Centers for Disease Control and Prevention, over 30 million people, or approximately 15% of the population in the United States, are estimated to have CKD and it is the ninth leading cause of death; by 2040, it is predicted to become the fifth leading cause of death. There is convincing evidence that both lower GFR and greater levels of albuminuria are independently related to mortality, cardiovascular events, and the rate of end-stage renal disease (ESRD). Therefore, both GFR and albuminuria have been integrated into a CKD staging system for more precise classification and prognostic information (Table 36.1).

Most patients with CKD, especially the elderly, will never progress to kidney failure during their lifetime. Risk prediction models have been developed to help with the prediction of kidney failure as well as cardiovascular disease or death among patients with CKD.

II. **RISK FACTORS**. Identification of clinical risk factors helps detect high-risk patients so interventions can be implemented early with the goal of preventing CKD or slowing down its progression. Patients with a history of diabetes, hypertension, and cardiovascular disease are considered at the highest risk for CKD. Hispanic and African-American descent portend a higher risk of progression of CKD compared to the non-Hispanic White population. While older age, smoking, nephrolithiasis, recurrent urinary tract infection, family history of CKD, and previous history of certain chronic illnesses (e.g., human immunodeficiency virus, hepatitis C) all are associated with an increased risk of CKD, more recent studies have identified obesity and childhood history of kidney disease as important risk factors. Finally, since renal tubular toxicity of heavy metals such as cadmium and lead has been recognized, the role of environmental toxins (e.g., air pollution, particulate matter) has recently been investigated. It has been proposed that environmental nephrotoxins may synergize with conventional risk factors and account for certain cases of CKD erroneously attributed to diabetes, hypertension, and obesity. Although hyperuricemia is a strong independent risk marker for incident CKD and hypertension, current available data do not support urate as a causal factor in these conditions. Table 36.2 summarizes risk factors for progression of CKD.

| TABLE 36.1 | Staging system for chronic kidney disease |

Glomerular filtration rate (mL/min/1.73 m^2)

G1	≥90
G2	60–89
G3a	45–59
G3b	30–44
G4	15–29
G5	<15
Urinary albumin/creatinine ratio (mg/g)	
A1	<30
A2	30–299
A3	>300

| TABLE 36.2 | Risk factors and interventions for CKD progression |

	Risk factors of CKD progress	Management
Demographic characteristics	Old age, male gender Hispanics and African Americans Family history of CKD, DM Low birth weight	Regular monitor renal function
Medical History of chronic illnesses	DM, HTN, CVD, hyperuricemia; human immunodeficiency virus, hepatitis C Underlying cause of kidney disease: nephrolithiasis, recurrent urinary tract infection; episodes of AKI	Manage the existing disorders
Environmental toxin Nephrotoxic agents	Heavy metals (cadmium) Environmental toxins (e.g., air pollution and particulate matter) Potentially nephrotoxic drugs	Stop or limit the exposure
Slow down the progression	Hypertension	RASi, diuretics, restrict salt intake
	Proteinuria	RASi, SGLT-2i
	Glycemic control	Insulin, SGLT-2i
	Metabolic acidosis	Sodium bicarbonate (daily dose of 0.5–1 mEq/kg)
	Miscellaneous: smoking, obesity, hyperlipidemia, high-protein diets	Smoking cessation, lose weight, dietary protein restriction

CKD, chronic kidney disease; DM, diabetes; HTN, hypertension; CVD, cardiovascular disease; AKI, acute kidney injury, RASi, renin–angiotensin–aldosterone system inhibitors; SGLT-2i, sodium-glucose cotransporter 2 inhibitors.

III. MANAGEMENT. In patients with CKD, renal function should be monitored closely (every 1 to 4 months, depending on the rate of progression) with periodic estimation of the GFR. The guidelines of the Kidney Disease Outcomes Quality Initiative recommend that patients with stage G4 CKD be referred to a nephrologist. Delayed referral of patients with late-stage CKD is associated with suboptimal outcomes, including increased mortality.

A. Interventions to Slow Down the Rate of Progression

1. **Hypertension.** Hypertension is present in approximately 80% to 85% of patients with CKD. The prevalence of hypertension increases in parallel with decreasing GFR. Control of systemic hypertension slows down the rate of progression of CKD both in patients who have diabetes and those who do not. Factors that contribute to hypertension in CKD are water and salt retention, increased activity of the renin–angiotensin–aldosterone system, enhanced activity of the sympathetic nervous system, impaired nitric oxide synthesis, defective endothelium- mediated vasodilatation, and concurrent use of erythropoietin. An angiotensin-converting enzyme inhibitor (ACE-I) or angiotensin receptor blocker (ARB) is considered the first line of therapy of hypertension in CKD although diuretics are also frequently needed to help optimize volume status and/or manage hyperkalemia especially in those patients with advanced renal dysfunction. Please see the section on Hypertension of this book for an in-depth coverage of this topic.

2. **Proteinuria.** Not only is proteinuria an independent cardiovascular risk factor, but it also can lead to progressive renal structural damage. A reduction in urinary protein excretion to less than 300 to 500 mg/day is associated with a slowing of progression of CKD. ACE-Is and ARBs are the first-line medications to manage proteinuria in CKD stage A2 to A3, and there is also evidence that they can prevent development of proteinuria in those patients with CKD stage A1. The potential decline in GFR that is related to the use of ACE-I or ARB (i.e., through reduction in intraglomerular pressure) is not associated with adverse renal or cardiovascular outcomes. Studies involving patients with diabetes and proteinuria have shown that spironolactone may have an additive effect in reducing proteinuria and blood pressure when combined with maximal doses of an ACE-I or an ARB. Sodium-glucose cotransporter 2 (SGLT-2) inhibitors can reduce intraglomerular pressure and proteinuria through activation of tubuloglomerular feedback and vasoconstriction of afferent arteriole. In patients with CKD (with or without diabetes), who are already receiving either an ACE-I or ARB, addition of these medications can slow the progression of kidney disease.

3. **Glycemic control.** Poorly controlled blood glucose levels are associated with an increased risk of CKD. In addition to cardiovascular risk reduction, glycemic control slows down the progression of albuminuria and loss of kidney function. In patients with type-2 diabetes, treatment with SGLT-2 inhibitors improves glycemic control by interfering with proximal tubular reabsorption of glucose. They also decrease cardiovascular mortality and reduce the risk of CKD progression.

4. **Metabolic acidosis.** Acid–base balance is normally maintained by the renal excretion of the daily acid load, derived mostly from the metabolism of sulfur-containing amino acids. A rise in ammonium excretion can prevent acidosis until the GFR is below 40 to 50 mL/min and non–anion-gap metabolic acidosis develops following reduction in renal ammonia synthesis. As the kidney function declines, reduction in titratable acid (phosphate)

excretion can also manifest as non–anion-gap metabolic acidosis, while progressive retention of organic acids will later lead to increased anion-gap metabolic acidosis. Metabolic acidosis accelerates bone loss, increases skeletal muscle breakdown, reduces albumin synthesis, and hastens progression of CKD. Alkali therapy to maintain the serum bicarbonate concentration at 22 to 26 mEq/L is recommended. Sodium bicarbonate (in a daily dose of 0.5 to 1 mEq/kg/day) is the drug of choice to treat acidosis, improve nutritional status, and slow the progression of CKD.

5. **Miscellaneous.** Smoking cessation and dietary protein restriction (see below Nutrition and CKD) are among other targets that would lead to improved renal outcome among other beneficial effects such as cardiovascular risk reduction. Losing weight in overweight or obese patients is also likely to slow CKD progression through the reduction of hyperfiltration.

B. Management of Complications

1. **Fluid overload.** Extracellular and total body fluid volume expansion generally becomes evident when GFR falls to less than 10 to 15 mL/min. At higher GFR levels, fluid overload can occur if the ingested amount of salt and water exceeds the potential for compensatory excretion. The combination of dietary salt restriction (e.g., less than 2.4 g/day) and the use of a loop diuretic is the key management strategy for fluid overload in CKD. Most patients with stage G4 will require a loop diuretic; if furosemide is used, it should be dosed twice daily to provide effective natriuresis.

2. **Hyperkalemia.** The ability to maintain potassium excretion at near-normal levels is generally preserved until the GFR falls to less than 20 to 25 mL/min or patients become oliguric. Common factors that predispose to hyperkalemia are high potassium intake, hypoaldosteronism, acidosis, and medications such as ACE-I and ARB. Patients with CKD and diabetes and/or heart failure are particularly prone to hyperkalemia. For those patients taking inhibitors of the renin–angiotensin–aldosterone system (RAAS), temporarily holding the agents or adding a diuretic often improves hyperkalemia. For others with chronic or recurring hyperkalemia, prescription of newly developed potassium exchangers (e.g., patiromer, sodium zirconium cyclosilicate) will help control serum potassium levels while patients continue to benefit from inhibition of RAS. Please see the section on Hyperkalemia of this book for in-depth coverage of this topic.

3. **Mineral and bone disorders.** Disorders of mineral and bone metabolism are common in patients with CKD. A tendency for phosphate retention begins early in the course of CKD due to reduced phosphate filtration. Parathyroid hormone secretion increases at this stage to enhance urinary phosphate excretion and keep serum phosphate levels within the normal range. More than half the patients with a GFR of less than 60 mL/min present with hyperparathyroidism, which is an independent risk factor for increased cardiovascular disease and mortality. Therefore, while phosphate retention takes place fairly early during the course of CKD and is a trigger for development of secondary hyperparathyroidism, hyperphosphatemia is a relatively late event and does not typically manifest before stage G4. Renal conversion of vitamin D to its active form (1,25-dihydroxyvitamin D) is also reduced in CKD resulting in decreased intestinal calcium absorption and a progressive tendency for low serum calcium levels. Hypocalcemia and decreased levels of active vitamin D further contribute to secondary hyperparathyroidism. Hyperphosphatemia also increases the production of fibroblast growth

factor 23 (FGF23) by osteocytes and osteoblasts. FGF23 binds to fibroblast growth factor receptor-1, and in the presence of the required coreceptor αKlotho, decreases type II sodium–dependent phosphate cotransporters NaPi2a and NaPi2c in the proximal tubule of the kidney, thereby inhibiting phosphate reabsorption. This phosphaturic hormone also inhibits the synthesis of active vitamin D and therefore can contribute to hyperparathyroidism.

Serum phosphate should be maintained less than 4.5 mg/dL in patients with CKD. Dietary phosphate restriction (less than 800 to 1,000 mg/day) and administration of oral phosphate binders to block absorption of ingested phosphate from the intestine may manage hyperphosphatemia and delay the development of secondary hyperparathyroidism. There are two types of phosphate binders: calcium-containing (e.g., calcium carbonate, calcium acetate) and non–calcium-containing (e.g., sevelamer, lanthanum carbonate). They should be taken with meals to bind dietary phosphorus. More recently, iron-containing phosphate binders (e.g., ferric citrate) have been developed to simultaneously provide iron supplementation and phosphate binding and reduce pill burden. The choice of phosphate binder can be informed by serum calcium concentration which should be maintained at the lower end of the normal range (8.4 to 9.5 mg/dL), with the goal of the "calcium × phosphate" product to be less than 55 mg^2/mL^2. The total dose of elemental Ca (including dietary sources) should not exceed 2,000 mg/day. Aluminum hydroxide, although a potent phosphate binder, should be avoided because of aluminum toxicity that manifests as osteomalacia, anemia, bone and muscle pain, and dementia. The target serum intact PTH should be 35 to 70 pg/mL for those with stage G3 CKD, 70 to 110 pg/mL for those with stage G4 CKD, and 150 to 300 pg/mL for those with end-stage renal disease. In addition to the strict control of hyperphosphatemia, the use of inactive compounds, ergocalciferol (vitamin D2) and cholecalciferol (vitamin D3) can initially help correct 25(OH) vitamin D deficiency. Later on, activated vitamin D (i.e., calcitriol) and vitamin D analogs (e.g., paricalcitol) can be used to lower PTH and manage renal bone disease; the risk of a rise in serum "calcium × phosphate" product is generally lower with vitamin D analogs. Calcimimetics, such as cinacalcet, increase the sensitivity of the calcium-sensing receptor in the parathyroid gland to calcium and reduce PTH secretion and hyperplasia of the gland. They can induce profound hypocalcemia and are not approved for use in CKD patients who are not treated with dialysis. Patients with symptomatic renal bone disease and with nonsuppressible serum PTH values should be offered parathyroidectomy. Indications for parathyroidectomy include serum PTH greater than 800 pg/mL refractory to medical therapy, hyperplastic parathyroid gland measuring greater than 500 mm^3, or glands larger than 1 cm in diameter.

4. **Anemia.** Anemia is common in patients with CKD, especially among those with diabetes, and its prevalence increases progressively as renal function declines. Hemoglobin should be checked at least annually in CKD stage G3a to G3b, and at least twice per year in those with CKD stage G4 to G5. Deficient erythropoietin synthesis, shortened red blood cell survival, and iron deficiency are among the most frequent reasons for anemia in this patient population. Iron supplementation is indicated for CKD patients who have a TSAT ≤20% and a serum ferritin concentration of ≤100 ng/mL. While most clinicians use oral iron for nondialysis CKD patients, studies have reported inconsistent findings concerning its efficacy. There have

been concerns regarding the safety of intravenous iron supplementation in nondialysis CKD patients that have not been confirmed in most recent studies. Erythropoiesis-stimulating agents (ESAs) can be administered (50 to 100 units/kg/week) to those patients whose hemoglobin remains less than 10 g/dL, despite adequate iron stores, to avoid red blood cell transfusion. The subcutaneous route is preferred in these patients to preserve their veins for future hemodialysis access. Caution should be exercised in those patients with recent or active cancer as well as those with a history of stroke. Hypoxia-inducible factor prolyl hydroxylase inhibitors (HIF-PHIs) are a novel class of oral ESAs that might represent an option for the treatment of anemia in nondialysis CKD patients in the future. Recommended management of complications of CKD is summarized in Table 36.3. Please refer to Chapter 39 for a detailed discussion of anemia management in CKD.

C. **Conservative Management**. In a subset of patients with CKD, renal function continues to decline and reach end-stage kidney. Such patients may elect to withhold dialysis especially if they are elderly or with significant debilitating comorbidities. Based on shared decision- making principles, conservative management of end-stage kidney disease (e.g., management of symptoms, nutritional interventions, advance-care planning) should be considered an option for all patients who decide not to pursue renal replacement therapy.

IV. SPECIAL TOPICS IN CKD

A. **Nutrition and CKD**. The nutritional status of patients with CKD often becomes disordered as the disease progresses; protein-energy wasting is a common finding at later stages. The appetite of the patients can become blunted with distorted taste and smell resulting from progressive accumulation of nitrogen-containing products from dietary and intrinsic protein catabolism. The gastrointestinal microbiome is also affected by uremia leading to disrupted nutrient absorption. This can lead to muscle and fat wasting especially in those with existing comorbidities (e.g., diabetes) and also in the elderly population.

A low-protein diet has been found to mitigate proteinuria both in animal models and human kidney disease possibly through reduction in intraglomerular pressure. It can also decrease urea generation with consequent improvement in oxidative stress, endothelial dysfunction, inflammation, and ultimately cardiovascular risk. The recommended protein intake for patients with an eGFR of less than 45 mL/min/1.73 m^2 is 0.6 to 0.8 g/kg/day, which can fulfill dietary needs, especially if half of the protein originates is of high biologic value (e.g., fish, eggs, dairy products). The safety of this approach will be further enhanced by providing adequate energy (i.e., 30 to 35 kcal/kg/day) and ongoing nutritional surveillance. Although low-protein diet decreases phosphorus intake, the quantity and bioavailability of phosphorus would depend on the type of protein (i.e., the phosphorus-to-protein ratio). For example, food additives include readily absorbable phosphorus and hence processed foods typically result in a higher phosphorus burden. Finally, nutritional interventions (e.g., low-protein diet, alkali therapy, supplementation of trace elements and vitamins) may be used for conservative management of uremia as a means of avoiding renal replacement therapy in selected patients.

Although obesity is an established risk factor for diabetes and hypertension, its role as an independent risk factor for CKD has been debated. Nevertheless, adopting a healthy lifestyle and aerobic exercise offers benefits with respect to body weight, fat mass, and markers of oxidative stress and inflammatory

TABLE 36.3	The recommendations for managing the complications of CKD			
Complications	**CKD stages, GFR (mL/min)**	**Suggestions for dietary restriction**	**Medication or operation**	**Therapy targets**
Fluid overload	<10–15 mL/min	Salt <2.4 g/day Water intake depends on urine volume	Loop diuretic (furosemide, bid)	Without edema, effusion, and heart failure
Hyperkalemia	<20–25 mL/min	High potassium intake	Stop RASi, correct acidosis, potassium exchangers	Normal range
Mineral and bone disorders	Hypocalcemia Monitoring intervals CKD 3: 6–12 mo CKD 4: 3–6 mo CKD 5: 1–3 mo	Total elemental Ca <2,000 mg/day (include medicine)	Calcium carbonate and calcium acetate Vitamin D supplement	8.4–9.5 mg/dL Avoiding hypercalcemia
	Hyperphosphatemia Monitoring intervals: same as serum calcium	Phosphate intake <800–1,000 mg/day	Phosphate binder: Calcium-containing (restricting the dose) Non-calcium-containing (avoiding the long-term use of aluminum)	Normal range <4.5 mg/dL "Calcium × phosphate" <55 mg²/mL²
	Hyperparathyroidism Monitoring intervals CKD 4: 6–12 mo CKD 5: 3–6 mo 1,25 (OH)D deficiency <60 mL/min	Correct hyperphosphatemia and hypocalcemia CKD 5D: calcimimetics, calcitriol, or vitamin D analogs Parathyroidectomy (fail to respond to medicine) First: inactive vitamin D2, D3 Later: calcitriol or paricalcitol		iPTH in CKD 3: 35–70 pg/mL; CKD 4: 70–110 pg/mL; CKD 5:150–300 pg/mL CKD 5D: 2–9 times the upper normal limit
Anemia	Check Hb period at least CKD 3: annually CKD 4–5ND: twice per year CKD 5D: every 3 mo Anemia not being treated with an ESA: every 1–3 mo	Oral iron (CKD-ND patients) Intravenous iron (HD patients); ESAs; HIF-PHIs Red cell transfusion (urgent condition)		Correct it as the general population recommendation TSAT ≤30%, ferritin ≤500 ng/mL: treatment with iron agents Hb ≤9–10 g/L, ESA therapy ESA treatment: Hb ≤11.5 g/L Stop ESAs: Hb >13 g/L

CKD, chronic Kidney disease; CKD-ND, CKD nondialysis; ESAs, erythropoiesis-stimulating agents; iPTH, intact parathyroid hormone; Hb, hemoglobin; TSAT, serum transferrin saturation; HIF-PHI, hypoxia-inducible factor-prolyl hydroxylase enzyme inhibitors.

response in those with CKD and obesity. Likewise, bariatric surgery could portend long-term benefits regarding development and progression of CKD both through management of risk factors of disease development (e.g., diabetes, hypertension) and possible mitigation of risk factors of disease progression (e.g., hyperfiltration, inflammation).

B. CKD of Unknown Cause in Agricultural Communities. Formerly called "Mesoamerican Nephropathy," this form of CKD was first noted among sugarcane workers in Central America and is now recognized in other parts of the world such as Sri Lanka and Central India. It typically affects young men between 20 and 50 years old with normal or slightly elevated blood pressure and normal blood glucose levels. The urinalysis shows no or mild proteinuria with a small number of red cells and leukocytes. It is not clear whether CKD results from repetitive episodes of acute kidney injury (intravascular volume depletion due to extreme heat in the fields and lack of appropriate hydration) or represents a chronic process (e.g., due to pesticides, heavy metals, infections). Renal biopsy is nonspecific and typically shows chronic interstitial disease, tubular atrophy, inflammation, and fibrosis. The kidney disease is commonly advanced (stages G3 or G4) by the time of diagnosis. In the absence of a proven etiology, preventive measures such as provision of adequate and safe hydration, rest, and shade for workers at risk have been proposed.

C. CKD and Illicit Drugs. Illicit drugs represent unique risk factors for CKD incidence and progression. Use of cocaine, heroin, or methamphetamine, has been linked with an increased risk of CKD progression and mortality among those patients with pre-existing CKD. However, studies have shown that past or present marijuana use may not be associated with an increase in the risk of CKD.

V. REFERRAL TO NEPHROLOGISTS. All patients with GFR less than 30 mL/min/1.73 m^2 (stage G4) should be referred to a nephrologist. Late referral (i.e., less than 3 months prior to the start of maintenance renal replacement therapy) is associated with higher mortality after the initiation of dialysis. On the other hand, timely referral to nephrologists is associated with lower costs as well as decreased morbidity and mortality.

Once referred, it is important for nephrologists to identify patients who may eventually require renal replacement therapy because adequate preparation can decrease morbidity. Early identification also allows for preparation of a functioning access and optimal timing of dialysis initiation.

VI. SUGGESTED READINGS

Gilbert S, Weiner DE. *National Kidney Foundation Primer on Kidney Diseases*. 7th ed. Elsevier; 2018.
Silver SA, Bell CM, Chertow GM, et al. Effectiveness of quality improvement strategies for the management of CKD: a meta-analysis. *Clin J Am Soc Nephrol*. 2017;12(10):1601–1614.
Whittaker CF, Miklich MA, Patel RS, et al. Medication safety principles and practice in CKD. *Clin J Am Soc Nephrol*. 2018;13(11):1738–1746.

Cardiovascular Complications of Chronic Kidney Disease

Ashutosh M. Shukla, Mark S. Segal

INTRODUCTION

Cardiovascular disease (CVD) is the largest cause of morbidity and mortality worldwide and assumes even greater significance in patients with chronic kidney disease (CKD). Despite this, CVD in CKD and end-stage kidney disease (ESKD) remains poorly investigated, as the vast majority of clinical studies involving CVD to date have avoided enrolling patients with significant CKD.

I. **EPIDEMIOLOGY.** Any level of CKD, commonly defined as estimated glomerular filtration rate (eGFR) below 60 mL/min/1.73 m^2 body surface area, henceforth referred to as mL/min, is associated with a near doubling, and severe CKD defined as eGFR below 30 mL/min is associated with more than tripling of the cardiovascular mortality compared to the general population. It is now also well established that proteinuria, specifically albuminuria, is also an independent predictor of cardiovascular outcomes, with a similar rise in the risk of cardiovascular mortality in those with Kidney Disease Improving Global Outcomes (KDIGO) A2 or A3 category albuminuria, compared to those with normoalbuminuria (A1 category). These associations and synergistic effects of albuminuria and low eGFR on all-cause and cardiovascular mortality exist in both patients with or without pre-existing CVD, and are reflected in the latest KDIGO guidelines that classify CKD not only based on eGFR (stages 1 to 5) but also by subclassifying each stage by the degree of albuminuria (categories A1 to A3). In 2003, the National Kidney Foundation and American College of Cardiology corecognized CKD as an independent CVD risk factor and a "coronary artery disease equivalent" for CVD outcomes.

II. **TYPES OF CARDIOVASCULAR DISEASE IN CKD.** The spectrum of CVD in CKD changes with the progressive decline in the renal function. CVD disease related to atherosclerosis rises early in the course of CKD, whereas a number of pathologies not easily lumped together, but loosely described in most renal literature as nonatherosclerotic CVD assumes greater significance as the CKD progresses.

III. **VASCULAR OR CARDIOVASCULAR DISEASE RELATED TO ATHEROSCLEROSIS AND ITS COMPLICATIONS**

A. **Myocardial Infarction.** Presentation of atherosclerotic CVD in CKD is often atypical. Progressive CKD and ESKD patients commonly have significant functional limitations, and thus, typical chest pain on exertion with attendant shoulder discomfort and radiation to the arm is uncommon. On the other hand, dyspnea at rest or on exertion is a common angina equivalence symptom. Sometimes, the only indication regarding the ongoing critical coronary syndrome is fatigue and lack of energy, and a high index of suspicion is required when evaluating these patients. Extracellular fluid volume increase and intradialysis hypotension are common among patients on hemodialysis (HD). These have the potential for masking underlying coronary disease. Sudden shifts in extracellular volume, hypokalemia, and hemodynamic instability are particularly of concern in HD patients with silent ischemia.

B. **Stroke.** Any level of discernible CKD, that is, eGFR ≤60 mL/min, is associated with an over 40% increase in the risk of stroke; the risk rises with progressive CKD and patients with ESKD have nearly 3 to 10 times higher risk of stroke compared to the general population, with the overall absolute incidence of stroke among ESKD being reported between 15 and 49 per 1,000 patient-years. The spectrum of stroke, ischemic (about 90%) versus hemorrhagic (about 10%), is similar in CKD and ESKD. Epidemiologic data show trends for a lower incidence of stroke in patients on peritoneal dialysis (PD) than those on HD; the latter conclusion is far from concrete.

C. **Other Vascular Disease.** While myocardial infarction (MI) and stroke are classic atherosclerosis-related CVD, the incidence of peripheral arterial disease and splanchnic disease is also high in patients with CKD and ESKD, with patterns for disease severity similarly correlating to the decline in eGFR and rising proteinuria. Overall, the outcomes of the revascularization surgeries in earlier stages of CKD are similar to those in the general population, while advanced CKD and ESKD patients have increased probabilities of the need for amputation and pathology beyond revascularization.

D. **Vascular Pathology in CKD.** Two types of vascular processes and, in turn, calcification patterns dominate in patients with CKD and ESKD, each likely impacted by a different pathogenesis.

E. **Atherosclerosis and Intimal Calcification.** The intimal calcification in CKD is likely secondary to increased atherosclerosis burden. The process appears to be similar in patients with CKD and ESKD as in those with normal renal function, albeit at a higher severity, due to greater severity of local, mechanical, and inflammatory forces. Additionally, medial calcification and resultant arterial stiffness further contribute to shear stress and atherosclerosis, further worsening intimal calcification.

F. **Vascular Stiffness and Medial Calcification.** Patients with CKD and ESKD have a unique vascular pathology that manifests itself with medial calcification, mainly due to a phenotype switch of vascular smooth muscle cells to osteoblast-like cells. While this contributes to worsening atherosclerosis, reduction in vascular compliance and increase in vascular stiffness resulting from medial calcification also has significant impact on the nonatherosclerosis cardiovascular outcomes in CKD. Bone and mineral abnormalities of CKD, inflammation, and a number of uremic toxins further contribute to the initiation and propagation of the medial calcification (see below).

CVD not directly related to atherosclerosis: Considering that many of the processes loosely lumped together as nonatherosclerotic CVD, below, are more common among those with vascular and structural heart disease, the true independence of these processes from the atherosclerotic process and their true incidence is uncertain.

G. Cardiac Arrhythmias and Sudden Cardiac Death. Nearly half of all ESKD deaths are related to CVD. However, only about 20% of those deaths are recorded as being directly related to atherosclerotic CVD. The remainder, is reported to be related to the occurrence of cardiac arrhythmias, with sudden cardiac death (SCD) as the dominant diagnosis. The risk of mortality is nearly threefold higher after the long-weekend interval in three times a week HD, and nearly 70% higher in the immediate postdialysis period. Use of low-K dialysate is also associated with a higher risk of death. These data signify the concerns related to electrolyte imbalance, including hyper- and hypokalemia, and rapid fluid shifts as important precipitating causes for SCD. The type of arrhythmias responsible for the SCD in ESKD is also under debate. Cohort studies in patients with in situ implantable cardiac monitors have shown that tachyarrhythmias, for example, ventricular tachycardia and ventricular fibrillation are dominant arrhythmias responsible for nearly 80% of SCD in ESKD; however, recent findings have raised doubts on this data with some reports showing a much greater proportion of deaths due related to bradyarrhythmias, with dialysis vintage and associated myocardial fibrosis as a prominent contributory factor.

H. Atrial Fibrillation. Progressive CKD is associated with an increasing incidence of conduction and rhythm disorders, with atrial fibrillation (AF) being the most common form of sustained arrhythmia in CKD and ESKD. AF prevalence estimates range from 16% to 21% in nondialysis CKD and 15% to 40% in ESKD.

I. Left Ventricular Hypertrophy in CKD. Left ventricular hypertrophy (LVH) is a common pathology in patients with CKD. Its prevalence rises progressively with the worsening CKD; about 50% to 70% of nondialysis CKD patients and about 90% of patients with ESKD on dialysis have LVH. LVH regresses, at least partially after kidney transplantation, suggesting the role of CKD-related factors in the pathogenesis of LVH.

J. Heart Failure. HF and CKD share a special interdependent relationship; recognition of both conditions is increasing, and they are mutually detrimental. The incidence of new-onset HF in nondialysis CKD is about 17% to 21%, with prevalence varying based on the degree of renal dysfunction, albuminuria, and presence of other comorbidities. The prevalence of HF rises to over 40% in ESKD patients, with the likelihood of HF being greater in patients on HD than those on PD. About 40% of the HF patients in ESKD have HF with reduced ejection fraction (HFrEF), while a quarter have HF with preserved ejection fraction (HFpEF); the remainder are undiagnosed or unspecified. Coronary artery disease is responsible for nearly two-thirds of all HFrEF, while it contributes to about a quarter of cases of HFpEF. Advancing age, diabetes, obesity, reduced physical fitness levels, and systemic inflammation have a strong influence on the pathogenesis of HFpEF. Several CKD- and ESKD-related variables discussed below further contribute toward the pathogenesis of both types of HF in CKD.

IV. RISK FACTORS AND PATHOPHYSIOLOGY OF CARDIOVASCULAR DISEASE IN CKD

A. Traditional Risk Factors. Traditional cardiovascular risk factors, such as older age, smoking, hypertension, dyslipidemia, and diabetes, are more prevalent in CKD populations. Analyses of large ESKD databases such as the United States Renal Data System (USRDS) have shown that over 60% of the ESKD patients have diabetes, with two-thirds of these patients having ESKD secondary to diabetes.

Similar analyses have also shown that hypertension is near ubiquitous, present in over 90% of advanced CKD and ESKD patients. Hyperlipidemia is unique in CKD, with the pattern of lipid abnormalities and its associations with cardiovascular mortality varying vastly across the spectrum of CKD. Patients in the earlier stages of CKD and with greater severity of proteinuria have a greater propensity for a more traditional lipid disorder with high levels of low-density lipoprotein cholesterol (LDL) and triglycerides with or without an associated reduction in the levels of high-density lipoprotein cholesterol (HDL). However, the pattern changes with CKD progression such that only a third of all ESKD have high levels of total cholesterol and LDL values, with patients on PD more likely to have these abnormalities compared to those on HD. Inflammation appears to be a prominent factor responsible for altering the traditional associations between hyperlipidemia and cardiovascular outcomes. Data also show that inflammation makes the CVD in CKD refractory to traditional therapies like statins. CKD also contributes to chemical modifications of the lipoprotein molecules, that is, oxidative changes and carbamylation, both of which have been shown to adversely impact the vascular pathology and atherosclerosis. Composition of the HDL molecule and their protective effects on atherosclerosis is also altered in CKD, thus, reducing the efficacy of the HDL's protective role. Finally, triglycerides occupy a central role in the CVD in CKD. Nearly half of all CKD patients have triglyceride levels above 200 mg/dL (2.26 mmol/L), both due to increased production related to low glucose tolerance and impaired degradation due to reduced activities of circulating lipases. A number of traditional cardiovascular risk factors appear to correlate with the severity of kidney dysfunction. Patients with CKD are also more likely to have metabolic syndrome (see below), further contributing to increased cardiovascular risk.

B. Nontraditional Risk Factors. Among the several nontraditional cardiovascular risk factors in CKD, some are directly related to the decline in renal function, that is, retention of uremic toxins, anemia, elevated levels of inflammatory cytokines, positive calcium balance, hyperphosphatemia, hyperparathyroidism, etc., while others, are related to the comorbidities and variables coexisting with CKD, that is, metabolic syndrome, inflammation with or without malnutrition, endothelial dysfunction, etc.

C. Inflammation. Chronic systemic inflammation plays a critical role in the pathogenesis of several systemic complications in patients with CKD, including progressive CKD and CVD. Patients with CKD commonly have increased levels of systemic markers of inflammation, such as high-sensitivity C-reactive protein (hsCRP), ferritin, and various inflammatory cytokines, including interleukin (IL)-1, IL-6, tumor necrosis factor (TNF)-a, and interferon-y among others. There also appears to be a trend toward worsening inflammatory state with the advancing CKD.

D. Endothelial Dysfunction and Vascular Stiffness. Reduced endothelial nitric oxide (NO) availability, and the resultant endothelial dysfunction and vascular stiffness make the vessels susceptible to atherosclerosis. Several additional CKD-related processes adversely impact vascular health. Abnormalities in bone mineral health, especially reduced circulating levels of αKlotho, increased fibroblast growth factor (FGF)-23, high phosphorus or calcium-phosphorus product, and reduced levels of vitamin D have been shown to be associated with and mechanistically causal to the endothelial dysfunction in CKD. Several uremic toxins also have been implicated in endothelial dysfunction. Principle among these is the increased levels of circulating asymmetrical dimethylarginine (ADMA), which is a direct endogenous inhibitor of endothelial nitric oxide synthase, the principal substrate contributing to healthy endothelial and vascular function.

E. **Metabolic Syndrome**. Metabolic syndrome is characterized by a combination of disorders, including impaired glucose tolerance, hyperinsulinemia, elevated blood pressure, dyslipidemia, obesity, etc. While the individual disorders have been shown to have negative impact on outcomes in CKD, two large cohort studies have shown that the presence of a combination of these in the form of metabolic syndrome substantially increases the probability of cardiovascular complications, by nearly 40% to 80%.

F. **Bone Mineral Disease of CKD**. The abnormalities of calcium, phosphorus, and PTH axis have been well recognized metabolic abnormalities in CKD for over half a century. Since the 1990s, it is now further recognized that these abnormalities are not only crucial for the CKD-associated bone disease but also significantly impact the cardiovascular outcomes in CKD. Vascular calcification in dialysis patients may be associated with positive calcium balance, hyperphosphatemia, increased serum calcium-phosphorus product, high PTH values, and high levels of FGF-23.

G. **Dialysis-Related Factors**. Type, frequency, and duration of dialysis have significant implications on fluid balance, electrolyte and acid–base fluxes, and overall cardiovascular health. While a number of therapeutic approaches have been shown to be useful in addressing challenges related to these factors, prospective evaluations of these in sufficiently powered, large intervention studies are needed.

V. **DIAGNOSTIC EVALUATION OF CARDIOVASCULAR DISEASE IN CKD**. Serologic markers of cardiac injury and stress: Increased levels of cardiac troponins I and T (cTnI and cTnT) are frequently encountered in asymptomatic CKD patients. Cohort studies have shown that these can signify cardiac hypertrophy or even subclinical myocardial stress, and portend worse long-term cardiovascular outcomes and survival. These troponins are also the preferred and now nearly ubiquitously used biomarkers for the diagnosis of acute MI. Like in the general population, a serial change in troponin levels over 3 to 6 hours should be used to define acute MI, rather than a single value obtained on presentation.

B-type natriuretic peptide (BNP) or N-terminal pro-BNP are other frequently used cardiac biomarkers to diagnose HF in patients with CKD. Worsening renal function is associated with increasing levels of both BNP and more specifically, N-terminal pro-BNP, as there is a reduced renal clearance of the molecules and increased prevalence of HF. Thus, similar to cardiac troponins, normal levels of BNP or its metabolites have a high negative predictive value, but their role in establishing the diagnosis is limited.

A. **Electrocardiographic**. The prevalence of electrocardiographic (ECG) abnormalities in CKD depends on the individual's age and the presence of comorbidities. Published reports suggest that some form of abnormality in ECG is prevalent in about 50% to 70% of CKD patients. The presence of an abnormal ECG has been correlated with increased rates of cardiovascular events and death in patients with nondialysis CKD and ESKD. As described before, the prevalence of AF is high in CKD and ESKD. Considering these, most dialysis units prefer obtaining a baseline ECG for most patients initiating renal replacement therapy, and ECG is a standard of care investigation for prospective renal transplant recipients.

B. **Transthoracic Echocardiography**. Patients with nondialysis CKD have been shown to have lower LV ejection fraction, higher prevalence of RV systolic impairment, higher LV mass index, higher LV and left atrium diameter, more regional wall motion abnormalities, and higher prevalence of RV hypertrophy or dilated RV. A recent cohort study showed that 87% of the incident ESKD patients starting on HD have major echocardiographic abnormalities; 54% have three or more abnormalities, and many of these have a significant negative impact on survival. Left atrial dilation (55%), LV hypertrophy (37%), and LV diastolic impairment (54%) are among the most common findings. These findings emphasize the need for universal evaluation of cardiac structure and function in all patients initiating renal replacement therapies. Obtaining this echocardiography after initial stabilization, at about 1 to 3 months, may allow a more accurate estimate of the long-term therapeutic needs of these patients.

C. **Imaging Strategies.** The accuracy of noninvasive stress imaging testing in patients with significant nondialysis CKD and ESKD is lower than that in the general population. Pharmacologic stress imaging is the procedure of choice for most advanced CKD and ESKD patients and provides among the highest area under the receiver operating curve for any noninvasive tests in most circumstances. Even among the stress imaging techniques, dobutamine stress imaging is preferred due to the concerns related to the thallium scintigraphy in patients with the uremic milieu. A recent study showed that the risk of acute kidney injury with the currently considered "gold-standard" investigation for coronary heart disease, that is, coronary angiography is low (about 12%), especially when used with low or isosmolar contrast, suggesting that it may be preferred in appropriately high-risk individuals.

VI. MANAGEMENT OF ATHEROSCLEROTIC HEART DISEASE IN CKD

A. **Statins.** The Study of Heart and Renal Protection (SHARP) trial demonstrated that hyperlipidemia treatment with a statin was associated with a 17% reduction in the major cardiovascular events and need for revascularizations. While the study employed ezetimibe with statins, its role in the outcomes is considered unclear. Similar data for statin benefits are also visible in the metaanalysis of trials that enrolled patients with CKD, showing that statin use is associated with a significant (about 19% to 24%) reduction in cardiovascular events and mortality. Unfortunately, these benefits appear to be reduced as renal failure advances, and statin therapy benefits on either cardiovascular events or mortality are unclear in the dialysis population. The current KDIGO guidelines recommend statin therapy for all patients with eGFR below 60 mL/min.

B. **Management of Hypertriglyceridemia.** The results from the Veterans Affairs High-Density Lipoprotein Intervention Trial (VA-HIT) showed that gemfibrozil reduced the risk of cardiovascular events by 27% in those with established CHD and HDL below 40 mg/dL. Similar results have been shown in another metaanalysis showing nearly 30% decline in cardiovascular events. Unfortunately, lower tolerance of fibrates, especially when used in conjunction with statins, does not allow for the use of fibrates or niacin in regular renal care to manage hypertriglyceridemia in CKD.

C. **Hypertension and Cardiovascular Disease.** A detailed discussion about the principles of management of hypertension in patients with or without CKD has been covered in Chapters 23 and 24.

D. **Antiplatelet Therapy.** While there is no randomized study examining the efficacy of aspirin on the cardiovascular outcomes in CKD patients, a large metaanalysis showed that the use of antiplatelet agents, largely aspirin, significantly reduced the incidence of fatal or nonfatal MI, though the effect size was limited (3 for every 1,000 patients treated). At the same time, antiplatelet therapy was also associated with a significant increase in the rate of major bleeding, 15 additional major bleeding events for every 1,000 patients treated. Antiplatelets had no effect on stroke or mortality, and the results were similar in patients of all CKD stages. Similar analyses of the P2Y12 inhibitors in acute MI or postpercutaneous coronary intervention have shown that the use of P2Y12 inhibitor is associated with a significant cardiovascular and survival advantage in patients with CKD, and these benefits occur with a limited and acceptable increase in the risk of major bleeding episodes when compared to the normal renal function population. Finally, a few recent analyses have shown that among the P2Y12 inhibitors, ticagrelor, an irreversible inhibitor, may hold a greater advantage in terms of risk reduction compared to the older and reversible inhibitor clopidogrel.

E. **Coronary Interventions in CKD.** Patients with CKD and ESKD are not only at high risk for the development of coronary heart disease, but CKD of any severity is also associated with increased probability for adverse outcomes after acute MI, percutaneous coronary intervention, and coronary artery bypass grafting compared to those with normal renal function. As such, these patients are at high risk of adverse outcomes with or without intervention, with 70% 1-year and only 25% 5-year survival reported in ESKD patients undergoing revascularization procedures.

Two overarching philosophies drive the decision making for revascularizations in CKD and ESKD.

1) Revascularization versus conservative management: Cumulatively, over the last 10 to 15 years, cohort-based analyses have repeatedly shown that in patients with CKD and ESKD, cardiac revascularization is associated with improved survival compared to the optimal medical management. Despite this, the probability of intervention in CKD and ESKD has continued to be lower than in those with normal renal function. However, a recent randomized study enrolling patients with advanced (primarily stage 4 and 5) CKD and ESKD showed that revascularization strategy, with a majority of patients (85%) receiving a percutaneous intervention, did not provide any survival advantage over the optimal medical management.

2) While the older data suggested a relative survival advantage for coronary artery bypass grafting (CABG) over percutaneous interventions, a number of analyses from the randomized studies and cohort-based data now show that percutaneous intervention with drug-eluting stents may provide equivalent outcomes compared to CABG. As such, most prognostic models include renal function in their short- and long-term outcome prediction.

F. **Anticoagulation Therapy in CKD.** The need for anticoagulation therapy in patients with CKD and ESKD is commonly based on the aggregate risk of stroke in this population. In this regard, it has been shown that the various available predictive models are less accurate in predicting the probability of stroke in CKD and ESKD. At present, we lack evidence to suggest any one predictive score model over the others though, the CHA2DS2-VASc appears most commonly used predictive score in routine clinical practice. Furthermore, though we lack randomized studies in advanced CKD and ESKD population, available data show that the efficacy of vitamin K antagonists, that is, warfarin in preventing stroke, reduces significantly as the renal function declines, and may not be effective at all in patients with ESKD. This combined with the available data showing increased risk for major bleeding episodes and increased vascular calcification, including probabilities of calcific uremic arteriolopathy, makes warfarin an un-desired intervention for patients with AF in the presence of CKD and ESKD. We also lack randomized studies comparing the efficacy of conservative care or warfarin therapy to the newer available direct oral anticoagulant therapy. In this regard, a few systematic reviews show that direct oral anticoagulant ther-apy may have greater efficacy in preventing stroke while reducing the chances of bleeding in patients with CKD, with a more favorable risk-benefit profile as the renal failure progresses. Given these, pending the conduct of randomized studies, major professional societies suggest a dose-adjusted direct oral antico-agulation therapy in patients with CKD and ESKD, when warranted for AF and venous thromboembolism. Despite these, the latest USRDS 2018 annual report shows that nearly a third of all ESKD patients with AF and/or venous thrombo-embolism are on warfarin therapy, and only about 10% are treated with direct oral anticoagulant therapy.

G. **Implantable Cardioverter Defibrillators and Pacemaker Outcomes in CKD.** Implantable cardioverter defibrillators (ICD) have been shown to reduce cardiovascular mortality and SCD in patients with structural heart disease and HF. However, early studies with ICD in HF largely excluded patients with significant CKD. Subgroup analyses of these initial HF clinical trials showed a possible survival advantage with ICD in patients with CKD and ESKD. However, several recent analyses have shown that the benefits of ICD in preventing cardiac death in patients with CKD are limited and of declining order as the renal failure pro-gresses. Concerns for the overestimation of SCD as a cause of death, advanced nature of the cardiac disease, and competing risk of mortality appear to be the major reasons for the lack of benefit.

H. **Upcoming Therapies.** A number of newer therapies are being evaluated or have been recently established for the CVD. These therapies are being explored for the management of CVD in CKD. Novel inhibitors of proprotein convertase sub-tilisin kexin 9 (PCSK9) and the anti-inflammatory agent canakinumab need fo-cused study in patients with significant CKD to determine their effectiveness.

VII. SUGGESTED READINGS

House AA, Wanner C, Sarnak MJ, et al. Heart failure in chronic kidney disease: conclusions from a Kidney Disease: Improving Global Outcomes (KDIGO) controversies conference. *Kidney Int.* 2019;95(6):1304–1317.

Kumar S, Lim E, Covic A, et al. Anticoagulation in concomitant chronic kidney disease and atrial fibrillation: JACC review topic of the week. *J Am College Cardiol.* 2019;74(17):2204–2215.

Sarnak MJ, Amann K, Bangalore S, et al. Chronic kidney disease and coronary artery disease: JACC state-of-the-art review. *J Am Coll Cardiol.* 2019;74(14):1823–1838.

USRDS Report United States Renal Data System (USRDS). A national data system that collects, analyzes, and distributes information about chronic kidney disease (CKD). https://www.usrds.org/media/1732/v2_c08_ESKD_cvd_18_usrds.pdf

38

Renal Disease in Patients with Liver Disease

Abhilash Koratala, Amir Kazory

Renal involvement in patients with liver disease results from the effects of chronic liver disease, infectious agents causing immunologic injury to the kidneys, or from systemic diseases that affect both the liver and kidneys (Table 38.1). Please refer to Chapters 5, 6, 7, and 13 for coverage of these topics. This chapter focuses on acute kidney injury (AKI) in a patient with advanced liver disease, with emphasis on hepatorenal syndrome (HRS).

HRS refers to development of AKI in a patient with cirrhosis due to hepatic dysfunction–induced circulatory derangement and maladaptive kidney perfusion. It is frequently considered a diagnosis of exclusion. Patients with cirrhosis and ascites have a probability of up to 40% of developing HRS within a 5-year period. There are two types of HRS based on different clinical presentations.

Type I HRS is the more severe form. It is defined as >50% reduction in creatinine clearance or a twofold increase in serum creatinine (sCr) (KDIGO stage ≥2 AKI) known or presumed to have occurred within the last 2 weeks. It typically follows a fulminant course with the development of oliguria, encephalopathy, and hyperbilirubinemia. The prognosis of patients with type I HRS is poor, with a median survival of few weeks to ≤3 months.

Type II HRS is a less severe form than type I HRS and is characterized by refractory ascites often resistant to diuretics and needing frequent large-volume paracentesis. Some patients progress to type I HRS after an acute precipitating event such as bacterial infection or gastrointestinal bleeding. The median survival is approximately 7 months.

HRS can occur in patients with advanced hepatic dysfunction, whether acute or chronic, and from any cause, including metastatic liver disease. It is less common in biliary cirrhosis. HRS is a functional reduction in the glomerular filtration rate (GFR) unaccompanied by structural renal parenchymal abnormalities. For example, if hepatic function is restored by liver transplantation, kidney function may return to normal.

I. **PATHOPHYSIOLOGY.** The term "hepatorenal physiology" is often used to describe the underlying mechanism of renal dysfunction in HRS. It essentially refers to AKI incited by portal hypertension-induced arterial vasodilatation and pooling of blood in the splanchnic circulation, ultimately leading to renal hypoperfusion. Systemic vasodilation and a reduction in peripheral vascular resistance are facilitated by increased production of vasodilators in the cirrhotic liver in response to shear stress in the portal vessels, in which nitric oxide is thought to play a central role. This creates arterial underfilling, which activates the renin–angiotensin–aldosterone and the sympathetic nervous systems, endothelin-1

TABLE 38.1	Involvement of kidneys in liver disease

Glomerular diseases in patients with liver disease
  Immunoglobulin A nephropathy, particularly in alcoholic liver disease
  Hepatic glomerulosclerosis
Glomerulonephritides in patients with hepatitis B and hepatitis C
  Membranous nephropathy (HBV)
  Polyarteritis nodosa (mainly HBV, rarely HCV)
  Cryoglobulinemic glomerulonephritis (mainly HCV, rarely HBV)
  Membranoproliferative glomerulonephritis without cryoglobulins (HCV)
Prerenal azotemia
  Gastrointestinal fluid losses (e.g., diarrhea from lactulose)
  Gastrointestinal bleeding
  Aggressive diuretic therapy
Renal venous congestion
  Volume overload from decreased renal-free water clearance and increased
    tubular sodium absorption
  Decreased cardiac output (cirrhotic cardiomyopathy) and high backward pressure
Acute tubular injury/necrosis (ATN)
  Prolonged ischemia from volume depletion
  Progressive HRS pathophysiology leading to lingering renal hypoperfusion
  Cholemic nephropathy (bile casts + associated tubular epithelial cell injury)
  Bacterial translocation and increased circulating inflammatory cytokines
Drug-induced acute interstitial nephritis
  Rifampin
  Trimethoprim/Sulfamethoxazole
  Acetaminophen
  Aspirin
  Allopurinol
  Nonsteroidal anti-inflammatory drugs
Others
  Intra-abdominal hypertension
  Wilson disease
  Preeclampsia
  Cystic diseases
  Granulomatous diseases
  Immunologic diseases
  Amyloidosis

secretion, renal vasoconstrictor prostaglandins such as thromboxane, and arginine vasopressin. Together, these cause intense renal vasoconstriction manifested by sodium and water retention. Furthermore, these patients can be simultaneously exposed to a number of potentially nephrotoxic elements such as hypovolemia, infections, bile acids, and nephrotoxic drugs.

Cirrhosis-associated cardiac dysfunction can in turn contribute to renal injury (cardiorenal syndrome). Splanchnic vasodilation initially results in a hyperdynamic circulation characterized by increased cardiac output, heart

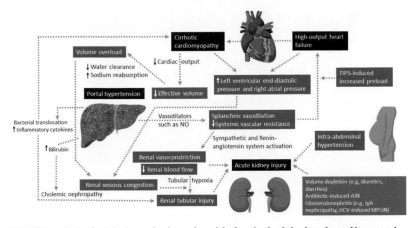

FIGURE 38.1: Pathophysiologic mechanisms of renal dysfunction in cirrhosis and portal hypertension. Portal hypertension-induced arterial vasodilatation with pooling of blood in splanchnic circulation is the central mechanism in cirrhosis-associated renal dysfunction. Splanchnic pooling results in excessive sympathetic nervous system (SNS) activity and activation of the renin–angiotensin–aldosterone system (RAAS) leading to renal vasoconstriction, reduced renal blood flow, and potentially ischemic tubular injury. It also contributes to the development of high cardiac output state, elevated filling pressures, which may ultimately culminate in overt heart failure or cirrhotic cardiomyopathy. Elevated right atrial pressure coupled with renal sodium and water retention in the setting of decreased effective circulating volume leads to renal venous congestion and impaired perfusion. True volume depletion from diuretics or diarrhea is another important cause of acute kidney injury in these patients. In addition, increased bilirubin levels, inflammatory cytokines, and bacterial translocation contribute to renal tubular injury. Further, intra-abdominal hypertension from ascites, certain forms of glomerulonephritis such as IgA nephropathy, hepatitis C–induced membranoproliferative glomerulonephritis and antibiotic or infection-induced acute interstitial nephritis (AIN) must be considered in the differential. NO, nitric oxide; TIPS, transjugular intrahepatic portosystemic shunt.

rate, and plasma volume. High-output cardiac failure may lead to elevated left ventricular end-diastolic pressure, right atrial pressure, and renal venous congestion. As the disease progresses, patients evolve from a state of high cardiac output to one of low output, characterized by blunted cardiac responsiveness, impaired diastolic function, and a variety of electrophysiologic conductance abnormalities termed "cirrhotic cardiomyopathy." This leads to both impairment in forward flow (renal hypoperfusion) as well as high backward pressure (renal venous congestion). The interactions between the liver, heart, and kidney in the context of cirrhosis are illustrated in Figure 38.1. Additionally, transjugular intrahepatic portosystemic shunt (TIPS) performed to alleviate portal hypertension in a subset of patients may predispose to cardiac dysfunction by increasing the preload due to shifting of blood from splanchnic bed into the systemic circulation.

II. CLINICAL PRESENTATION AND DIAGNOSIS. HRS presents with oliguria, a benign urine sediment, avid sodium retention, and a progressive rise in sCr. Renal dysfunction is often characterized by failure to excrete a water load, a reduction in the urinary sodium (typically <10 mEq/L, though not an absolute criterion), increased urine osmolality, and progressive hyponatremia. Patients

T A B L E 38.2	Diagnostic criteria of hepatorenal syndrome[a]

End-stage liver disease with ascites

Increase in sCr ≥0.3 mg/dL or an increase in sCr ≥1.5-fold from baseline

No sustained improvement in kidney function after 2 days of IV volume expansion with albumin (1 g/kg/day) and diuretic withdrawal

Absence of shock

Absence of nephrotoxin exposure (NSAIDs, aminoglycosides, iodinated contrast media, etc.)

Absence of overt hematuria(>50 RBCs/HPF), proteinuria (>500 mg/day), or obstructive nephropathy

[a]Based on the revised consensus recommendations of the International Club of Ascites (2015).

become drowsy, nauseated, and thirsty. In advanced HRS, the blood pressure often drops, coma deepens, and urine volume falls further. The onset of AKI is frequently insidious, but can be precipitated by factors such as gastrointestinal bleeding, infection, or excessive use of diuretics. Spontaneous bacterial peritonitis often triggers progressive HRS in patients with preexisting renal insufficiency. The diagnostic criteria of type I HRS are outlined in Table 38.2.

It is of note that these criteria eliminated the absolute sCr cutoff values that can be found in the older versions (e.g., sCr >1.5 mg/dL). The main reason is that sCr as a biomarker of renal function has several limitations since it is influenced by body weight, race, age, and gender. Moreover, muscle wasting leading to decreased creatinine production, increased renal tubular secretion of creatinine, and increased volume of distribution diluting the sCr are frequently observed in cirrhotic patients and can result in underestimation of the severity of renal dysfunction.

A low-fractional excretion of urinary sodium (FE_{Na} <1%) and low urinary sodium (<10 to 20 mEq/L) are commonly seen in HRS-1 (reflecting neurohormonal activation), while a FE_{Na} >2% or a urinary sodium >40 mEq/L favors intrinsic tubular injury. Low FE_{Urea} may be used instead of FE_{Na} when the patient is on diuretics. However, urine studies should not be used in isolation to establish the diagnosis of HRS. For instance, low FE_{Na} and FE_{Urea} can be observed in volume depletion as well as abdominal compartment syndrome in the context of tense ascites. A focused assessment of the heart, lungs and the inferior vena cava using point-of-care ultrasonography (POCUS) may aid in the diagnosis by excluding overt hyper or hypovolemia.

III. **TREATMENT.** Because treatment of established HRS is challenging, emphasis is placed on prevention by measures such as cautious use of diuretics, intravenous albumin therapy in patients with spontaneous bacterial peritonitis, and norfloxacin therapy in selected patients with ascites and Child–Pugh score class C. Repeated low-volume paracentesis is more effective and better tolerated than aggressive diuretic therapy in the treatment of refractory ascites. Patients should be placed on a low-salt diet (<2 g/day) and fluid restriction (1 to 1.5 L/day).

Treatment of suspected HRS in hospitalized patients usually starts by removal of the offending agents (e.g., diuretics, lactulose, nonsteroidal anti-inflammatory drugs) and volume expansion through administration of intravenous albumin (1 g/kg/day) for 2 to 3 days, as appropriate unless the patient is hypervolemic by physical examination or POCUS. If there is no adequate response and other renal parenchymal and structural diseases are excluded by appropriate investigations, the treatment is aimed at restoring the deranged hemodynamics of cirrhosis.

Vasoconstrictors are administered to address the arterial underfilling, typically in combination with albumin to optimize effective circulatory volume.

A. **Albumin.** While the recommended dose is 1 g/kg/day (100 g maximum) for a minimum of 2 days, a commonly used dosing regimen is 25 g of 12.5% albumin intravenously every 6 hours for the first 24 hours followed by 20 to 25 g/day; thereafter, titrated per clinical response. Albumin should be given in combination with midodrine and octreotide, norepinephrine, or terlipressin.

B. **Midodrine and Octreotide.** Oral midodrine (selective alpha 1–adrenergic agonist) and subcutaneous octreotide (somatostatin analog) are commonly used in combination with albumin although there is no large-scale prospective controlled trial supporting their current widespread use. Midodrine can be started orally at 7.5 mg three times a day and octreotide at 100 mcg subcutaneously three times a day. The dose can be increased to 12.5 mg and 200 mcg three times a day, respectively.

C. **Norepinephrine.** Norepinephrine is a potent vasoconstrictor and is usually reserved for critically ill patients in the ICU. Some experts advocate that it should be favored over midodrine–octreotide combination therapy for anybody with HRS based on the available evidence. It is given as an intravenous infusion (0.5 to 3 mg/hour) titrated to the goal of mean arterial pressure, which is typically a 15 mm Hg rise from the baseline value.

D. **Terlipressin.** Terlipressin, a vasopressin analog with greater affinity for the vascular V1a receptor than for the renal V2 receptor, is the standard treatment for HRS-1 in many European and Asian countries. It is not available in the United Sates currently. Interestingly, in studies outside the United States, Terlipressin (intravenous bolus, 1 to 2 mg Q4–6 hours) treatment has been associated with overall reversal rates of ~40% to 80% in patients with HRS-1. Vasopressin (starting at a dose of 0.01 unit/min) may be used as an alternative, although the evidence demonstrating its efficacy is sparse.

E. **Renal Replacement Therapy.** Dialysis does not improve the survival in patients with HRS unless they receive hepatic transplantation. However, it should be considered in patients with acute reversible hepatic failure and in those awaiting hepatic transplantation. Continuous renal replacement therapies may be superior in removing excessive fluid and correcting electrolyte abnormalities without causing hemodynamic instability. Selected patients with HRS-1 awaiting liver transplantation may benefit from TIPS as a rescue therapy albeit weighing the risk of periprocedural hepatic encephalopathy.

F. **Transjugular Intrahepatic Portosystemic Shunt.** The TIPS procedure has been successfully used to treat refractory ascites. Although patients with HRS are often too ill to undergo TIPS, there tends to be an improvement in renal function that can occur over weeks when it has been utilized.

G. **Liver Transplantation.** The definitive treatment of HRS is liver transplantation. Approximately 65 to 75% of patients experience resolution of HRS-1 after liver transplantation, with low recovery for those on dialysis at the time of transplantation. Therefore, in patients requiring dialysis for more than 6 weeks, combined liver–kidney transplantation should be considered. Nonetheless, widespread implementation is limited by the imbalance between the incidence of type I HRS and organ availability.

IV. SUGGESTED READINGS

Ginès P, Solà E, Angeli P, et al. Hepatorenal syndrome. *Nat Rev Dis Primers*. 2018;4(1):23.

Kazory A, Ronco C. Hepatorenal syndrome or hepatocardiorenal syndrome: revisiting basic concepts in view of emerging data. *Cardiorenal Med*. 2019;9(1):1–7.

Salerno F, Gerbes A, Gines P, et al. Diagnosis, prevention, and treatment of hepatorenal syndrome in cirrhosis. *Gut*. 2007;56(9):1310–1318.

Velez JCQ, Therapondos G, Juncos LA. Reappraising the spectrum of AKI and hepatorenal syndrome in patients with cirrhosis. *Nat Rev Nephrol*. 2020;16(3):137–155.

Wadei HM, Mai ML, Ahsan N, et al. Hepatorenal syndrome: pathophysiology and management. *Clin J Am Soc Nephrol*. 2006;1(5):1066–1079.

39 Anemia of Chronic Kidney Disease

Robert J. Rubin

I. DEFINITION. The Kidney Disease Improving Global Outcomes (KDIGO) recommends an evaluation when hemoglobin (Hgb) is less than 12 g/dL in females and <13.5 g/dL in males.

Anemia of chronic kidney disease (CKD) occurs because the diseased kidneys are unable to produce adequate erythropoietin, which stimulates erythroid precursor cells. It is characterized by a normocytic, normochromic anemia with a low corrected absolute reticulocyte count. Typically, the anemia of CKD develops when the glomerular filtration rate (GFR) declines to <30 mL/min. In large population-based studies, GFR <30 (CKD 4 and 5 by definition) has been associated with an anemia prevalence of 44%. The minimum workup of anemia in a patient with CKD should include Hgb/Hct, red blood cell indices, reticulocyte count, stool guaiac for evaluation of occult gastrointestinal blood loss, vitamin B_{12}, folate, thyroid function, and iron studies. Iron deficiency is present in about 58% of men and 70% of women with CKD 3–5 not on dialysis. Serum erythropoietin levels are not helpful in the workup of anemia of CKD. An algorithm is presented in Figure 39.1.

A. Target Hemoglobin/Hematocrit. A number of observational studies have suggested an association between anemia and cardiovascular morbidity, especially left ventricular hypertrophy in patients with renal failure. Four major studies, the Normal Hematocrit Cardiac Trial in 1998, the Correction of Hemoglobin and Outcomes in Renal Insufficiency CHOIR) and the Normalization of Hemoglobin Level in Patients with Chronic Kidney Disease (CREATE) in 2006, and A Trial of Darbepoetin Alfa in Type 2 Diabetes and Chronic Kidney Disease (TREAT) in 2009, showed an increased risk of cardiovascular events in hemodialysis and nonhemodialysis patients in those allocated to the treatment goal of a normal Hgb using erythropoietin-stimulating agents (ESAs).

In the light of these and other trials, KDIGO amended its guidelines in 2012 as follows for dialysis and nondialysis patients receiving ESA:

1. The Hgb level should be maintained between 9 and 11.5.
2. The Hgb level should not exceed 13 g/dL.

B. Evaluation of Iron-Deficiency Anemia in Chronic Kidney Disease. KDIGO recommends checking serum ferritin and transferrin saturation to assess the management of anemia in CKD and end-stage kidney disease (ESKD) patients. Serum ferritin <100 ng/mL reflects *absolute iron deficiency* in CKD patients. Transferrin saturation (TSAT) is the serum iron/total iron-binding capacity (TIBC) and reflects iron circulating in blood that is available for erythropoiesis. A TSAT value <20% defines *functional iron deficiency* in a patient receiving ESA therapy.

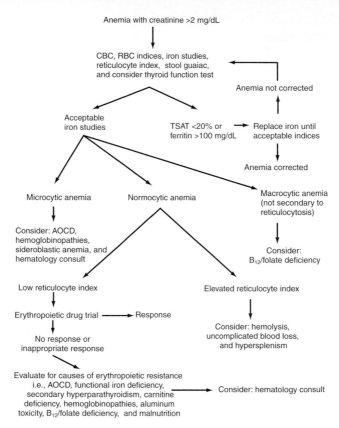

FIGURE 39.1: Approach to the patient with anemia of chronic kidney disease. AOCD, anemia of chronic disease; CBC, complete blood cell count; RBC, red blood cell; TSAT, transferrin saturation.

The reticulocyte hemoglobin content (CHr) reflects the iron availability to bone marrow. A cutoff of <32 pg has been recommended for iron therapy in studies comparing CHr with ferritin. Another form of functional iron deficiency is *reticuloendothelial blockade* or *anemia of chronic disease* (AOCD). This complication of inflammation is indicated by a TSAT <20% and a ferritin >800 ng/mL.

The response to ESA treatment is a guide to distinguish between functional deficiency and AOCD. Serum ferritin generally decreases after ESA therapy in functional iron deficiency but increases in AOCD. If the diagnosis is unclear and the ferritin is <800 ng/mL, the Hgb/Hct may be monitored after a trial of intravenous (IV) iron. If the ferritin is >800 ng/mL and TSAT >50%, iron therapy is usually withheld. In the Dialysis Patients' Response to IV Iron with Elevated Ferritin Study, anemic dialysis patients who were given ferric gluconate despite elevated ferritin (500 to 1,200 ng/mL) had an improvement in Hgb. However, the conclusions were confounded because the dose of ESA was increased in all patients prior to initiation and there was no long-term follow-up to determine whether this effect of iron therapy persisted beyond 6 weeks. Consequently, the KDIGO guidelines have not been changed based on this study.

TABLE 39.1	Oral iron preparations		
Iron preparation	# of Pills required to provide 200 mg of iron	Tablet size (mg)	Amount of elemental iron (mg/pill)
Ferrous sulfate	3	325	65
Ferrous gluconate	S	325	38
Ferrous fumarate	3	200	66
Iron polysaccharide	2	150	150
Ferric citrate	1	1,000	210

II. **MONITORING OF IRON LEVELS.** After initiation of erythropoietic therapy, the TSAT and serum ferritin should be checked every month in patients not receiving IV iron, and at least once every 3 months in patients receiving IV iron.

III. **TREATMENT GUIDELINES**
A. **Oral Iron.** Oral iron supplementation should be given to CKD patients not yet at ESKD either 1 hour before meals or 2 hours postprandial, as food tends to reduce gastrointestinal iron absorption. At least 200 mg of elemental iron should be given daily in two to three doses (Table 39.1). Oral iron therapy is not recommended for dialysis patients because of the high level of ongoing iron losses (approximately 25 to 100 mg weekly) and poor utilization of oral iron.
B. **Intravenous Iron.** The usual dose of IV iron is 1 g of iron dextran or ferric gluconate given as eight doses of 125 mg, or 10 doses of iron sucrose (iron saccharate,) of 100 mg each given with each dialysis session. Other iron preparations may have different dosing schedules. Delayed adverse reactions of arthralgias and myalgias are dose related above 100 mg. There is a small incidence of anaphylactoid reactions, which are more common in patients with a history of multiple drug allergies. Thus, a small test dose (25 mg) of IV iron is given 15 to 60 minutes before the first dose of any iron preparation. Iron sucrose may be given to patients with a prior history of an allergic reaction to iron dextran. Pretreatment with a histamine H2 receptor blocker and 50 to 100 mg of hydrocortisone usually prevents these reactions, which are likely due to histamine release.
C. **Epoetin Alfa (Epogen, Procrit, Retacrit).** Epoetin alfa (Epogen/Procrit) is a 165-amino acid recombinant glycoprotein (30.4 kd). Epoetin alfa-epbx (Retacrit) is a biosimilar to epoetin alfa. Most ESKD patients receive epoetin intravenously during dialysis. The revised label suggests a starting dose of epoetin of 50 to 100 IU/kg three times a week in adult patients with ESKD or in CKD patients prior to ESKD. Epoetin should be given as a weekly subcutaneous injection to CKD and peritoneal dialysis patients initially at 80 to 120 IU/kg/wk. The Hct/Hgb should be measured 3 to 4 weeks after initiation of treatment and 2 weeks after a dosage adjustment. It should be monitored every 4 weeks. Epoetin therapy is contraindicated in the presence of uncontrolled hypertension. Based on recent studies in cancer, surgical, and CKD patients, the Food and Drug Administration has issued the following *black box warnings*:

> Patients experienced greater risks of death and serious cardiovascular events when administered ESAs to target higher hemoglobin levels (13.5 g/dL nondialysis, 14.0 g/dL dialysis). Dosing should be individualized to achieve and maintain hemoglobin levels between 10 and 12 g/dL.

D. **Darbepoetin Alfa (Aranesp).** Darbepoetin alfa (Aranesp) is a recombinant erythropoiesis-stimulating glycoprotein with a half-life that is threefold longer after IV dosing and twofold longer after subcutaneous dosing than that of epoetin. The recommended starting dose is 0.45 mcg/kg subcutaneously every week or double the dose every other week. The side-effect profile is similar to that of epoetin.

E. **Micera (Methoxy Polyethylene Glycol-Epoetin Beta).** Micera (methoxy polyethylene glycol-epoetin beta) is a longer-acting ESA and is given every 2 weeks at a dose of 0.6 mcg/kg. It has a similar side-effect profile to darbepoetin.

F. **Future Agents.** Hypoxia-inducible factor activators (HIFs): There are three HIFs currently in phase 3 trials. These drugs are oral in contrast to the three ESAs described above which are given either IV or SC. HIFs have a different mechanism of action than ESAs, upregulating the intestinal absorption of iron, transferrin receptor as well as erythropoietin and its receptor. Studies have shown HIFs noninferiority to ESA, however, long-term safety data are currently not available

G. **Erythropoietin-Stimulating Agent Hyporesponsiveness.** ESA hyporesponsiveness has various definitions. It is usually defined as the failure to respond or to maintain an Hgb response within the recommended dosing range. If the patient has TSAT <50% and ferritin <800 ng/mL, a trial of iron supplementation is suggested. In the iron-replete patient, inflammation, infection, folate and vitamin B_{12} deficiency, aluminum toxicity, and hyperparathyroidism should all be evaluated and corrected if present as these are all causes of resistant anemia.

IV. SUGGESTED READINGS

Bazeley J, Wish JB. The evolution of target hemoglobin levels in anemia of chronic kidney disease. *Adv Chronic Kidney Dis.* 2019;26(4):229–236.

Besarab A. The effects of normal as compared with low hematocrit values in patients with cardiac disease who are receiving hemodialysis and epoetin. *N Engl J Med.* 1998;339(9):584–590.

Coyne DW. Ferric gluconate is highly efficacious in anemic hemodialysis patients with high serum ferritin and low transferrin saturation: results of the dialysis patients' response to IV iron with elevated ferritin (DRIVE) study. *J Am Soc Nephrol.* 2007;18(3):975–984.

Drueke TB. Normalization of hemoglobin level in patients with chronic kidney disease. *N Engl J Med.* 2006;355(20)2071–2084.

Fishbane S. *CJASN.* 2009;4(1):57–61.

Gupta N. Hypoxia-inducible factor prolyl hydroxylase inhibitors: a potential new treatment for anemia in patients with CKD. *Am J Kidney Dis.* 2017;69(6):815–826.

Kliger AS, Foley RN, Goldfarb DS, et al. KDOQI US Commentary on the 2012 KDIGO clinical practice guideline for anemia in CKD. *Am J Kidney Dis.* 2013;62(5):849–859.

Kidney Disease Improving Global Outcomes. KDIGO clinical practice guideline for anemia in chronic kidney disease. *Kidney Int Suppl.* 2012;2(4):1–335.

Pfeffer MA. A trial of darbepoetin alfa in type 2 diabetes and chronic kidney disease. *N Engl J Med.* 2009;361(21):2019–2032.

Singh A. Correction of anemia with epoetin alfa in patients with chronic kidney disease (CHOIR Study). *N Engl J Med.* 2006;355(20):2085–2098.

40 Nutrition in Renal Failure

Danielle F. Aycart, Jeanette M. Andrade

Nutritional requirements vary with the degree of renal insufficiency. The diet is modified to reduce uremic symptoms from the accumulation of toxic metabolites, to address acid–base imbalances, to facilitate electrolyte and water homeostasis, and to prevent renal osteodystrophy. Patients with advanced chronic kidney disease (CKD) may develop protein-calorie malnutrition (PEM) and require dietary supplementation. Other factors such as mental health status, low socioeconomic status, and multiple medications are associated with PEM. PEM also occurs with concurrent illnesses, depletion of micronutrients (electrolytes, trace elements, and vitamins) that are removed with dialytic procedures, inadequate dialysis, and consequences of uremia (fatigue, muscle cramps, anorexia, nausea, vomiting, stomatitis, altered sense of taste, altered mental status, insulin resistance, increased catabolic hormones, gastroparesis, and malabsorption).

The nutritional assessment of CKD patients is vital for predicting clinical outcomes. The use of the subjective global assessment (SGA) has been recommended by the National Kidney Foundation (NKF) Kidney Disease/Dialysis Outcomes and Quality Initiative (KDOQI) to detect malnutrition through its seven components. In 2001, the Malnutrition-Inflammation Score (MIS) was developed for patients with renal disease. The MIS includes the seven components of the SGA and also body mass index, serum concentration of albumin, and serum concentration of total iron-binding capacity. Other methods to evaluate the nutritional status of the patients used are the normalized protein equivalent of nitrogen appearance (nPNA), anthropometric measurements (e.g., skinfold thickness, waist circumference, body weight), and conicity index.

I. GENERAL NUTRITIONAL CONCEPTS

A. **Energy (Caloric) Requirements.** Patients with uncomplicated renal insufficiency have normal basal energy expenditure and caloric requirements of 25 to 35 kcal/kg body weight. For edematous patients, the calculation should be based on their usual or estimated "dry" weight. For obese patients, calculate the "adjusted" body weight from the ideal body weight plus 25% of the excess weight. Patients who are catabolic or have proteinuria have greater energy requirements and without additional carbohydrates, their fat and protein stores will be depleted. Portable indirect calorimeters are available to ascertain actual energy expenditure, respiratory quotients (PCO_2/PO_2), and oxygen consumption (VO_2). However, indirect calorimetry measurements may be unreliable as a consequence of cardiovascular shunting. Therefore, practitioners often rely on predictive equations (i.e., Schoenfeld, Mifflin-St Jeor) for the estimation of energy requirements despite these equations either over- or underestimating the energy requirements of CKD patients.

B. Macronutrients

1. **Protein.** Stable patients with renal disease have the same minimum daily protein requirements as does the general healthy population (0.8 g/kg ideal body weight). As the kidney prior to disease progresses, a low-protein diet (0.55 to 0.6 g/kg ideal body weight) or a very low–protein diet (0.28 to 0.43 g/kg ideal body weight) is recommended. Renal patients with diabetes require a higher dietary protein (0.8 to 0.9 g/kg ideal body weight) to maintain a stable nutritional status and glycemic control. Patients on dialysis require a higher protein amount ranging from 1.0 to 1.5 g/kg ideal body weight. The quantity of protein necessary to prevent PEM depends on the food's biologic value (ratio of essential to nonessential AA). Fish, eggs, and milk are of higher biologic value (HBV) than poultry or beef, especially when compared with grains.

   The amount of protein prescribed is based on the patient's renal function, proteinuria, type of dialysis, and body weight (Table 40.1). Patients are in a negative protein balance if their intake is restricted to less than 0.5 g protein/kg/day unless they are provided with essential AA supplementation. Alpha ketoanalogs (ketoacids) are experimental supplements that contain no nitrogen yet undergo liver transamination into the corresponding AA. There are several high essential AA products available commercially in both enteral (Renalcal™, Nepro™) and parenteral (Aminosyn-RF, NephrAmine™, RenAmin™) products. Intensive and repeated dietary counseling is helpful to improve compliance for protein restriction.

   The loss of albumin or total protein can be calculated using various methods. A 24-hour urine collection is considered the reference standard method. Dietary protein intake (eDPI) could be estimated by 24-hour urinary urea nitrogen (UUN), nonurea nitrogen excretion, and urinary protein losses (taken in consideration when the loss is greater than 5 g/day) using the following formula:

   $$eDPI\ (g/day) = 6.25 * [UUN\ (g/day) + 0.031 \times weight\ (kg) + proteinuria\ (g/day)]$$

   For example, to calculate the protein intake of a lean, nonedematous 70-kg man, with a UUN of 5 g and a proteinuria loss of less than 5 g/day:

   $$eDPI = 6.25 * [5 + (0.031 \times 70)] = 44.81\ g/day$$

   In patients with significant proteinuria, the amount of protein lost in the urine is considered, and the dietary protein prescription is adjusted. Because stool contains about 1 g of nitrogen per 300 mL, significant losses may occur in patients with diarrhea. Urinary nitrogen should be collected on ice (to minimize errors introduced by microbial contamination). If patients are hematuric, precise nitrogen assays will not be possible.

2. **Carbohydrates.** Carbohydrates are a major source of calories in renal patients with multiple dietary restrictions and, thereby, are protein sparing. Sugars also permit the complete oxidation of fatty acids, which avoids ketone production. Dietary goals are to consume 45% to 65% of total calories from carbohydrates, mainly from complex carbohydrate sources. Grains, vegetables, and fruits are common sources of carbohydrate and have the added benefits of dietary fiber. Dietary fiber recommendations for patients with renal disease are the same as the general healthy population, 20 to 35 g/day. Excessive carbohydrate can lead to hypertriglyceridemia and

TABLE 40.1 Special recommendations for CKD patients

Patients with	Macronutrients				Micronutrients and fluid				
	Total calories (kcal/kg/day)	CC % of total calories	Protein (g/kg/day)	Fats (per day) % of total calories	Sodium (g/day)	Potassium (g/day)	Phosphorus (g/day)	Fluid (L/day)	Others
Nephrotic syndrome	35	45–65%	0.8	≤7%; SF <30%; P/SF 2:1; CHO <200 mg	2–3	Dependent on GFR	<1.5		25(OH) precursors
AKI without Dialysis	20–30	3–5 (maximum 7) g/kg/d EAA (<1.7 g/kg/d)	0.8–1.0 (noncatabolic AKI) 1.0–1.5 (with RRT) <1.7 (hypercatabolic AKI, CRRT)	Fat: 0.8–1.0 g/kg/d	Oliguric 1–2	Oliguric 0.6–1.0; Based on individual needs	≤1.0	1–1.5	Trace elements
CKD predialysis	25–35	40–60%	0.6–0.8 Monitor UUN	Mostly poly or monounsaturated LC n-3PUFA	<3	4.7 (<3 if hyperkalemia)	<0.8	0.1–0.9 + 24-hr output	Calcium 0.8–1.0 g/day, Vitamin D
HD	25–35	35–50%	1–1.2 Monitor PCR, albumin	30%; P/SF 2:1 Mostly poly or monounsaturated, LC n-3PUFA	<3	<3	<0.8	1–1.5	Calcium <0.8 g/d, Water-soluble vitamins, vitamin D vitamin K

Parenteral nutrition: 10–20% dextrose (<5–7 mg/kg/min in adult, <15–20 mg/kg/min in neonates); 1.5
10% AA; 20% lipids (<0.11 g fat/kg/hr)

(*continued*)

TABLE 40.1 Special recommendations for CKD patients (*Continued*)

Patients with	Macronutrients					Micronutrients and fluid				
	Total calories (kcal/kg/day)	CC % of total calories	Protein (g/kg/day)	Fats (per day) % of total calories	Sodium (g/day)	Potassium (g/day)	Phosphorus (g/day)	Fluid (L/day)	Others	
PD	25–35[a]	No evidence	1.2–1.5	30%; P/SF 2:1 Mostly poly or monounsaturated	2–4	<3	<0.8			
Kidney transplant	25–35	Emphasize on CC and dietary fiber intake	1.5 (early phase ≤4 wks) 0.8 (Long term)	Limit saturated fat intake	Restrict if BP indicates	<4.7 (<3, if hyperkalemia)	DRI	Depends on kidney function	Calcium 1 g/ day. Dietary modification[b]	

[a]Peritoneal dialysate solution would provide approximately 231 kcal/2 L.
[b]Dietary modification for control hyperlipidemia, electrolyte imbalances associated with immunosuppressive therapy (i.e., cyclosporine and hyperkalemia/hypomagnesemia, mycophenolate and hypophosphatemia, tacrolimus, and hypercalcemia/hyperkalemia).
AKI, acute kidney injury; CC, complex carbohydrates; CRF, chronic renal failure; HD, hemodialysis; DRI, dietary reference intake; PD, peritoneal dialysis; SF, saturated fat; P/SF, polyunsaturated to saturated fat ratio; CHO, cholesterol; PCR, protein catabolic rate; EAA, essential amino acids.

hyperglycemia, which can increase morbidity (immunocompromise, steatosis, and hypercapnia).

Although glucose (dextrose) or glucose polymers are the most common carbohydrate sources, many other carbohydrate products are available, including parenteral glycerol and fructose, which do not require insulin action for metabolism. In the setting of insulin insensitivity or resistance, insulin has been associated with profound antinatriuretic activity and microalbuminuria.

3. **Lipids.** Hyperlipidemia occurs in more than 50% of patients with CKD and is of great concern because of the high mortality due to atherosclerotic cardiovascular disease. Causes of hypercholesterolemia and hypertriglyceridemia are multifactorial and include proteinuria in the nephrotic range, depressed lipoprotein lipase activity, decreased metabolism of remnant lipoproteins, and impaired cholesterol transport. Initiation of dialysis does not correct these disorders. During peritoneal dialysis, hypertriglyceridemia worsens due to the absorption of large quantities of dextrose from the dialysate. Most patients require pharmacologic therapy to achieve the increasingly stringent cholesterol levels.

Dietary lipid guidelines and goals for renal patients are the same as the general healthy population, 20% to 30% of the total caloric requirement with an increased consumption of unsaturated fatty acids and limited amounts of saturated and trans fats. Renal patients are recommended to consume 1.3 to 4 g/day of polyunsaturated fatty acids (PUFAs) to reduce triglycerides, LDL cholesterol and to raise HDL cholesterol levels.

Plant-based oils, nuts, and seeds are good sources of unsaturated fatty acids, which has a wide range of effects on the cardiac system and modulating the inflammatory response. The essential PUFAs present in plant-based oils, seeds, and nuts are linoleic acid (LA 18:2, n-6) and α-linolenic acid (ALA 18:3 n-3), while long-chain n-3 PUFA such as eicosapentaenoic acid (EPA 20:5 n-3), docosapentaenoic acid (DPA 22:5 n-3), and docosahexaenoic acid (DHA 22:6 n-3) are present in fish, seaweed, and flaxseed oil.

Reducing low-density lipoprotein (LDL) cholesterol levels is especially important in patients with cardiovascular risk factors because of the now well-established increased mortality risk with poorly controlled lipid levels. However, it may be difficult to design a diet that provides adequate calories with the concurrent fat and protein restrictions. Fruits (limited by their potassium content), sugars, and syrups are often useful, but these foods contain high amounts of simple sugars, which increase certain lipid levels. The goal for LDL cholesterol reduction is controversial, with low levels not of proven benefit in high-risk patients already on chronic dialysis.

Carnitine is an important intermediate in fatty acid metabolism, and its deficiency has been associated with diverse and poorly characterized organ dysfunctional syndromes, including cardiomyopathy, infections, muscle weakness, and anemia refractory to erythropoietin. Supplementation of carnitine is given to dialysis patients to improve symptoms such as muscle weakness, intradialytic cramps, and hypotension, but there is not enough data to support supplementing with L-carnitine in CKD patients.

C. **Micronutrients.** Virtually every anabolic and catabolic process in humans is intimately related to micronutrients. Electrolytes are responsible for the seemingly limitless metabolic reactions, play key roles in structure, and maintain acid–base balance. Acid–base considerations must be assessed before any electrolytes can be provided to patients. If a patient is alkalemic, acid salts (chloride, phosphate, and sulfate) should be used, whereas an acidemic patient will require the use of bicarbonate precursors such as acetate, citrate, gluconate, or lactate. Each salt must be carefully selected with pathophysiologic insight. In CKD patients, the main concern remains deficiency of micronutrients, although there is a potential concern of micronutrient accumulation and toxicity due to the compromised renal function. Deficiencies occur due to specific dietary recommendations, comorbidities, medication, impaired intestinal absorption, changes in the metabolism, and excessive losses through the urine or dialysate.

D. Electrolytes

   1. Sodium and chloride. Most patients, in the later stages of renal insufficiency develop salt retention. This can be a management problem in patients with nephrotic syndrome or oliguric renal failure. The dietary prescription is commonly expressed in either milliequivalents of NaCl or grams of sodium (100 mEq NaCl contain 2.3 g of sodium and 3.5 g of chloride). Many patients with acute renal failure (ARF) have an initial oliguric phase, when salt must be restricted, and then a polyuric phase, in which salt must be supplemented.

   In general, patients consume fresh fish, poultry, and either fresh or frozen fruits and vegetables and avoid consuming high sodium processed foods, cured meats, and luncheon meats. Instead of the use of salt for seasoning, patients should use fresh seasonings (such as garlic, onion, lemon juice) and either fresh or dried herbs and spices.

   2. Potassium. The recommendation is to adjust dietary potassium intake to maintain serum potassium at normal range (3.5 to 5.1 mEq/L). In most patients, a diet limited to 1 mEq of potassium/kg body weight/day will prevent hyperkalemia. Additional potassium may need to be prescribed because of peritoneal dialysate or gastrointestinal (GI) losses (nasogastric losses or diarrhea). The impact of acid–base must also be appreciated with respect to potassium. For every 0.1 unit acute decline in pH, serum potassium rises about 0.5 mEq/L. Since 40 g of oral protein contains 1 g (26 mEq) of potassium, a high-protein diet would preclude severe potassium restriction. The fiber found in plant-based foods affects the degree of potassium absorption. Patients should consume low-potassium fruits such as apples, berries, and pears, and vegetables such as asparagus, carrots, and cucumbers and avoid consuming high-potassium fruits such as bananas, oranges, and dried fruit and vegetables such as avocados, Brussels sprouts, and deep-colored leafy greens.

   3. Phosphorus. Hyperphosphatemia and secondary hyperparathyroidism develop with advance renal insufficiency unless dietary phosphate is restricted concurrent with the use of oral phosphate binders. Dietary phosphorus recommendations are between 800 and 1,000 mg/day or 10 to 12 mg phosphorus per gram of protein. Patients on diets that are high in animal protein will have an obligatory source of phosphorus and may require higher doses of binders. The recommendation is to adjust the dietary phosphorous intake to maintain serum phosphorous at normal range (0.8 to 1.5 mEq/L).

   Hypophosphatemia is rare in patients with renal failure unless accompanied by poor nutritional intake. It must be remembered, however, that conventional high-flux hemodialysis removes up to approximately 800 mg of phosphorus per 4-hour treatment, compared with 400 mg by daily peritoneal dialytic procedures. It is important to monitor patients for the occurrence of hypophosphatemia because it is becoming a more frequent finding with the relatively large phosphate clearance seen with high-flux dialyzer membranes and high-volume continuous renal replacement protocols (such as continuous venovenous hemodialysis [CVVHD]).

The animal-based phosphate absorption in the intestinal tract is higher than with plant-based phosphate. Thus, patients should be encouraged to consume low-phosphorus fresh fruits such as apple, grapes, and pears, and fresh vegetables such as cauliflower, celery, and green beans and avoid consuming high-phosphorous dairy products such as milk, cheese, and yogurt, nuts, and beverages such as cocoa, beer, and dark cola drinks.

4. **Magnesium.** Because renal insufficiency decreases magnesium excretion, magnesium-containing laxatives and antacids should be avoided. Dietary magnesium requirements are between 8 and 16 mmol (200 to 400 mg) daily.

E. **Trace Elements**

1. **Iron.** Iron deficiency has become quite common in renal patients because of the increased utilization during erythropoietin therapy. Repetitive, albeit small, blood losses during hemodialysis also contribute to the iron deficit. Oral repletion is difficult in renal patients because of poor dietary intake of iron and decreased absorption when administered with phosphate-binding antacids. Even when oral iron is given in high doses (65 to 150 mg of elemental iron) between meals, additional parenteral administration is often necessary because yearly requirements may exceed 2 g and bioavailability of oral iron is only 10% to 20%. Animal-based foods such as beef, liver, and sardines may be good sources of iron, although they are often limited in the diet of CKD patients due to phosphorus content. Patients should be encouraged to consume plant-based foods such as chickpeas, beans, and spinach along with a citrus to enhance the absorption of nonheme iron.

2. **Zinc.** Zinc may become deficient in patients with advanced renal insufficiency because of decreased intake and absorption. This can be one of many causes of dysgeusia, alopecia, or impotence, and these conditions may at least partially respond to zinc supplementation. However, there is not enough evidence to recommend a zinc supplementation for CKD patients exceeding the dietary recommendation for the healthy general population of 8 to 11 mg/day. Excess zinc supplementation may not be desirable for several reasons. Zinc can antagonize copper absorption and result in sideroblastic anemia. Parenteral zinc supplementation can exacerbate the mild acute phase reaction in ICU patients, as evidenced by a significantly higher febrile response.

F. **Vitamins.** Vitamin status is complex in patients with renal insufficiency as deficiencies may be seen, whereas others accumulate to the point of toxicity. The fat-soluble vitamins (A, E, and K) do not require supplementation and dietary recommendations are the same as the general healthy population. Excess vitamin A and K can be toxic in dialysis patients. Vitamin D deficiency is of great concern and is discussed elsewhere (Chapter 41). The water-soluble vitamins, however, can become deficient because of losses into dialysate and decreased availability from the restricted diet, anorexia, or abnormal metabolism. For most water-soluble vitamins, supplementation should follow the recommended daily intake (RDI). Vitamin C is not supplemented beyond the normal recommended daily requirement because its metabolite (oxalate) accumulates and contributes to secondary oxalosis in dialysis patients. For B-complex vitamins, homocysteine levels rise with advancing renal failure and persist after initiation of dialysis. Studies have shown that although supplemental pyridoxine (vitamin B_6), cobalamin, and, perhaps, folate can lower homocysteine levels in healthy patients, these agents have a much attenuated effect in the end-stage renal disease population. It is unclear whether this resistance can be overcome with higher vitamin doses, and results from the use of two to five times the RDI of vitamin B_6 and folate has not been shown. It has been also suggested that hyperhomocysteinemia may arise from the shrinking of endogenous nitrogen pools as a result of decreased protein intake or stress-induced losses. It has been proposed that increased total homocysteine may result from the attempt of the malnourished and/or stressed body to preserve methionine homeostasis.

Dietary needs are typically met with a variety of foods, especially plant based. If supplements are required, a specific formula for this population is prescribed: folic acid 1 mg; B_6 10 mg; thiamine 1.4 to 1.6 mg; riboflavin 1.6 to 2.0 mg; pantothenic acid 5 to 10 mg; and ascorbic acid 60 mg.

II. **SPECIFIC RECOMMENDATIONS.** Table 40.1 contains the specific nutritional requirements for patients with AKI, nephrotic syndrome, CKD prior and on hemodialysis, patients on peritoneal dialysis, and those after a renal transplant. However, special consideration is needed when considering the nutrition of critically ill patients in an ICU setting. These patients are typically hypermetabolic and have increased caloric requirements as well as catabolic rates. Serial measurements of the PCR will best reflect their nutritional needs because protein requirements can vary widely and may exceed four times their basal values. Intradialytic parenteral nutrition with solutions of 10% to 20% dextrose, 10% AA, and 20% lipids (avoiding infusions of greater than 0.11 g fat/kg/hr) is reserved for those whose gut is not functioning. Intradialytic administration of carbohydrate should not exceed hepatic oxidative rates (5 to 7 mg carbohydrate/ kg/min in adults or 15 to 20 mg/kg/min in neonates). Rapid infusion of intravenous lipid over short intervals that are used in intradialytic feeding has been associated with free fatty acid shower, hypertriglyceridemia, and cholecystokinin stimulation (all of which normalize with longer infusion times). Cholesterol intake should be guided by periodic lipoprotein analyses. For anabolic patients gaining weight, calories must be increased with the use of fats and simple carbohydrates. As parenteral nutrition supplementation often necessitates the administration of large fluid volumes, continuous renal replacement modalities (such as CVVHD) are sometimes superior to intermittent hemodialysis to assure volume removal and thereby permit adequate nutrition. Most patients can be fed adequately with 1.5 L of parenteral feeding per day.

With regard to micronutrients and fluid, sodium, potassium, and fluid restriction will depend on the residual renal function and urine output. Anuric patients typically require a daily restriction of 2 to 3 g of sodium (77 to 110 mEq), 70 mEq (1 mEq/kg) of potassium and 1 to 1.5 L of fluids. Adherence to fluid restriction is important to avoid volume-dependent hypertension and adverse postdialytic symptoms associated with excess fluid removal (such as intradialytic hypotension or cramping). Phosphate is limited to 0.81 g/day (8 to 10 mM).

Dialysis patients should receive supplements of water-soluble vitamins because of the potential for their increased removal, especially during high-flux dialysis. For most water-soluble vitamins, supplementation should be 100% of the RDI. The removal of fat-soluble vitamins by hemodialysis is negligible, and their supplementation is generally not recommended. Exceptions include treatment with vitamin D for renal osteodystrophy and possible supplementation of vitamin K in patients on long-term antibiotics.

III. SUMMARY. In summary, nutrition in the renal failure patient must be carefully assessed, prescribed, and monitored to minimize morbidity and mortality. Energy mix can be empirically achieved to a range between 35 and 45 kcal/kg/day. Synthetic AA or protein must be empirically adjusted to a dose of 0.6 to 1.5 g protein/kg ideal body weight/day, depending on the patient and, if utilized, the dialytic procedure. Much remains to be learned about preferred carbohydrate sources (i.e., fructose, glycerol, or xylitol that are associated with different insulin actions) and fat sources (i.e., polyunsaturated versus saturated ratios, omega-6 versus omega-3 ratios). Overall, though, plant-based proteins contain complex carbohydrates and fats that reduce complications associated with renal disease.

An empiric approach is similarly used for micronutrient supplementation. After acid–base assessment, the salt is selected and electrolytes are dosed depending on tolerance. Deficiencies of chromium (hyperglycemia), selenium (muscle pain, cardiomyopathy, low triiodothyronine), and zinc (alopecia, delayed wound healing, depression) are dosed as per symptomatology and loss quantification, while copper and manganese are primarily excreted through the biliary system. Iron is generally not used or needed with recombinant erythropoietin or darbepoetin therapy in the critically ill renal patient. Trace elements and vitamins can generally be dosed as per the RDI (which is the oral requirement). Fat-soluble vitamin supplementation can be deleterious (i.e., vitamins A and K can be osteolytic), and excesses should be avoided in the renal failure patient.

IV. SUGGESTED READINGS

Carrero JJ, González-Ortiz A, Avesani CM, et al. Plant-based diets to manage the risks and complications of chronic kidney disease. *Nat Rev Nephrol.* 2020;16(9):525–542. doi:10.1038/s41581-020-0297-2

Chadban S, Chan M, Fry K, et al. The CARI guidelines. Protein requirement in adult kidney transplant recipients. *Nephrology (Carlton).* 2010;15(Suppl 1):S68–S71.

Ikizler TA, Burrowes JD, Byham-Gray LD, et al. KDOQI clinical practice guideline for nutrition in CKD: 2020 update. *Am J Kidney Dis.* 2020;76(3)(suppl 1):S1–S107.

Kalantar-Zadeh K, Fouque D. Nutritional management of chronic kidney disease. *N Engl J Med.* 2017;377(18):1765–1776.

Kalantar-Zadeh K, Kopple JD, Block G, et al. A malnutrition-inflammation score is correlated with morbidity and mortality in maintenance hemodialysis patients. *Am J Kidney Dis.* 2001;38(6):1251–1263. doi:10.1053/ajkd.2001.29222

Kellum AJ, Lameire N, KDIGO AKI Guideline Work Group. Diagnosis, evaluation, and management of acute kidney injury: a KDIGO summary (part 1). *Crit Care.* 2013;17(1):204.

Kidney Disease: Improving Global Outcomes (KDIGO). KDIGO clinical practice guideline for acute kidney injury. *Kidney Inter.* 2012;2:1–138.

National Academy of Medicine. *Dietary Reference Intakes for Sodium and Potassium.* National Academies Press (US); 2019.

National Kidney Foundation, Academy of Nutrition and Dietetics. Clinical Practice Guideline for Nutrition in Chronic Kidney Disease: 2019 Update. https://www.kidney.org/sites/default/files/Nutrition_GL%2BSubmission_101719_Public_Review_Copy.pdf

41 Renal Bone Disease

Michael Lipkowitz

I. **DEFINITION.** Mineral and bone disorder in chronic kidney disease (CKD-MBD) comprises abnormalities in bone structure and metabolism/dynamics as well as dysregulation of metabolic factors including calcium (Ca), phosphorus (P), 25-OH (vitamin D) and 1,25 dihydroxy vitamin D (calcitriol), parathyroid hormone (PTH) fibroblast growth factor 23 (FGF23), and the calcium sensing receptor (CaSR).

II. **RENAL OSTEODYSTROPHY.** Renal osteodystrophy comprises the histomorphometric changes on biopsy of bone structure and dynamics. There are four major types of bone findings on biopsy (Table 41.1):

a. Osteitis fibrosa cystica or hyperparathyroid bone disease usually seen in the presence of prolonged severe hyperparathyroidism. This is a hyperdynamic bone lesion characterized by increased numbers and activation of both osteoblasts and osteoclasts with increased osteoid (unmineralized bone matrix). There is decreased cortical bone with an increased risk of fractures thought to be due to increased bone turnover.

b. Osteomalacia: This results from an increase in osteoid production without mineralization. This has become rare in CKD and was likely due to aluminum deposition in bone preventing mineralization.

c. Adynamic bone disease: This is a low turnover bone disease with a decrease in osteoblasts and osteoclasts, as well as loss of osteoid formation. It is most commonly due to pharmacologic oversuppression of the parathyroid glands, but there is also evidence of resistance to PTH in CKD.

d. Mixed uremic osteodystrophy (MUO): There is a mix of findings of high and low turnover bone disease on biopsy.

The proportions of the four different types of bone disease currently present in the CKD and dialysis populations are uncertain, as few large bone biopsy studies have been done. In addition based on the KDIGO guidelines of 2017, the therapy is changing to limit the use of PTH suppressing medications predialysis and to liberalize the acceptable upper level of PTH. The rationale for this change is that adynamic bone disease is the most common abnormality and may, in large part, be due to medications that suppress bone formation. Osteitis fibrosa cystica and MUO may be slightly less common, and osteomalacia is rare.

III. **PATHOPHYSIOLOGY.** The likely initiating factor in the cascade of events that cause MBD is the decreased excretion of phosphorus, resulting in increased FGF23 levels, decreased ionized Ca, decreased calcitriol levels, and decreased expression of vitamin D receptors (VDRs), CaSR, and FGF23 receptors,

TABLE 41.1	Renal osteodystrophy

Condition	Clinical findings	Lab findings	Pathology
Normal	Normal	Normal	Moderate lamellar osteoid, many osteoblasts, minimal reabsorption, and osteoclasts
Osteoporosis	Low BMD, fragility fractures	Low Ca or vitamin D	Normal bone turnover, normal osteoid, decreased bone volume
Osteitis fibrosa cystica	Low BMD, bone pain or fragility fractures, proximal muscle weakness, pruritus	High PTH, high P, low or normal Ca	High bone turnover, both formation and reabsorption. Woven osteoid and normal mineralization. Increased reabsorbing osteoclasts, fibrotic marrow
Adynamic bone disease	Low BMD, bone pain, fragility fractures	PTH <2× ULN, nl or high Ca	Decreased bone formation and reabsorption, few osteoblasts or osteoclasts, minimal osteoid that is not mineralized
Mixed uremic osteodystrophy	Low BMD, bone pain, fragility fractures	Increased PTH, low vitamin D, Ca, and P	High bone turnover with increased reabsorption and secretion, increased osteoid formation, and impaired mineralization
Osteomalacia	Low BMD, fragility fractures	High aluminum levels, low vitamin D, Ca	Low bone turnover. Wide osteoid seams, minimal mineralization, few reabsorbing osteoclasts, aluminum deposition at the mineralization front

BMD, bone mineral density; Ca, calcium; P, phosphate; PTH, parathyroid hormone; ULN, upper limit of normal.

particularly in the parathyroid glands. This ultimately results in secondary hyperparathyroidism.

a. Phosphate excretion: As CKD worsens phosphate reabsorption by proximal tubule NaP cotransporters declines, resulting in phosphaturia.

The earliest sign of this is likely an increase in FGF23, which regulates P reabsorption within the kidney. If plasma P increases, it binds Ca, lowering serum levels, which then triggers rises in calcitriol and PTH. FGF23 increases, calcitriol decreases, and PTH increases, decreasing P absorption from the gut and excretion by the kidney to normalize levels. As CKD worsens to GFRs <40, there is increasing likelihood that P levels will exceed the normal range.

b. FGF23: FGF23 is produced in bone by osteoclasts and osteoblasts and in conjunction with a coreceptor klotho binds to FGF receptors in the proximal tubule and parathyroid glands. In the kidney, FGF23 results in the decrease in expression of NaP cotransporters, increasing P excretion. It also inhibits 1-α hydroxylase inhibiting the formation of calcitriol from 25-OH vitamin D. The reduction in calcitriol inhibits intestinal absorption of phosphorus. There is a reduction in klotho in CKD that inhibits FGF23 action. FGF23 also inhibits PTH secretion; the high levels of PTH in CKD may in part be due to loss of FGF receptor and klotho in the parathyroid glands and resulting resistance to FGF23.

   i. FGF23 has also been implicated in cardiovascular disease in CKD. Higher levels predict an increased incidence of cardiovascular events. In animal models, overexpression of FGF23 causes cardiac hypertrophy.

c. Calcitriol: Calcitriol levels fall early on CKD (GFR <60). This is likely due to inhibition of 1-α hydroxylase by both increased P load in the tubule and elevated levels of FGF23. The resulting low levels of calcitriol stimulate PTH secretion both directly and indirectly. Low levels of calcitriol result in a decrease in Ca absorption from the intestine and release from bone, resulting in hypocalcemia, which stimulates PTH secretion via the CaSR. Calcitriol also acts directly via VDR on parathyroid cells to suppress transcription. Low levels result in increased transcription as well reduced expression of VDR. This is likely a cause of increased parathyroid gland mass and nodularity.

d. CaSR: The CaSR is expressed at high levels on cells in the parathyroid glands and are sensitive to minute changes in calcium levels. There are data that suggest that receptor expression is decreased in CKD, reducing responsiveness to Ca levels and promoting hyperparathyroidism.

e. PTH: Parathyroid hormone is secreted in response to Ca levels, and is also upregulated by FGF23 in response to increased P and downregulated by VDR in response to calcitriol. There is evidence that high P may also independently increase PTH secretion. PTH acts on proximal tubule NaP cotransporters to reduce P reabsorption by decreasing the activity and number of transporters. In thick ascending limb (TAL) and thick ascending limb (DCT), it causes an increase in Ca reabsorption. PTH also increases 1-α hydroxylase activity resulting in increased calcitriol levels, but this effect is lost as CKD advances. In bone, PTH initially releases Ca from skeletal stores, but eventually releases calcium via bone reabsorption, which if unchecked results in osteitis fibrosa cystica.

IV. DIAGNOSIS OF MBD.   The definitive diagnosis of the form of MBD is made by bone biopsy; however, this has in general been done only at academic medical centers and requires skilled personnel to perform and analyze the biopsy. Although laboratory values can suggest the nature of the MBD, there are situations where biopsy may be optimal if available to best guide therapy.

a. Symptoms: MBD is not usually symptomatic until disease is severe, and consists of fragility fractures and undiagnosed bone pain.

b. Bone biopsy: This procedure measures the dynamics of bone formation by labeling the mineralization front with tetracycline administered for 2 to 3 days at two time periods 21 days apart, followed by a core biopsy of the iliac crest. The mineralized bone is detected by tetracycline, which fluoresces and has a high affinity for mineralized bone. Osteoid (unmineralized bone) is stained with a different material. The results are quantitated for TMV: bone turnover, mineralization, and volume. In normal bone, there is a distinct separation of the two tetracycline mineralization fronts, with a layer of osteoid on the surface of the more recent front, as well as many osteoblasts but few osteoclasts. In osteitis fibrosa cystica, there are increased osteoclasts and signs of reabsorption as well as increased tetracycline labeling signifying increased bone formation. In adynamic bone disease, there is minimal mineralization labeling, thin osteoid, and decreased osteoblast and osteoclast numbers and activity. In osteomalacia, there is increased osteoid but no mineralization. Mixed uremic osteodystrophy is similar to osteitis fibrosa cystica with increased osteoid.

c. Imaging: There are no imaging studies that can definitively determine the nature of bone disease. On bone x-rays or CT, subperiosteal reabsorption, particularly seen in middle phalanges, and reabsorption of bone in distal clavicles, distal phalanges, and skull can be seen in hyperparathyroid bone disease.

i. Dual x-ray absorptiometry (DEXA) measure of bone mineral density (BMD): There are data to suggest that bone disease in early stages of CKD (G1–2) may be similar to osteoporosis in the non-CKD population if metabolic parameters such as PTH, Ca, P, etc. are normal, although there is an increased fracture rate in CKD. In this setting, BMD measurements can be used to estimate fracture risk and determine need for antiresorptive therapy such as bisphosphonates, etc. For more advanced CKD stages G3a–5D, there is still an association of DEXA BMD with fractures, although DEXA cannot diagnose the underlying form of bone disease. It is recommended that DEXA be performed in this more severe disease if the results will be used to guide therapy, particularly with antiresorptive drugs, although there is an increased risk of complications from therapy as bisphosphonates can worsen adynamic bone disease and denosumab can cause prolonged hypocalcemia. If available, bone biopsy may be a better choice to guide therapy.

d. Laboratory tests: The earliest abnormality in CKD-MBD is a rise in FGF23, although this is not usually measured. Ca and P begin to become abnormal as GFR falls below 30 to 40 mL/min, resulting in increased PTH secretion. Current guidelines recommend measuring Ca, P, PTH, vitamin D, and alkaline phosphatase (AP) beginning at CKD G3a. For CKD G3, measurements can be done at 6- to 12-month intervals for Ca and P, and for PTH if abnormal. Frequency increases to 3 to 6 months for Ca and P, and 6 to 12 for PTH at G4. AP is measured yearly if PTH is elevated. In G5-5D, Ca and P should be measured every 1 to 3 months and PTH every 3 to 6 months. If there are abnormalities in the measurements, frequency is increased to guide therapy. Vitamin D testing and therapy as for the general population is recommended as this may lower PTH levels and increase calcitriol levels. Currently, recommendations are for therapy based on trends in the levels of these parameters and not on individual tests, in particular, as there are large day to day and diurnal variability in P and PTH levels (e.g., rise on P over time). Therapy is aimed at correcting these parameters before severe osteodystrophy develops.

Once there is evidence of bone disease, the best predictor of adynamic bone disease versus osteitis fibrosa cystica is PTH. Levels below 2× the upper limit of normal, especially in the presence of high Ca and low bone-specific alkaline phosphatase (BSAP) is more suggestive of adynamic bone disease. PTH levels above 9× the upper limit of normal predict high turnover bone disease; high BSAP is often also seen in this setting.

Measurement of bone turnover markers such as *n*-telopeptide and others is not recommended as they are affected by low GFR and are not reliable markers o bone turnover in this setting.

V. THERAPY FOR CKD-MBD (TABLE 41.2)

a. Phosphate levels: Treatment in this setting should be implemented if serial assessments of Ca, P, and PTH taken together confirm abnormal levels, and should attempt to decrease P levels toward normal. There are no data that define an ideal P level in CKD at this time, nor optimal therapy, although trials are in progress to answer some of these questions.

  i. Dietary restriction: Low-P diet can affect P levels, and is recommended. Diets high in vegetable protein may have less absorbable P than meat-based diets, but care must be taken in that many foods have P-containing additives. It is also difficult to maintain such a diet the setting of other restrictions such as for K and for diabetes. This is best done in conjunction with a nutritionist.

  ii. Phosphate binders: these medications bind P in the intestine and prevent absorption. All have significant GI side effects that limits adherence. Current guidelines suggest limiting Ca-based binders, but the data to support this remains weak. Further, Ca-based binders are much cheaper than other choices, and may be the only viable choice for uninsured or underinsured patients.

  iia. There are data that suggest that Ca-based binders (calcium carbonate or acetate) increase Ca balance and may promote vascular calcification and are associated with increased mortality. Current guidelines recommend restricting the use of Ca-based binders, however they are the most affordable agents and may need to be used if cost is a factor.

  iib. Sevelamer is a polymer that exchanges either Cl (sevelamer HCl) or bicarbonate (sevelamer carbonate) for P in the intestine. It can bind bile salts lowering cholesterol, and may lower FGF23 in comparison to Ca binders. There are studies suggesting a mortality benefit versus Ca binders, but the data are generally weak.

  iic. Lanthanum carbonate may decrease FGF23; and in some studies, may provide a mortality benefit, although again data are weak. There are no studies on the long-term effects of lanthanum accumulation in the body.

  iid. Sucroferric oxyhydroxide and ferric citrate are newer P binders that both provide iron and bind P. They are effective P binders

Treatment	Mechanism	Advantages	Disadvantages
Low-P diet	Prevents P absorption from intestine	Few side effects, inexpensive	Difficult to avoid P and maintain healthy diet especially if other requirements; e.g., diabetic
Ca carbonate or acetate	Forms insoluble Ca–P complexes	Least-expensive binders	GI side effects, hypercalcemia, Ca load may promote calcification, low turnover bone disease
Sevelamer HCl or carbonate	Exchange Cl or carbonate for P	No Ca load, may lower cholesterol	GI side effects, expensive, limit fat soluble vitamin absorption
Lanthanum carbonate	Forms insoluble La–P complexes	No Ca load, fewer pills	GI side effects, expensive, La accumulates, long-term effects unknown
Ferric citrate	Forms insoluble Fe–P complexes	No Ca, provide Fe-raising Fe stores	GI side effects, expensive, long-term risks especially for Fe-overload undetermined
Sucroferric oxyhydroxide	Exchanges hydroxyl for P	No Ca, low pill burden, may not affect Fe stores	GI side effects, expensive, uncertain as yet effect on Fe stores
Vitamin D	Raises vitamin D levels	Decreases PTH slightly	May cause hypercalcemia and increase calcification
Calcitriol and analogs	Active 1,25 vitamin D. Suppresses PTH via VDR, raises Ca levels by intestinal absorption and renal tubule reabsorption	Can raise Ca if low, lowers PTH	Increased Ca absorption, increased P absorption, hypercalcemia, potential for adynamic bone disease due to PTH oversuppression
Cinacalcet	Calcimimetic-allosteric activation of CaSR in parathyroid to decrease PTH secretion, in tubule to decrease Ca reabsorption, and on osteoblasts to promote mineralization	Decreases PTH, improves mineralization. Decreases FGF23 and may decrease cardiovascular mortality in dialysis	Expensive, GI side effects, hypocalcemia, may only be relevant in dialysis patients
Etelcalcetide	Parenteral calcimimetic–see cinacalcet for mechanism	Decreases PTH, improves mineralization. Decreases FGF23, effect on mortality as yet uncertain. May be more effective than cinacalcet	Expensive, GI side effects, hypocalcemia, IV administration. Best protocols for use as yet undefined.
Parathyroidectomy	Decrease secreting parathyroid tissue	Resolves unremitting hyperparathyroidism	Total parathyroidectomy requires long-term Ca and calcitriol, intrathoracic glands can be missed or difficult to remove, severe hypocalcemia due to "hungry bone" syndrome can be difficult to manage in the short term

Ca, calcium; P, phosphate; Fe, iron; La, lanthanum; PTH, parathyroid hormone; CaSR, calcium sensing receptor; FGF23, fibroblast growth factor 23; VDR, vitamin D receptor.

that may decrease FGF23 in part by correcting Fe deficiency. While the increase in iron stores is beneficial in dialysis, it is unclear what the long-term effects in CKD without anemia will be.

    iie. Tenapanor is an experimental drug that blocks sodium–hydrogen exchanger 3 in the intestine causing a secondary change in cell junctions that decreases paracellular P absorption.

  iii. Dialysis: In CKD 5D, dialysis effectively removes P. Within the limits, dialysis dose can be adjusted to increase P removal.

b. Ca levels: Current guidelines recommend preventing hypercalcemia and keeping Ca in normal range. This is based on evidence that hypercalcemia may be associated with vascular calcification, which has been linked to mortality. In dialysis patients, mild hypocalcemia can be tolerated based on the finding that mild asymptomatic hypocalcemia with the use of calcimimetics was not harmful in the EVOLVE trial.

    i. Current recommendations suggest avoiding Ca-based phosphate binders in adults, but to use in children, who need to absorb Ca to build bone during growth, on Ca levels and intake.

    ii. A common cause of hypercalcemia in CKD is the use of vitamin D, calcitriol, and calcitriol analogs such as paricalcitol and doxercalciferol. In the latest guidelines, calcitriol and analogs are not recommended to be routinely used until dialysis is initiated, although can be used for severe or worsening hyperparathyroidism. However, they are still one of the recommended therapies for hyperparathyroidism in dialysis. In the setting of hypercalcemia, these agents should be reduced or stopped and the hyperparathyroidism addressed with other measures. In dialysis patients, calcimimetics may also reduce Ca levels in this setting.

  iii. The level of Ca in dialysate can also affect serum Ca levels. Current guidelines recommend using dialysate Ca concentrations of 2.5 and 3.0 mEq/L, which are standard available dialysate concentrations. Use of lower Ca concentrations has been linked to arrhythmia and heart failure in several observational studies, so they should be avoided.

  iv. In the absence of Ca-lowering medications, hypocalcemia might result from either hyper P or vitamin D deficiency. In the setting of vitamin D deficiency, hyper P should be treated before vitamin D supplementation, as raising Ca in this setting could result in increased vascular calcification. Vitamin D supplementation may also raise calcitriol levels which in turn might increase P absorption from the intestine.

c. PTH levels/secondary hyperparathyroidism: The ideal PTH level in CKD has not been defined for any level of GFR. However, levels below 2× the upper limit of normal have been associated with adynamic bone disease, and levels greater 9× the upper limit of normal with osteitis fibrosa cystica. Elevated PTH levels may initially be beneficial by increasing P excretion by the kidney and overcoming bone resistance to PTH that is present in CKD. Guidelines do not recommend treatment unless levels are persistently elevated or increasing on repeated measurements. Of note, due to variability in serum levels and assay results, as many as 26 measurements at a given time point may be needed to define a truly accurate PTH level, so a single abnormal level should not be treated.

i. For elevated PTH levels in CKD 3–5, nondialysis patients, it is recommended that factors that can cause increases in PTH including hyper P, high phosphate intake, hypo Ca, and vitamin D deficiency be assayed and treated, and that calcitriol and active analogs not be routinely used.

ia. For "severe" or worsening hyperparathyroidism, calcitriol and active vitamin D analogs may be necessary to control secondary hyperparathyroidism.

ib. The use of calcimimetics in nondialysis CKD G3–G5 has not been recommended due to the high incidence of symptomatic hypocalcemia. There have been few clinical trials to evaluate calcimimetics in CKD 3–5. Several trials suggest that cinacalcet lowers PTH, these trials are confounded by high use of Ca-containing P binders and activated vitamin D analogs to prevent the hypocalcemia, and there are no data to indicate that there are either bone or cardiovascular benefits from calcimimetic use.

ii. For hyperparathyroidism in dialysis (CKD 5D) patients' current recommendations recommend use of either calcitriol, activated vitamin D analogs, calcimimetics, or a combination to maintain PTH in the range of 2 to 9× the upper limit of normal of intact PTH assay.

iia. Some studies have proposed benefits of individually activated vitamin D analogs such as paricalcitol over calcitriol, but the data have not been definitive at this time.

iib. Calcimimetics have been shown to decrease FGF23, which has been linked to cardiovascular disease in CKD. The randomized controlled EVOLVE trial in 3,800 dialysis patients with PTH >300 did not show a benefit for the primary outcome of mortality and major cardiovascular events; however, a prespecified secondary analysis showed reduction of FGF23 levels that were associated with lower rates of cardiovascular death and nonatherosclerotic cardiac events. However, the data are only significant in subgroup analyses and have not been replicated in other controlled studies. In these studies, mild asymptomatic hypocalcemia was well tolerated.

iic. Parenteral versus oral calcimimetics: Etelcalcetide is a recently developed small peptide intravenous calcimimetic. It has been shown to be superior to cinacalcet in reducing PTH in on study by the manufacturer. There are no clear mortality data yet, although PTH and FGF23 levels are reduced. One of the significant side effects of cinacalcet is GI intolerance; there are similar GI side effects with etelcalcetide, although perhaps in a lower percentage of patients. The renal community is still developing strategies on how to best utilize parenteral agents; suggested indications might include nonadherence or poor response to oral regimens.

iii. Parathyroidectomy: In patients with severe hyperparathyroidism unresponsive to medical therapy and dialysis, parathyroidectomy should be considered. Patients with PTH >9× the upper limit of normal with hypercalcemia not induced by medications, fragility fractures, bone and joint pain, myopathy, or severe itching are relatively clear candidates for surgery. In the absence of symptoms, there are no clear targets for surgery, but usually PTH >1,000 is utilized. Usually, all the parathyroid glands are hypertrophied and nodular, although adenomas can be found as well.

    iiia. Surgical procedure: The most common procedures are partial/subtotal parathyroidectomy where all glands except for a portion of one gland are removed, or total parathyroidectomy with autotransplantation of a part of one gland near the sternocleidomastoid muscle or in the forearm.

    iiib. Hungry bone syndrome: In the majority of dialysis patients with parathyroidectomy, particularly for total removal, hypocalcemia develops. This needs to be monitored carefully postoperatively and is usually treated with initial infusions of high doses of calcium and calcitriol followed by oral dosing. It can be severe and results in about a 15% readmission rate for symptoms.

    iiic. Recurrent hyperparathyroidism can occur either as a result of hypertrophy of the remaining parathyroid tissue (an argument for autotransplantation which facilitates further surgery) or due to additional glands usually located in the chest cavity that can be difficult to identify and remove.

  d. Tertiary hyperparathyroidism: In some cases of secondary hyperparathyroidism, parathyroid glands develop autonomous function that does not respond to medical therapy. This is likely the result prolonged stimulation of parathyroid cell growth by hyper P, low calcitriol, and low Ca coupled with a decreased density of VDR and CaSR on the cells. The glands become nodular; and in some cases, there is monoclonal transformation that can result on adenomas. Development of hypercalcemia in dialysis patients with high PTH in the absence of medications that raise Ca raises suspicion of tertiary hyperparathyroidism. Treatment is parathyroidectomy since, by definition, there is a lack of response to medical therapy.

  e. Vitamin D deficiency: Current recommendations call for vitamin D supplementation for elevated PTH and for vitamin D deficiency (levels below 15 ng/L). There are data that such supplementation can decrease PTH levels. However, there is no convincing evidence that supplementation prevents bone or cardiovascular disease. Although many large observational studies showed an association of vitamin D with cardiovascular outcomes, the recently reported VITAL randomized controlled trial in 25,000 subjects did not show a benefit for cardiovascular disease. Subgroup analyses for CKD are expected to be performed.

VI. MINERAL AND BONE DISEASE IN TRANSPLANT. Kidney transplant patients have a significant incidence of MBD, both from abnormalities experienced in the course of CKD and dialysis, and subsequently from immunosuppressive medications.

  a. Monitoring for MBD:

    i. In the immediate posttransplant period, frequent/weekly monitoring of Ca and P until stable

    ii. For CKD G1-3bT (GFR from normal to 30 mL/min), Ca, P, and PTH every 6 months and then depending on levels and changes

     iii. For CKD G4T, Ca and P every 3 to 6 months and PTH every 6 to 12 months.

     iv. For CKD G5T, Ca and P every 1 to 3 months and PTH every 3 to 6 months

     v. Measurement of AP is done yearly for patients with elevated PTH

    Management of abnormalities can be treated as for CKD. Vitamin D insufficiency should similarly be assayed and treated.

b. BMD measurement: DEXA measurements are recommended if results are expected to change management. The correlation of BMD and fractures is similar in transplant as in CKD.

c. In the first 12 months after transplant, treatment should be guided by the presence or absence of abnormalities of Ca, P, PTH, and vitamin D. If osteoporosis is suggested, treatment with vitamin D, Ca, and antiresorptive agents is suggested. After 12 months, there are no sufficient data for the guidelines to recommend therapies. If the nature of the bone disease is unclear, bone biopsy can be performed to guide therapy.

d. Posttransplant hyperparathyroidism: This is a common finding, in as many as 40% to 50% of patients, and is more common in patients who have had poorly controlled PTH levels on dialysis. The majority of patients resolve over time but up to 10% have been found to have persistent disease after several years. Severe hypercalcemia can occur, and result in polyuria, graft artery vasoconstriction, and allograft loss. Hypophosphatemia that can be severe and symptomatic also occurs. Treatment varies depending on symptoms and severity of PTH.

     i. Many transplant centers recommend parathyroidectomy prior to transplant for patients with refractory hyperparathyroidism and TPH levels >800.

     ii. For patients who have mild hypercalcemia (<11 mg/dL) and who are asymptomatic, treatment can be initiated with calcimimetics and Ca, P and PTH monitored over time for improvement. Of note, treatment with calcimimetics has not been shown to improve bone disease. If there is a poor response to calcimimetics, parathyroidectomy is indicated. For severe hypercalcemia or if there are clinical signs such as bone pain, fractures, or calciphylaxis, parathyroidectomy may be the first choice based on a small observational study, although a trial of cinacalcet can be initiated followed by parathyroidectomy if needed.

     iii. Hypophosphatemia, if asymptomatic, is initially treated by treating hyperparathyroidism with Ca, vitamin D, or calcitriol to decrease the phosphaturic effect of PTH. Severe and symptomatic low P (<1 mg/dL) will require oral phosphate supplements. If severe hypophosphatemia persists, parathyroidectomy may be necessary.

     iv. High PTH with normal Ca: The first step in therapy is to measure and replete vitamin D levels. If PTH remains elevated and Ca is normal, calcitriol can be used. If PTH is unresponsive to these measures, other causes such as use of diuretics that increase Ca excretion, low Ca intake, and high-dose steroids should be examined. Cinacalcet and parathyroidectomy are not indicated for isolated elevated PTH.

VII. VASCULAR CALCIFICATION. There is increased vascular calcification in CKD. The origins of calcification are complex and in addition to the endothelial calcification, seen in non-CKD, there is medial calcification. Increased calcification is related to increased mortality in CKD, although coronary calcium scores are less useful than in individuals with normal renal function. This calcification is also the underlying pathology for calciphylaxis, or uremic calcific arteriolopathy, which cause small vessel occlusion and tissue necrosis. Although no studies have definitively shown a difference in mortality related to specific binder use, there are data that suggest increased Ca load, such as from Ca-based binders or activated vitamin D, increases vascular calcification. Calcification is increased both in hyperparathyroid, hyperdynamic bone disease and adynamic bone disease.

There are no specific recommendations to treat this vascular calcification at this time other than to control PTH, Ca, and P levels. Lateral abdominal x-rays can be used to screen for calcification and focus clinicians on optimal control of MBD in these high-risk patients.

VIII. SUGGESTED READINGS
Barreto CF, Barreto DV, Massy ZA, et al. Strategies for phosphate control in patients with CKD. *Kidney Int Rep.* 2019;4(8):1043–1056. doi: 10.1016/j.ekir.2019.06.002

Gutierrez O, Isakova T, Rhee E, et al. Fibroblast growth factor-23 mitigates hyperphosphatemia but accentuates calcitriol deficiency in chronic kidney disease. *J Am Soc Nephrol.* 2005;16(7): 2205–2215. doi: 10.1681/ASN.2005010052

Isakova T, Nickolas TL, Denburg M, et al. KDOQI US commentary on the 2017 KDIGO clinical practice guideline update for the diagnosis, evaluation, prevention, and treatment of chronic kidney disease–mineral and bone disorder (CKD-MBD). *Am J Kidney Dis.* 2017;70(6):737–751. doi: 10.1053/j.ajkd.2017.07.019

Kidney Disease: Improving Global Outcomes (KDIGO) CKD-MBD Update Work Group. KDIGO 2017 clinical practice guideline update for the diagnosis, evaluation, prevention, and treatment of chronic kidney disease–mineral and bone disorder (CKD-MBD). *Kidney Int Suppl.* 2017;7(1):1–59.

Moe SM, Chertow GM, Parfrey PS, et al. Cinacalcet, fibroblast growth factor-23, and cardiovascular disease in hemodialysis: the evaluation of cinacalcet HCl therapy to lower cardiovascular events (EVOLVE) trial. *Circulation.* 2015;132(1):27–39. doi: 10.1161/CIRCULATIONAHA.114.013876

Scialla JJ, Kendrick J, Uribarri J, et al. State-of-the-art management of hyperphosphatemia in patients with CKD: an NKF-KDOQI controversies perspective. *Am J Kidney Dis.* 2021;77(1):P132–P141. doi: 10.1053/j.ajkd.2020.05.025

Dialysis

42

Hemodialysis and Continuous Therapies

Mohammad A. Hashmi, Keiko I. Greenberg

Hemodialysis is defined as a primary diffusion-based therapy in which solute from the patient's blood crosses a semipermeable membrane (the dialyzer) into the dialysate. Removal of excess fluid is accomplished by ultrafiltration, in which hydrostatic pressure causes the bulk flow of plasma water through the membrane. With advances in vascular access, anticoagulation, and the production of reliable and efficient dialyzers, hemodialysis has become the predominant method of treatment for acute and chronic kidney failure.

I. **INDICATIONS FOR HEMODIALYSIS.** Most patients with acute kidney injury are successfully managed without dialysis (see Chapter 35). For chronic kidney disease (CKD) patients, the National Kidney Foundation has developed practice guidelines to assist in the management of complications of CKD, choice of kidney replacement therapy modality, creation of vascular access, administration of erythropoiesis-stimulating agents (ESAs), nutrition, bone and mineral metabolism, and timing of the initiation of dialysis. These Kidney Disease Outcomes Quality Initiative clinical practice guidelines have had a profound impact on the treatment of CKD patients. Factors to be considered before initiating hemodialysis in patients with CKD should also include comorbid conditions and patient preference. Timing of therapy is dictated by serum chemistries and symptoms. Hemodialysis is usually started when estimated glomerular filtration rate decreases to approximately 10 mL/min/1.73 m^2. However, more important than the absolute laboratory values is the presence of uremic symptoms. Generally, all patients are offered dialysis unless they have a terminal disease such as metastatic cancer or have significant neurologic or psychiatric disease that would make dialysis dangerous to themselves or others (Table 42.1). The indications for acute or emergent dialysis include severe hyperkalemia, acidosis, and volume overload not amenable to conservative medical therapies, as well as uremic pericarditis and severe encephalopathy. Dialytic therapies can also be used to correct certain other urgent electrolyte problems including hypercalcemia, hyperphosphatemia, and hyperuricemia (such as that seen in tumor lysis syndrome), as well as to treat some toxin or drug overdoses.

II. **VASCULAR ACCESS.** Provision of dialysis requires reliable repeated access to the patient's circulation that can provide blood flow of approximately 300 to 450 mL/min. Ideally, the access should be created well before the need for chronic dialysis, typically when the estimated glomerular filtration rate falls below approximately 15 to 20 mL/min/1.73 m^2, depending on the tempo of kidney deterioration.

TABLE 42.1	Indications and contraindications for hemodialysis

Indications
   Relative
      Symptomatic azotemia including encephalopathy
      Dialyzable toxins (drug poisoning)
   Absolute
      Uremic pericarditis
      Hyperkalemia, severe (see Chapter 18)
      Diuretic unresponsive fluid overload (pulmonary edema)
      Intractable acidosis
Contraindications
   Relative
      Hypotension unresponsive to vasopressors
      Terminal illness
      Advanced neurologic diseases (such as dementia)

A. Acute Vascular Access. Internal jugular or femoral vein catheters are the preferred method to obtain temporary vascular access for emergent dialysis and are used until a more permanent access is established. Subclavian vein catheterization is now avoided for temporary access in all patients with CKD due to higher risk of central venous stenosis, which may later cause problems establishing permanent dialysis access. Temporary or nontunneled catheters can often be used in the internal jugular location for 2 to 3 weeks. Femoral vein catheters, in comparison, are typically used for less than 1 week. Temporary catheters are associated with high risk of infection. Other risks associated with dialysis catheters include bleeding, thrombosis, or stenosis of the vessel, pneumothorax, hemothorax, and air embolus. Dialysis catheters should not be used as routine intravenous lines because breaks in sterile technique greatly increase the risk of infection and catheter thrombosis. Catheters obstructed by clot can often be successfully cleared using thrombolytic agents (e.g., tissue plasminogen activator). In the presence of bacteremia, temporary dialysis catheters should be removed, the appropriate cultures taken, and systemic antibiotics administered. Empiric antibiotic therapy includes vancomycin to cover methicillin-resistant *Staphylococcus aureus*, and cefepime (or third-generation cephalosporin, carbapenem, or beta-lactam/beta-lactamase combination) for coverage of gram-negative bacilli. Monitoring of vancomycin is recommended.

B. Chronic Vascular Access

   1. Arteriovenous fistula. The arteriovenous (AV) fistula is the preferred vascular access for chronic hemodialysis and may last for years. When progression to end-stage kidney disease is imminent, efforts should be made to spare the nondominant arm from venipuncture and arterial puncture. Fistulae are created by the surgical anastomosis of an artery and vein, most commonly the radial or brachial artery to the cephalic vein. Typically, a new primary fistula should be allowed to mature for 2 to 4 months, during which time the vein enlarges ("arterializes") sufficiently to provide sufficient blood flow for dialysis. Examination of the functioning AV fistula reveals a palpable pulsation ("thrill") and a bruit by auscultation.

2. **Arteriovenous grafts.** When a patient's vessels are inadequate to create an AV fistula, polytetrafluoroethylene grafts (e.g., Gore-Tex®) are typically used to form a conduit from artery to vein. AV grafts should be placed at least 2 to 4 weeks before the anticipated need for hemodialysis. Use of early cannulation grafts may be appropriate in some circumstances. For patients with failed accesses or central venous stenosis, a Hemodialysis Reliable Outflow (HeRO) graft may be an option.

3. **Tunneled catheters.** Tunneled cuffed catheters are often used as a bridge to the development of a mature AV fistula if a mature fistula is not in place at the time of initiation of chronic hemodialysis. Most often, they are configured as dual-lumen devices (with a single exit site, tunnel, and venotomy), which then split into separate catheters once inside the large central vein. Due to the risk of catheter-related complications, it is preferable to develop permanent vascular access with an AV fistula. Tunneled devices are often placed in patients with acute kidney injury if dialysis is still needed after 3 weeks of using a temporary catheter.

4. **Assessment of vascular access.** To optimize dialysis delivery, it is important to ensure that the access blood flow meets that of the desired extracorporeal pump rate. Inadequate blood supply will cause recirculation and reduce solute clearance. Regular monitoring of dialysis access is crucial for detection of stenosis, thrombosis, and other complications of AV fistulas and grafts. Monitoring includes physical examination, laboratory studies, and angiographic studies when indicated. Complications of chronic vascular access are discussed further in Chapter 45.

III. **HEMODIALYSIS: THE PROCEDURE.** The hemodialysis machine prepares the dialysate, regulates dialysate and blood flow past a semipermeable membrane, and monitors functions involving the dialysate and extracorporeal blood circuit. Blood and dialysate are perfused on opposite sides of the semipermeable membrane in a countercurrent direction for maximal efficiency of solute removal via diffusion. Heparin is typically required for systemic anticoagulation. Dialysate composition, the characteristics and size of the membrane in the dialyzer, and blood and solute flow rates all affect solute removal.

A. **Dialysate Composition.** Sodium, potassium, magnesium, and calcium concentrations are prescribed as the clinical situation dictates. The electrolyte composition of the dialysate is chosen with great care because ion fluxes (potassium in particular) can induce arrhythmias. Low-calcium baths may be used in the acute and chronic therapy of hypercalcemia. Bicarbonate is used as the base buffer, and its concentration can be changed as needed. The standard dextrose concentration of dialysate is 100 mg/dL.

B. **Dialyzers.** Dialyzers are composed of thousands of small hollow fibers through which blood flows. Commonly used membranes include cuprophane, cellulose acetate, and several high-porosity synthetic copolymer membranes (e.g., polyacrylonitrile, polymethylmethacrylate, and polysulfone). Use of nonsynthetic cellulosic membranes has become uncommon because they are bioincompatible—they can activate the alternative complement pathway and lead to leukocyte agglutination and cytokine release. For the vast majority of treatments, synthetic polymer membranes are used—they exhibit better biocompatibility, improved ultrafiltration characteristics, and increased solute clearance, especially in the middle molecule (molecular mass 300 to 2,000 dalton) range; they are also less thrombogenic, allowing dialysis without heparin when indicated. These membranes are also used in high-flux dialysis and hemofiltration. A disadvantage of synthetic membranes is their high cost. Dialyzer reprocessing or reuse to improve dialyzer biocompatibility and reduce hypersensitivity reactions to ethylene oxide sterilization was once common but infrequently done today.

IV. AIMS OF DIALYTIC THERAPY. Incomplete understanding of the pathogenesis of uremic symptoms has made it difficult to define an optimal dialysis prescription. Although a predialysis blood urea nitrogen (BUN) concentration of <80 mg/dL was once an aim of therapy, correlation of toxic manifestations of uremia with BUN is often poor. Historically, time-averaged concentrations of urea (i.e., achieving less than 50 mg/dL) were utilized to guide dialysis dosing, and this was followed by the development of more comprehensive mathematical approaches for urea kinetic modeling. Key concepts in one model include the protein catabolic rate (a measure of the dietary protein intake), residual kidney function, and the dimensionless parameter, Kt/V urea. The latter term expresses the fractional urea clearance, where K is dialyzer urea clearance, t is dialysis treatment time, and V is body urea distribution volume. This ratio determines the magnitude of decline of BUN during a dialysis, and it serves as a measure of the dose of dialysis related to urea removal. In practice, this parameter should be at least 1.2 (minimum 1.2, target 1.4) to minimize uremic symptoms and is calculated using a complex set of equations. The more simplistic urea reduction ratio (i.e., target of a 65% reduction in BUN levels) is also used to assess dialysis adequacy. New technology for the continuous monitoring of urea losses into dialysate may overcome the pitfalls of basing adequacy determination on just blood levels. Even though a switch to high-flux dialysis can be shown to provide significantly higher clearances, it still does not yield the dramatic increases needed to approach that of native kidney function.

V. ULTRAFILTRATION. The process in which fluid is removed from blood through a microporous filter is called ultrafiltration. As blood flows through the filter, the pressure gradient drives fluid (the ultrafiltrate) across the membrane which is discarded. In this process, solutes with low molecular weight (e.g., sodium and potassium) are removed from the blood along with the water (solvent drag), whereas suspended solids and solutes with high molecular weight are retained. Most hemodialysis treatments involve both dialysis and ultrafiltration. There has been increasing focus on avoiding high ultrafiltration rates (UFRs) during dialysis due to studies linking high UFR to increased mortality. UFR should be <13 mL/kg/hr whenever possible, although data suggest that UFRs as low as 8 to 10 mL/kg/hr are also associated with increased mortality.

There are clinical scenarios, such as congestive heart failure, in which isolated ultrafiltration is employed without concurrent dialysis. During isolated ultrafiltration, all clearances are driven by convective forces, without diffusive solute losses. Small electrolytes are removed in nearly the same concentration as plasma, and therefore, electrolyte shifts generally do not occur. Consequently, with this technique, it is possible to use low blood flows to remove a significant amount of fluid, while minimizing adverse electrolyte or hemodynamic consequences. However, it should be noted that ultrafiltration still carries all the technical risks and complications associated with any extracorporeal treatment (e.g., bleeding, infection). Importantly, inadvertent excessive removal of fluid from the intravascular space could potentially compromise renal perfusion, leading to acute kidney injury.

VI. EXTRACORPOREAL THERAPIES IN THE INTENSIVE CARE UNIT SETTING. Critically ill, hemodynamically unstable intensive care unit (ICU) patients are often challenging to treat with conventional dialytic modalities. The intermittent volume and solute fluxes may cause significant morbidity, which includes worsening of hypotension and arrhythmias. ICU patients may also have significant obligate fluid intake that makes volume management very difficult with intermittent dialysis. As a result, continuous kidney replacement therapy is frequently used for the management of patients with hemodynamic instability, cardiogenic shock with pulmonary edema and inadequate urine output, diuretic-refractory congestive heart failure, and for patients who need parenteral nutrition.

The modalities of continuous kidney replacement are: continuous venovenous hemofiltration (CVVH), continuous venovenous hemodialysis (CVVHD), and continuous venovenous hemodiafiltration (CVVHDF). CVVHD is similar, conceptually, to traditional hemodialysis but enhances patient stability by slow fluid and solute fluxes accomplished at low blood-flow rate (usually 250 to 350 mL/min) and dialysate flow rates (usually 20 to 25 mL/kg/hr). CVVH relies on convective solute clearance (rather than diffusion) by using hydraulic pressure to drive ultrafiltration of bulk fluid across a high-porosity hemofilter membrane. This approach necessitates the generation of very large volumes of ultrafiltrate (20 to 25 mL/kg body weight/hr), which has a composition similar to that of plasma water. The quantity of solute removed (the kidney replacement "dose") is thus a function of the amount of ultrafiltrate generated. These losses must be replaced by a balanced electrolyte solution in amounts determined by desired fluid and electrolyte losses or gains. The replacement fluid may enter the extracorporeal circuit before the dialyzer (prefilter CVVH) or after the dialyzer (postfilter CVVH). Solute removal may be further enhanced by combining these two modalities into hemodiafiltration (CVVHDF). There are a variety of dialysate and replacement fluid options available commercially or prepared locally. The base buffer can be either bicarbonate or citrate. The latter can also serve as a regional anticoagulant, but its use necessitates the careful monitoring and replacement of calcium as indicated. At high pump speeds, the daily solute and fluid clearance rates can match or even exceed those of daily conventional hemodialysis, which is particularly appropriate for very catabolic patients (i.e., those with sepsis or burns) who require high-dose or high-volume parenteral nutrition. The disadvantage of these modalities includes use in the ICU setting only, poor emergent treatment for hyperkalemia and acidosis, and access-site infection. AV fistulas and grafts are not used for continuous kidney replacement therapy due to risk of needle dislodgement and bleeding; dual-lumen dialysis catheters are required. To prevent thrombosis in the extracorporeal circuit, anticoagulation is usually required and can be accomplished with either systemic heparin or regional anticoagulation with citrate. These machines may also be used for fluid removal alone (slow continuous ultrafiltration) in select patients with severe congestive heart failure and inadequate urine volume.

The optimal dialysis therapy for the management of acute kidney injury is unknown; options include thrice weekly hemodialysis, daily intermittent hemodialysis (which provides a higher total dialysis dose, improved volume control, and, possibly, improved mortality in the ICU setting), CVVH, CVVHD, CVVHDF, or slow, low-efficiency hemodialysis via prolonged treatments with conventional machines. With a paucity of outcomes data clearly favoring one modality, the choice is determined by local machine resources (expense and availability of new equipment), nursing care availability (requires training large numbers of ICU staff), cost (equipment, custom sterile fluids, nursing), anticoagulation technique (none, heparin, or citrate), or even schedules for other patient procedures (slow, continuous modalities are not usually portable outside of the ICU).

VII. COMPLICATIONS OF HEMODIALYSIS. Several complications can occur during hemodialysis, ranging in frequency from common to very rare and in severity from mild to life-threatening.

A. **Intradialytic Hypotension.** Intradialytic hypotension is the most frequent complication during hemodialysis. It can occur in the setting of rapid or excessive ultrafiltration, atherosclerotic heart disease, autonomic neuropathy, and incorrect dry weight. Patients may be asymptomatic or experience lightheadedness, nausea, vomiting, chest pain, or muscle cramps. Ultrafiltration should be stopped or the rate slowed depending on the severity of the hypotension and symptoms. A small fluid bolus and/or albumin may be required in severe cases. Measures to prevent intradialytic hypotension include: accurately determining dry weight, lowering dialysate temperature, lowering blood flow, avoiding administration of antihypertensive medications prior to dialysis, avoiding eating during dialysis, and administering midodrine before dialysis.

B. **Muscle Cramps.** Muscle cramps occur commonly during rapid, high-volume ultrafiltration, due to plasma volume contraction and rapid sodium fluxes. Lowering the ultrafiltration rate is likely to be the most effective measure to prevent cramps. Other measures with varying levels of evidence and/or limited practical utility include: administration of fluids (normal saline, hypertonic saline, or 50% dextrose) to promote shifting of fluids into the vascular space, sodium modeling, quinine (no longer available in the United States), and carnitine.

C. **Hypoxemia.** Hypoxemia during dialysis is important in patients with compromised cardiopulmonary function. Research implicates membrane incompatibility, acid–base changes induced by the dialysate base buffer, and hypoventilation. Predisposed patients should be given supplemental oxygen and dialyzed with synthetic copolymer membranes using dialysate with an appropriately adjusted bicarbonate concentration.

D. **Arrhythmias.** Hypoxemia, hypotension, removal of antiarrhythmic agents during dialysis, and rapid changes in serum bicarbonate, calcium, magnesium, and potassium (especially in patients taking digoxin) all contribute to arrhythmias in predisposed patients. Recent studies using implantable loop records have shown that bradyarrhythmias are more common in dialysis patients than ventricular tachycardias. In the inpatient setting, continuous electrocardiogram monitoring during dialysis may be warranted in high-risk patients.

E. **Dialyzer Reaction.** Hypersensitivity reactions can rarely occur in response to dialyzer membrane constituents (such as cuprophane or polysulfone/polyethersulfone) or disinfectants used to sterilize the membrane (such as ethylene oxide or formaldehyde). Reactions are categorized as type A and type B based on the timing of symptom onset. Type A reactions occur within minutes of starting dialysis. Signs and symptoms include pruritus, urticaria, laryngeal edema, bronchospasm, chest pain, hypotension, and cardiac arrest. Management includes stopping dialysis without returning blood to the patient and fluids, antihistamines, corticosteroids, and vasopressors if needed. Type B reactions occur later in the treatment and are less severe. Symptoms include chest and back pain, nausea, and vomiting; cessation of dialysis may not be required. If a dialyzer reaction is suspected, a different dialyzer should be used for the next treatment. Rising the dialyzer with normal saline may be appropriate for less severe reactions.

F. **Dialysis Disequilibrium Syndrome.** This syndrome is believed to result primarily from less rapid clearance of urea and other osmoles from the brain than from the blood, which results in an osmotic gradient between these compartments. This osmotic gradient leads to a net movement of water into the brain that results in cerebral edema. The syndrome is uncommon and is usually seen with the first dialytic treatments in severely azotemic patients. Other predisposing factors include severe metabolic acidosis, older age, pediatric patients, hyponatremia, liver disease, and the presence of other central nervous system disease, such as a preexisting seizure disorder. Symptoms, which can occur during or after the procedure, include headache, lethargy, nausea, muscular twitching, and malaise, with rare progression to mental status changes, seizures, and even cardiorespiratory arrest. Preventive measures include the use of lower blood flow rates, smaller-surface-area dialyzers, and shorter dialysis times with the goal of reducing BUN by no more than 40% over a short period of time. Use of continuous kidney replacement therapy should be considered in patients with severely elevated BUN. The use of higher dialysate sodium and intradialysis mannitol infusion (25 to 50 g) has been reported to reduce the risk of this syndrome.

G. **Pericarditis.** Two distinct patterns of pericarditis are encountered in patients with kidney failure. Pericarditis can occur in uremic nondialyzed patients and in those already receiving dialysis therapy. Uremic pericarditis usually responds to intensive daily dialysis, and a correlation between resolution of pericarditis and improvement in the uremia has been shown. Conversely, pericarditis that occurs in patients already on hemodialysis may be related to occult inadequate dialysis or concurrent illnesses, such as systemic lupus erythematosus or viral pericarditis. Treatment is intensive dialysis without anticoagulation. The patient should be monitored clinically and by echocardiography for features suggestive of pericardial tamponade. Patients need to be intensively monitored to detect hemodynamic instability, changes in pericardial friction rub, and pulsus paradoxus. If pericardial tamponade develops, percutaneous pericardiocentesis, placement of a pericardial window, or pericardiectomy may be necessary.

H. **Air Embolism.** Air embolism occurs when air is introduced into the patient's bloodstream. Mechanisms include improper administration of fluids or medications, inadequate priming of the dialyzer, poor connection between arterial needle and the circuit, and defects in tubing. Air embolism is a rare complication as current hemodialysis machines have air detectors and the blood pump is stopped when air is detected. Clinical manifestations depend on the size of the air embolism and affected organ(s). Embolism to the right side of the heart and pulmonary artery can increase pulmonary arterial pressure, causing hypoxia, hypotension, and cardiac arrest. Emboli that reach the left side of the heart can cause ischemic injury including stroke. Management includes supplemental oxygen, fluids, and vasopressors when needed. Hemodialysis (HD) should be stopped and blood in the extracorporeal circuit should not be returned to the patient.

I. **Bleeding.** Severe complications and even death can occur if bleeding from a dialysis access goes undetected or uncontrolled. One cause of blood loss is venous needle dislodgement. If the access is not clearly visible (e.g., covered by blankets), dislodgement of the venous needle may not be immediately detected. As blood is flowing through the extracorporeal circuit at a rate of 300 to 450 mL/min, significant blood loss can occur within minutes. It is necessary to properly cannulate AVF/AVGs and monitor them throughout dialysis.

Management of hemorrhage includes fluids, vasopressor support, and transfusions as needed. Using proper technique to secure needles/tubing, keeping access and tubing visible, and avoiding inappropriate adjustment of venous pressure alarms are some of the measures that can be taken to prevent needle dislodgement and detect needle dislodgement early.

Vascular access hemorrhage can also occur due to rupture of an AV fistula or AV graft. Ruptures occur at aneurysms and pseudoaneurysms, which develop when an access is repeatedly cannulated in the same location. High blood flow, recurrent stenosis, and infections may also increase risk of aneurysm/pseudoaneurysm formation. The majority of vascular access hemorrhages occur in the patient's home. Direct pressure should be applied to the site until emergency medical personnel arrive. Ruptured accesses are surgically ligated. Rotation of cannulation sites and regular examination of the dialysis access are crucial for preventing development of aneurysms and pseudoaneurysms.

J. Hemolysis. Red blood cells in the hemodialysis circuit are exposed to shear stress. Significant hemolysis can occur when additional factors that increase red blood cells fragility are present. These include mechanical factors such as very negative arterial pressure, high blood flow though small gauge needle, needle malposition, and obstructed/kinked tubing. Contamination of dialysate with chemicals such as chloramine, copper, and nitrates has also caused hemolysis, as has high dialysate temperature and use of hypotonic dialysate. When significant hemolysis occurs, the blood in the extracorporeal circuit appears "cherry red." Dialysis should be stopped immediately and the blood in the circuit should not be returned to the patient. Hemolysis can result in hyperkalemia due to release of potassium from hemolyzed cells. Other complications include arrhythmia, acute coronary syndromes, severe necrotizing pancreatitis, and death.

K. Water Contamination. Dialysate is made by adding dialysate concentrate to purified water. Dialysis patients are exposed to large amounts of dialysate weekly—improper water purification can result in patients being exposed to significant amounts of potentially toxic substances. Adverse events related to exposures to chemicals such as chloramine, fluoride, aluminum, copper, hydrogen peroxide, and formaldehyde have been reported. Dialysate can also be contaminated with microorganisms, which can lead to bacteremia and pyrogenic reactions. When multiple patients exhibit similar symptoms in a short time frame, water contamination should be suspected. Strict adherence to protocols for monitoring the water system is important in preventing such complications.

L. Infections. Infection is a common complication of hemodialysis. Patients are at risk of contracting viral infections such as hepatitis B, hepatitis C, and human immunodeficiency virus from other patients in the same dialysis facility. Prevention of hepatitis B starts prior to a patient starting hemodialysis—hepatitis B vaccination is recommended for patients with CKD stage 4 or higher (it is also recommended for all patients with diabetes). All patients are screened for hepatitis B prior to acceptance to a dialysis facility. Testing includes hepatitis B surface antigen, hepatitis B surface antibody, and hepatitis B core antibody. Patients who are not immune to hepatitis B through prior vaccination or infection should be vaccinated. Hepatitis B vaccine induces seroconversion in only 40% to 70% of hemodialysis patients. Nonimmune patients should be tested monthly for hepatitis B surface antigen. Patients who are hepatitis B surface antigen positive must be dialyzed in a separate space using a dedicated machine; staff that care for a hepatitis B–positive patient should not care for other patients during the same shift. Hand hygiene, use of personal protective

TABLE 42.2	Common drugs and toxins removed by hemodialysis or hemoperfusion, or both

Acetaminophen
Alcohols (ethanol, methanol, isopropyl alcohol, ethylene glycol)
Amphetamines
Antiarrhythmics (procainamide and N-acetyl-procainamide, sotalol)
Antihypertensives (angiotensin-converting enzyme inhibitors, beta-blockers)
Antimicrobials (many)
Antineoplastics (busulfan, cyclophosphamide, 5-fluorouracil)
Arsenic
Aspirin
Barbiturates
Carbamazepine
Lithium
Mannitol
Monoamine oxidase inhibitors
Theophylline
Valproic acid

equipment, and disinfection of equipment and surfaces are crucial to prevent transmission of pathogens from patient to patient. Such measures are also key to preventing bacterial infections. Patients are at risk for bloodstream infections when their AV fistula, AV graft, or catheter is accessed for hemodialysis. Prior to cannulation, the AV fistula or graft should be disinfected with alcohol-based chlorhexidine, povidone iodine solution, or alcohol. For patient with tunneled catheters, proper disinfection of the exit site and scrubbing of the hub at the time of catheter connection and disconnection are essential.

VIII. EXTRACORPOREAL THERAPIES FOR DRUG OVERDOSE. Hemodialysis and a related technique, hemoperfusion, are indicated for the management of overdose due to certain toxins (Table 42.2). Small molecules with low protein-binding and low volume of distribution are most likely to be effectively removed by hemodialysis. Charcoal hemoperfusion uses coated or uncoated charcoal particles to adsorb toxins or drugs. Complications are due to its bioincompatibility and include thrombocytopenia.

Antidepressants and benzodiazepines are poorly removed by dialytic techniques. Dialysis for poisoning should be considered only when there are significant acid–base or electrolyte disturbances, supportive measures are ineffective, or there is impending irreversible organ toxicity.

IX. OTHER CONSIDERATIONS IN THE CARE OF DIALYSIS PATIENTS. The following are important practical aspects in the care of hemodialysis patients that must be emphasized:

■ Fluid intake should be limited to 1 to 1.5 L/day to avoid fluid overload as most patients are oliguric/anuric. For dietary therapy, refer to Chapter 40.
■ Phosphate binders, such as calcium carbonate, calcium acetate, sevelamer hydrochloride or carbonate, and lanthanum carbonate should be administered with meals.

- Many drugs, such as antibiotics and antiarrhythmics, are removed by hemodialysis. Therefore, dosage adjustments, administration of supplemental doses, and monitoring of blood levels are frequently required. This may be especially problematic in patients undergoing hemofiltration or frequent dialysis.

- Patients are often on medications such as ESAs, vitamin D analogs, or calcimimetics as outpatients. These are often continued or dose-adjusted upon hospitalization.

- Magnesium-containing antacids and laxatives or phosphorus-based (Fleet®) enemas should be avoided in dialysis patients to prevent hypermagnesemia and hyperphosphatemia, respectively.

- If blood transfusions are required, they should be administered during hemodialysis to avoid fluid overload and hyperkalemia.

- As dialysis patients are immunosuppressed and frequently hypothermic, there should be a low threshold for an intensive workup if they present with features suggestive of infection.

- Specific dialysis treatment goals, such as the ultrafiltration volume or hemodynamic parameters (i.e., pulmonary capillary wedge pressure), should be discussed with the nephrologist to permit the appropriate setting of the extracorporeal device.

- Protection of the vascular access arm is crucial. This includes avoidance of blood pressure determination, venipuncture, and arterial puncture in this extremity. If access is still in the planning stage, protection of the nondominant arm is indicated. Protection involves informing the patient and hanging a sign above the hospital bed.

X. SUGGESTED READINGS

Daugirdas JT, Blake PG, Ing TS, eds. *Handbook of Dialysis*. 5th ed. Lippincott Williams & Wilkins; 2014.

Eknoyan G, Beck GJ, Cheung AK, et al. Effect of dialysis dose and membrane flux in maintenance hemodialysis. *N Engl J Med*. 2002;347(25):2010–2019.

Golper TA, Fissell R, Fissell WH, et al. Hemodialysis: core curriculum 2014. *Am J Kidney Dis*. 2014;63(1):153–163.

National Kidney Foundation. Kidney disease outcomes quality initiative. Clinical practice guidelines. Accessed September 20, 2020. https://www.kidney.org/professionals/guidelines

Nissenson AR, Fine RN, eds. *Handbook of Dialysis Therapy*. 5th ed. Elsevier; 2017.

43 Peritoneal Dialysis

Ashutosh M. Shukla

INTRODUCTION

Peritoneal dialysis (PD) was first described by George Cantor in 1923 and established as a method to treat acute kidney injury during World War II. Use of a flexible silicone tube for permanent access was introduced later for continuous ambulatory PD (CAPD) for the management of end-stage kidney disease (ESKD).

I. PERITONEAL DIALYSIS APPARATUS. PD catheters are flexible silicone tubes with intra- and extraperitoneal segments. Intraperitoneal catheters have many side-openings for fluid drainage and can have a straight, curled, or coiled ending. Extraperitoneal segments commonly have two dacron cuffs, one affixing the catheter to the peritoneum at the fascia transversalis, and the other to the subcutaneous space about 4 to 5 cm proximal to the exit site to anchor the catheter. The exit site of the PD catheter is conventionally positioned in the lower abdomen away from the beltline. However, in overweight and obese patients, it is in the upper abdomen to facilitate care. PD catheters can be placed by open surgical, laparoscopic, or fluoroscopy-guided methods. The external end of the PD catheter is connected to a titanium adapter and thereby to a connecting tube. Dialysis is provided by the parietal peritoneum that is a semipermeable membrane with an average surface area of about 1 to 1.3 m^2 comprising the capillary endothelium, interstitium, and the parietal mesothelium. Transport across the barrier is described by "3-pore model." The most abundant are the "small pores," about 40 to 50 Å that make the major contribution to the solute and fluid clearances. The ultrasmall pores are composed of acquaporin-1 that transports about 40% of the water. Large pores participate only minimally.

II. PERITONEAL TRANSPORT. PD relies on osmosis and convection to achieve the goals of solute and fluid clearance. Conventional PD dialysate utilizes dextrose as the osmotic agent for the convective force and fluid constitution to facilitate net loss of minerals and electrolytes retained in ESKD (Table 43.1). Uremic solutes travel down their gradient from blood to the PD fluid until equilibrium is reached; while the dextrose in the PD fluid travels in the reverse direction, thereby progressively diluting the PD fluid. Thus, the solvent drag, or ultrafiltration volume per unit of time, falls progressively during the PD dwell. There is also a constant resorptive fluid flux due largely to lymphatic absorption, but also driven by the oncotic gradient. The net result of the two forces is ultrafiltration and resorption that eventually reach equilibrium that is prolonged with increasing osmotic strength of the PD fluid. The speed of diffusion for each molecule depends on its size, charge, and its nonprotein-bound concentration and also on the characteristics of the peritoneal membrane that can

TABLE 43.1	Peritoneal dialysate composition

Dialysate component	Concentration options
Dextrose monohydrate	1.5%, 2.5%, or 4.25%
Osmolality	344, 394, or 483 mOsm/L
Sodium	132 mEq/L
Calcium	2.5 or 3.5 mEq/L
Magnesium	0.5 or 1.5 mEq/L
Chloride	102 mEq/L
Lactate	35 or 40 mEq/L

be determined by a peritoneal equilibration test (PET). The PET uses a 4-hour dwell and is performed ~6 to 8 weeks after PD initiation. It classifies the function of the peritoneum as low, average, and high transport status based on the dialysate/plasma creatinine ratio ($d/p_{creatinine}$) and the dissipation of dextrose that is examined by the ratio of dialysate glucose at 4 hours versus the beginning of the dwell ($d/d_{0glucose}$). About two-thirds of the ESKD population have average transport status. Conventional PD fluids also use lactate buffer and have lower than physiologic pH to avoid precipitation of calcium. Alternate PD fluids with an amino acid as osmotic agent (Nutrineal™) and more physiologic pH with a separate compartment for bicarbonate- and calcium-containing fluids (Physioneal™) are not yet proven to be superior. However, icodextrin (Extraneal™) is a varying-length glucose polymer with minimal transmembrane transport. It is designed to maintain a slow, but sustained, ultrafiltration profile for up to 12 to 14 hours.

III. TYPES OF PERITONEAL DIALYSIS. CAPD involves manual exchanges of 2 to 3 L of PD fluid three to five times daily. It uses most of the 24 hours for the dialysis. CAPD with one to two exchanges a day, especially using icodextrin, is also used in patients with heart failure requiring ultrafiltration but with minimal clearance. Automated peritoneal dialysis (APD) uses multiples of 5 to 6 L bags, a complex multiconnecting tubing set, and a cycler machine that performs automatic exchanges, usually overnight. Clustering of the exchanges over 8 to 10 hours reduces individual dwell time, and causes greater loss of water compared to solutes.

IV. PERITONEAL DIALYSIS TARGETS AND PRESCRIPTION. The urea-based clearance parameter of KT/V is widely used for dialysis dose measurements. Unfortunately, increases in KT/V have not been shown to confer significant benefits. Compared to HD, PD provides a slower rate of urea clearance but has better clearance of middle molecules. Both modalities provide equivalent long-term survival. The CANUSA cohort study in CKD reported that the risk of death was reduced by 12% for each 5 L/wk/1.73 m^2 increment in GFR and by 36% for each 250 mL/day increment in urine output. However, similar benefits were not seen for PD clearance or ultrafiltration. The ADEMEX study reported that patients randomized to a high weekly KT/V of 2.27 did not have significant survival benefit. However, cohort studies suggest that lowering the KT/V urea below ~1.5 to 1.7 can reduce survival, especially in those with poor residual renal function (RRF). The International Society for PD guidelines recommend a total (peritoneal + renal) KT/V of 1.7 as the target. However, KT/V provides an excellent goal for tailoring prescriptions for individual patients. The continuous nature of PD allows for the daily KT/V to be summarized to reach the weekly target-delivered dose of PD. The inherently longer dwell times of CAPD provides greater clearance of both small and middle molecules than APD. Ultrashort (less than 60 to 80 minutes) cycles provide greater water (than solute) clearance, and thus, should be avoided. Available data indicate that CAPD and various forms of APD provide equivalent survivals and outcomes. Nocturnal intermittent PD without a day dwell is not desirable for anuric ESKD patients since longer dwells allow for better clearance of the middle molecules. Overall, the choice of the type of PD usually can be left to individual patients.

V. **INFECTIOUS COMPLICATIONS OF PERITONEAL DIALYSIS.** PD patients suffer from exit-site infection, tunnel infection, and peritonitis. Exit-site and tunnel infections predispose to peritonitis and thus require routine hygiene with regular application of antimicrobial (mupirocin or gentamycin) agents. Downward looking exit sites and avoidance of suture at the exit site provide some protection against infection. The number of episodes of PD peritonitis for at-risk individual units has a target below 0.5 per year. The spectrum of infectious organisms responsible for exit-site and tunnel infections and peritonitis are generally similar. Gram-positive organisms comprise the majority of PD peritonitis: coagulase-negative *staphylococcus* and *Staphylococcus aureus* that colonizes the skin are the most prominent, highlighting the importance of touch contamination and hand hygiene in PD procedures, while streptococcus spp. is also frequent and can originate from the oral cavity. Coliforms are the dominant gram-negative organisms. They can originate from touch contamination or transluminal migration during periods of gastrointestinal (GI) disturbances such as ischemia or infection. About 10% to 20% of episodes of PD peritonitis are culture negative. Fungal infection can occur after the use of systemic antibiotics and is a major cause of PD catheter removal and technique failure.

Diagnosis of peritonitis is established by at least two of the three features: symptoms compatible with peritonitis (fever, abdominal pain, cloudy dialysis effluent); abnormal and cloudy effluent with white-cell count >100/μL (with >50% neutrophils) after at least 2 hours of dwell; and positive dialysis culture. Intraperitoneal antibiotics generally are preferred for the treatment of PD peritonitis, while oral management is adequate for most exit-site or tunnel infections. Many systemic antibiotics achieve therapeutic serum levels. Intraperitoneal administration of antibiotics permits treatment of complicated exit-site or tunnel infections. Empirical therapy for peritonitis usually includes coverage for gram-positive and gram-negative organisms after ensuring that there is no exit-site or tunnel infection or occult impacted hernia. The results of the PD fluid culture guide the definitive therapy. Most infections require 2 to 3 weeks of intraperitoneal antibiotics. PD patients who receive systemic antimicrobials are at an increased risk for subsequent development of fungal peritonitis, likely related to esophageal candidiasis. Nystatin mouthwash and swallow are recommended during each extended courses of antimicrobial administration in PD patients. Catheter removal and temporary or permanent transition to HD may be needed for *stenotrophomonas* and fungal infections, GI perforations, etc. Some semi-invasive procedures including dental procedures,

GI endoscopy, and gynecologic procedures can precipitate PD peritonitis, and thus, require prophylactic antimicrobial administration. A detailed discussion of the PD related infections is available at https://ispd.org/ispd-guidelines/.

VI. NONINFECTIOUS COMPLICATIONS OF PERITONEAL DIALYSIS: OUTFLOW/INFLOW CONCERNS. Catheter flow obstruction is quite common and usually presents with slow outflow and incomplete drainage. Most episodes are related to constipation, and respond to lactulose, senna, or polyethylene glycol with electrolyte solution. Outflow problems also can relate to migration of the PD catheter tip, blockage of the catheter by fibrin or clot, or omental wrapping. Inflow pain with a well-functioning catheter is usually due to cold dialysate or the acidic nature of the fluid that responds to tidal PD where small amount of PD fluid (~5% to 20%) are left undrained with each cycle of the dwell.

VII. RAISED INTRA-ABDOMINAL PRESSURE. PD patients can suffer from several complications related to the elevation of intra-abdominal pressure. PD fluid leaks around the catheter are common (~4% to 10%) in the early period after insertion and usually resolve by resting PD for 2 to 4 weeks. Late abdominal wall leaks are associated with hernia or abdominal wall defects and are less amenable to resting PD. PD fluid may travel through pleuroperitoneal communications to cause hydrothorax, or through a patent processus vaginalis to cause hydrocele. Long-term elevation of intra-abdominal pressure predisposes PD patients to hernias. Most hernia require surgical repair that can often be managed without changing PD to intermittent HD.

VIII. COLORFUL EFFLUENT. While infectious peritonitis is the most important cause of cloudy effluent, 10% to 30% of new PD patients develop a noninfectious eosinophilic peritonitis. This is largely self-limiting; but if severe, may require systemic corticosteroids. Hemoperitoneum or bloody/red effluent is generally a benign condition; but in women, occasionally represents malignancy, endometriosis, or tuberculous peritonitis.

IX. ENCAPSULATING PERITONEAL SCLEROSIS. Encapsulating peritoneal sclerosis (EPS) is a rare manifestation of PD with annual incidence rates of 0.14% to 2.5%, increasing with the duration of PD. It usually presents with progressive malnutrition and/or intestinal obstruction. Peritonitis and low pH, high glucose, and advanced glycation end products in the PD fluid have been implicated. Diagnosis is suspected from symptoms or recurrent episodes of hemoperitoneum, and confirmed by findings of tethered small loops of intestine with enveloping peritoneum that is thickened and may be calcified. Management is generally by transfer to HD, unless there is an acute abdomen. EPS has a high annual mortality of ~30% with a majority of deaths related to abdominal surgery.

X. OUTCOMES AND FUTURE OF PERITONEAL DIALYSIS. A focus on small solute-based clearance, and the relative ease of developing a healthcare system around HD have led to the establishment of in-center HD as the default treatment for ESKD. Cohort-based data have reported that PD provides survival similar to in-center HD but patients may have better quality of life. There has been a shift in approach to making the less expensive PD the default choice for renal replacement therapy. However, patients with unaddressed leaks, or with significant history of abdominal/GI surgery and high likelihood of peritoneal fibrosis are not good candidates for PD, whereas ostomies, abdominal hernias, polycystic kidney disease, and physical dependency are often feasible for PD if adequate support is available. Assisted PD has expanded in geriatric patients and medically frail populations. It can be used for patients who are blind or cannot hear. An observation study from Canada reported that over 80% of the incident ESKD patients are medically eligible for home-based treatments. Both providers and patients who receive proper education often select PD.

XI. SUGGESTED READINGS

Brown EA, Blake PG, Boudville N, et al. International society for peritoneal dialysis practice recommendations: prescribing high-quality goal-directed peritoneal dialysis. *Perit Dial Int.* 2020;40(3):244–253. https://doi.org/10.1177/0896860819895364

Crabtree JH, Shrestha BM, Chow KM, et al. Creating and maintaining optimal peritoneal dialysis access in the adult patient: 2019 update. *Perit Dial Int.* 2019;39(5):414–436. https://doi.org/10.3747/pdi.2018.00232

Li PK-T, Szeto CC, Piraino B, et al. ISPD peritonitis recommendations: 2016 update on prevention and treatment. *Perit Dial Int.* 2016;36(5):481–508. https://doi.org/10.3747/pdi.2016.00078

Szeto CC, Li PK-T, Johnson DW, et al. ISPD catheter-related infection recommendations: 2017 update. *Perit Dial Int.* 2017;37(2):141–154. https://doi.org/10.3747/pdi.2016.00120

44 Home Hemodialysis

Judit Gordon-Cappitelli

Home hemodialysis (HHD), as the name indicates, is hemodialysis (HD) done in the patient's home. Most patients have a care partner who assists them with the dialysis treatment, but some dialyze without a care partner (solo HHD). HHD was developed in the 1960s when the availability of in-center HD was very limited and the use of HHD was encouraged due to its lower costs. About one-third of patients with end-stage kidney disease (ESKD) in the United States were on HHD in the early 1970s. After the Medicare End-Stage Renal Disease program was created in 1972, increased funding for HD led to the proliferation of in-center HD units and to a decline of HHD. In recent years, there has been a resurgence in HHD due improved outcomes and availability of more patient-friendly HHD systems. However, only 2% of HD patients in the United States were on HHD in 2017.

I. **DIALYSIS SYSTEMS USED FOR HOME HEMODIALYSIS.** There are two types of HHD systems—in-center HD machines adapted to home use, and smaller, more portable machines designed for HHD. In-center machines are larger and require separate water purification systems that use reverse osmosis to generate water for dialysate. These allow patients to be treated with prescriptions similar to in-center HD (i.e., high dialysate flow rates). The first more compact unit developed was NxStage Medical, Inc's System One that received FDA approval for use for HHD in 2005. Its water system uses deionization to purify water. Dialysate is made in batches prior to treatment. Bagged dialysate is also available for use during travel or in the event of water-system malfunction. The maximum dialysate flow rate is lower than conventional HD machines at 300 mL/min. The majority of HHD patients in the United States use this system. HHD should be possible in virtually any home, although some plumbing and electrical modifications may be needed, particularly for systems that use reverse osmosis to purify water.

II. **PATIENT RECRUITMENT, EVALUATION, AND TRAINING.** Only a minority of patients are unsuitable for HHD because of inability to safely carry out treatments due to psychiatric, neurologic, or other conditions (such as illicit drug use). Therefore, HHD should be offered as an option to most patients with advanced chronic kidney disease and those who are already on HD. Patients who express interest in HHD should meet with the nephrologist and HHD clinic staff to discuss the training process and the expectations for the patient and their care partner. The evaluation of the potential HHD patient should include a home visit. Thereafter, a training schedule is developed in the dialysis unit that usually takes 4 to 6 weeks. Patients who value flexibility, autonomy, and the potential health benefits of HHD are the most likely recruits.

III. HOME HEMODIALYSIS PRESCRIPTION. The vascular access may be an arteriovenous fistula (AVF), arteriovenous graft (AVG), or catheter. AVF or AVG are strongly preferred. The blood flow rate is typically 350 to 450 mL/min for shorter treatments and 200 to 300 mL/min for longer treatments (i.e., nocturnal HHD). The dialysate flow rate for conventional HD systems adapted to home use may be 600 to 800 mL/min; but for low dialysate flow systems, the rate is typically 150 to 300 mL/min. The efficient use of dialysate for HHD is a priority to limit treatment costs and to minimize water bills. Low-flow dialysate systems use a reduced potassium concentration of 1 or 2 mEq/L due to the reduced solute clearance. The NxStage System One uses a lactate-based buffer whereas conventional systems use a bicarbonate-based buffer.

The frequency and duration of treatments in HHD is variable. Some patients dialyze thrice weekly for 3.5 to 4 hours similar to patients on in-center HD. They require a minimum delivered single pool Kt/V of 1.2 per HD session. Patients who use a low dialysate flow system will not meet this target with thrice-weekly dialysis and require alternate days, four times weekly or more frequent dialysis. The duration of the dialysis treatment decreases with increasing frequency of treatment, to a limit of 2.5 hours per session. Urea clearance can be added to Kt/V for patients who retain residual kidney function. Some patients opt for nocturnal HHD.

The HHD prescription can be customized, but alternate day or more frequent dialysis avoids the 2-day gap between treatments that has been associated with increased mortality and cardiovascular events. Increasing time on HD reduces the need for high UF rates that are associated with increased mortality. Frequent HD (four or more times a week) has been reported to improve outcomes in these randomized controlled trials: the Frequent Hemodialysis Network (FHN) Daily Trial, the FHN Nocturnal Trial, and the Alberta Nocturnal Hemodialysis Trial (Table 44.1).

IV. BENEFITS OF FREQUENT HEMODIALYSIS
A. Cardiovascular Outcomes. Cardiovascular disease is the leading cause of death in ESKD. Left ventricular hypertrophy is highly prevalent in the ESKD population and is an independent risk factor for mortality. The adjusted mean left ventricular mass (LVM) decreased by 16.4 ± 2.9 g at 12 months in those randomized to the frequent HD group compared to 2.6 ± 3.2 g in the conventional HD group (P < .001) in the FHN Daily Trial. The Alberta Nocturnal Trial also confirmed a greater decrease in LVM in those randomized to frequent HD compared to conventional HF.

The better control of hypertension with HHD may contribute to the regression of LCM. The weekly average predialysis systolic blood pressure decreased in the FHN Daily Trial by 10 mm Hg after 12 months in the frequent HD group but increased 2 mm Hg after 12 months in the conventional HD group (P < .001), accompanied by a greater decrease in the number of antihypertensive medications.

Intradialytic hypotension (IDH) also has been associated with increased risk of death and hospitalization for cardiovascular events. In the FHN Daily Trial, the incidence of IDH was lower in the frequent compared to the conventional HD group, perhaps related to a reduced ultrafiltration rate. Unfortunately, these randomized trials lacked the power necessary to evaluate the impact of frequent HD on mortality.
B. Hyperphosphatemia. The management of hyperphosphatemia remains challenging despite the availability of phosphorus binders. Abnormalities in bone

T A B L E 44.1	Randomized controlled trials of frequent hemodialysis				
Trial	**Primary outcome(s)**	**Arm**	**N**	**Dialysis frequency (days/wk)**	**Time per session (hrs)**	**Weekly standard Kt/V**

Trial	**Primary outcome(s)**	**Arm**	**N**	**Dialysis frequency (days/wk)**	**Time per session (hrs)**	**Weekly standard Kt/V**
FHN Daily Trial	Coprimary end points: death or 12-month change in left ventricular mass, and death or 12-month change in physical-health composite score	Conventional: thrice weekly dialysis, 2.5–4 hrs/session	120	2.9 ± 0.4	3.6 ± 0.5	2.5 ± 0.3
		Frequent: six times a week dialysis, 1.5–2.75 hrs/session	125	5.2 ± 1.1	2.6 ± 0.4	3.5 ± 0.6
FHN Nocturnal Trial	Coprimary end points: death or 12-mo change in left ventricular mass, and death or 12-mo change in physical-health composite score	Conventional: thrice weekly dialysis for <5 hrs/session	42	2.9 ± 0.2	4.3 ± 1.1	2.6 ± 0.7
		Frequent: six nights a week dialysis for ≥6 hrs/session	45	5.1 ± 0.8	6.3 ± 1.0	4.7 ± 1.2
Alberta Nocturnal Trial	Change in left ventricular mass	Conventional: thrice weekly dialysis	25		Not reported	
		Frequent: five to six nights per week dialysis for minimum 6 hrs/night	26		Not reported	

FHN, frequent hemodialysis network.

mineral disease in ESKD have been linked to LVH and vascular calcification. In all of these randomized trials, frequent HD was associated with a modest decrease in predialysis phosphorus compared to no change in the conventional HD group.

C. Quality of Life. In the FHN Daily Trial, the physical-health composite score increased relative to the conventional HD group. Poor quality of life in HD patients is very common. It has been linked to poor sleep quality. Frequent HD has been associated with observational studies with a reduction in restless leg syndrome and improved sleep quality.

D. Other Benefits. Other benefits of frequent HD seen in observational studies include a shortened postdialysis recovery time, an increased exercise capacity, a decrease in requirements for erythropoiesis-stimulating agents, a reduction in inflammatory markers, and a liberation from dietary restrictions.

E. Populations that May Benefit from Frequent Hemodialysis. The potential benefits of more frequent HD suggest that patients with left ventricular hypertrophy, difficult to control hypertension, reduced cardiac function, chronic hyper-phosphatemia, sleep disorders, and pregnant women may receive the greatest benefit from HHD. It should be noted that the FHN Trials and Alberta Nocturnal Trial were conducted using conventional HD machines with high dialysate flow rates. Thus, these results may not be applicable to patients who use the low-flow dialysate system commonly used in the US.

V. COMPLICATIONS OF HOME HEMODIALYSIS. Potential complications of HD are described in Chapter 42. A particular complication of HHD is patient and car-egiver burnout. Patients can be provided with the option to dialyze in the home unit or in-center temporarily to provide a respite. Nocturnal HD may result in hypokalemia or hypophosphatemia necessitating supplementation. Frequent HD has been associated with increased risk of vascular access interventions and hospitalization due to infection, as well as more rapid loss of residual kidney function.

VI. FUTURE OF HOME HEMODIALYSIS. Recent initiatives in the United States aimed at reducing the costs associated with caring for patients with CKD and ESKD have encouraged the growth of home dialysis modalities. As a result, the use of HHD is expected to continue to grow in the near future.

VII. SUGGESTED READINGS

Culleton BF, Walsh M, Klarenbach SW, et al. Effect of frequent nocturnal hemodialysis vs conventional hemodialysis on left ventricular mass and quality of life: a randomized controlled trial. *JAMA.* 2007;298(11):1291–1299.

FHN Trial Group; Chertow GM, Levin NW, et al. In-center hemodialysis six times per week versus three times per week. *N Engl J Med.* 2010;363(24):2287–2300.

Rocco MV, Lockridge RS, Beck GJ, et al. The effects of frequent nocturnal home dialysis: the frequent hemodialysis network nocturnal trial. *Kidney Int.* 2011;80(10):1080–1091.

Special Issue: an open-source practical manual for home hemodialysis supported by an unrestricted educational grant from Baxter Healthcare. *Hemodialysis Int.* 2015;19(S1):S1–S134.

45

Dialysis Access

Olanrewaju A. Olaoye, Mark S. Segal

I. **OVERVIEW OF TYPES OF DIALYSIS ACCESS.** General nephrology ambulatory management of progressive/advanced chronic kidney disease (CKD) ideally includes CKD education, dialysis access planning, and referral for kidney transplantation evaluation. If an advanced CKD patient decides on nonconservative management after the clinical trend suggests an inevitable course toward initiation of renal replacement therapy (RRT), a dialysis access should be planned based on the mode of RRT chosen (hemodialysis or peritoneal dialysis), the life expectancy of the patient, and other comorbidities. The goal as outlined in the most recent Kidney Disease Outcome Quality Initiatives (KDOQI) guidelines is based on achieving the "*right timing* for the *right access* in the *right patient*."

A. **Hemodialysis.** Hemodialysis access options include autologous fistula designated primary arteriovenous fistula (PAVF simply referred to as AVF); arteriovenous graft (AVG); and endovascular arteriovenous fistula (Endo-AVF), which is the newest advancement in hemodialysis access creation. Endo-AVF utilizes catheter-based approaches to percutaneously create an anastomosis between an autologous artery and its neighboring vein using thermal or radiofrequency ablation energy (Ellipsys and WavelinQ), without an open surgical incision, and hemodialysis catheters (nontunneled temporary and transitional/ tunneled dialysis catheters). Common fistula sites include radio-cephalic, brachio-cephalic, brachio-basilic, and axillo-axillary fistula—each site mentioned incorporates the names of the artery involved hyphenated with the anastomosed vein, respectively. Temporary and tunneled hemodialysis catheters are placed in order of preference in the right internal jugular (IJ), left IJ, and femoral veins. The subclavian vein should be avoided, when at all possible, due to the incidence of venous stenosis.

B. **Peritoneal Dialysis.** Peritoneal dialysis catheters typically require 4- to 6-week postplacement prior to routine use. However, a peritoneal dialysis catheter can be used immediately after insertion in what is called "urgent start" requiring the patient to be in a supine position continuously while small volumes of peritoneal dialysis fluid are exchanged. This requires the patient be able to come to the dialysis unit daily or 4 to 6 times a week until the insertion site fully matures. Peritoneal dialysis catheters are classified based on the intraperitoneal segment of the catheter and they include straight, coiled, straight with silicone discs, and T-fluted PD catheters. The intraperitoneal segment of any type of peritoneal dialysis catheter placed should rest within the pelvis when the patient is lying supine. The externalization sites include the right or left lower abdominal quadrant; the epigastrium; and the chest-wall and is guided by the patient's body habitus and the ease of access for catheter-tube connections.

II. FISTULAS. Since it may take 6 to 12 months to allow for creation of a PAVF, including the time to referral to a vascular surgeon, clearance for surgery, and 6 to 12 weeks of fistula maturation, the timing of creation is an art requiring the prediction of a future need for RRT.

A. Suitable Candidates/Creation. Suitability for a particular fistula is currently guided by the preoperative clinical, diagnostic, and ultrasound evaluations with emphasis on the quality of the artery and its most proximal vein. Historically, this contrasts with previously held factors such as prioritizing the most distal vessels within the nondominant limb of the patient.

B. Timing of Creation to Usability. PAVF: 6 to 12 months and AVG: 2 to 4 weeks.

C. Examination. Dialysis access examination, which should be done at every encounter, has been shown to be sensitive and specific for detecting any underlying pathology with the access.

   The examination is focused on detecting causes of dysfunction of the hemodialysis access: stenosis of the arterialized venous outflow tract; stenosis of the arterial/inflow tract; thrombosis; access accessory versus collateral veins; aneurysm (saccular outpouching of an access containing all the layers of the wall)/pseudoaneurysm; superficial versus periaccess deep infections; and ischemic/infarction-related monomelic neuropathy.

   Step 1: Visual examination: Observing for any aneurysm or infected or thinning overlying skin or coolness in the distal extremity.

   Step 2: Characterization of the pulse: The three core parameters for evaluating a hemodialysis access include *pulse, thrill, and bruit* (see Table 45.1).

   The *pulse* is best appreciated using fingertips, and a pulse that is forceful with increased intensity is usually suggestive of a *stenotic lesion*, especially when it is present anywhere upstream away from the arterial anastomosis in the fistula.

   Step 3: Special maneuvers:

   Pulse augmentation (see Fig. 45.1) is used to assess arterial blood inflow. The steps include (a) occlusion of the outflow vein, the part of the fistula/graft at a point away from the arterial anastomosis, and (b) finger-tip palpation assessment of the intensity of the pulses transmitted by the inflow of blood

T A B L E **45.1**	Basic parameters for examining hemodialysis access and the features signifying corresponding abnormalities	

Parameter	Examining tool	Normal	Abnormality concerning for stenosis
Pulse	Fingertips	Soft and easily compressible along the entire access	Forceful; not easily compressible
Thrill	Palm	Soft; diffuse; continuous/machinery like	Turbulent; localized to site; discontinuous; systolic phase only
Bruit	Stethoscope	Low-pitched; diffuse; continuous with systolic and diastolic phases	High pitched; localized to site; discontinuous; systolic phase only

Adapted from Asif A, Agarwal AK, Yevzlin AS, Wu S, Beathard GA. *Interventional Nephrology 2012 Edition.* McGraw Hill/Medical; 2012.

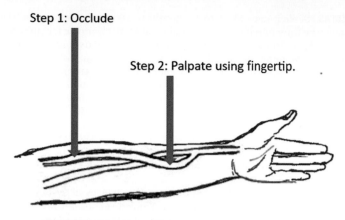

FIGURE 45.1: Pulse augmentation.
Step 1: Occlude at a point away from arterial anastomosis.
Step 2: Palpate using fingertip to assess augmented quality of inflow.

through the arterial anastomosis. It is normal for intensity of the pulses to be increased (augmented) with occlusion of the outflow vein. If augmentation does not occur, an inflow stenosis is suspected.

Access arm elevation (see Fig. 45.2): The arm with the fistula is elevated and if there is normal outflow, the fistula collapses. However, if there is an upstream stenosis in the upstream venous system, the fistula will remain distended for a prolonged period.

Step 4: Characterize the thrill and bruit:

Thrill and bruit are parameters assessed using palm and stethoscope, respectively. A thrill is a palpable sense of vibration. One can discriminate between the two types—diffuse versus local—with incredibly careful assessment techniques. A soft and continuous thrill suggests that blood flow within an access is adequate. Other abnormal findings related to stenotic lesions are depicted in Table 45.1.

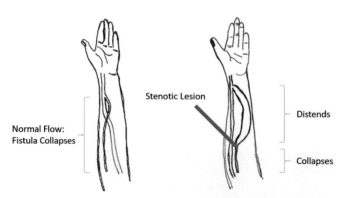

FIGURE 45.2: Access-arm elevation. Without a flow-restrictive lesion, fistula collapses. With stenotic/flow-restrictive lesion, distal segment distends and proximal segment collapses.

D. Maintenance. The primary patency rate of AVF after 5 years following placement is over 50% while that of AVG is approximately 10%. The primary failure rate is higher in AVF, contributing to frequent use of CVC placement, although AVF is still considered superior to AVG when considering thrombosis, morbidity, and mortality. Neointimal hyperplasia remains the main pathophysiology leading to intrafistula or intragraft stenosis, and research continues to evolve with the goal of defining the best way to prevent or manage this in terms of pharmaceutics and mechanical interventions, but with limited success. Long-term *monitoring and surveillance* techniques are invaluable in detecting stenosis and avoiding thrombosis of the vascular access. An optimally functioning vascular access should be able to "supply" the extracorporeal circuit with a nominal blood flow rate of 400 to 500 mL/min, and a mature permanent vascular access routinely delivers this rate. *Monitoring* of vascular access includes the physical examination, as detailed above; looking for an elevation of dynamic venous pressure (DVP) during dialysis; recirculation; inadequate dialysis delivery; and prolonged bleeding after needle withdrawal.

E. Troubleshooting. When monitoring suggests access dysfunction, vascular access *diagnostic testing*, such as the gold standard angiography, should be utilized. The goal of the diagnosis is to delineate progressive stenotic lesions for intervention before they become unmanageable/intractable, leading to thrombosis, and loss of the access. Findings that support the diagnosis of a stable stenotic lesion within the access, that is clinically insignificant, should not be intervened upon.

III. HEMODIALYSIS CATHETERS. Dialysis catheters are placed in central veins or right atrium thereby providing free flow of blood for optimal hemodialysis. Temporary central venous catheters available for hemodialysis are referred to as dialysis or trialysis catheters based on the number of lumens present—two or three, respectively; trialysis catheters are popularly used in intensive care units so as to provide additional central venous access for other therapies in addition to the two lumens dedicated for performance of hemodialysis. TDC are typically cuffed and the placement technique incorporates a tunneled segment proximal to the actual entry into a central vein. Both the cuff incorporation, which allows for ingrowth of native fibrous tissue leading to optimal anchor and providing a sealing barrier to the exterior, as well as the tunneling technique, are aimed to reduce the risk of central line associated bloodstream infection (CLABSI).

A. Suitable Candidates/Creation. All that is required is an open central vein. Hemodialysis catheters are the preferred access to provide RRT emergently with acute kidney injury patients and ESKD patients in need of emergent RRT.

B. Timing of Creation to Usability. Once placed, the access is ready for immediate use.

C. Examination. Temporary, or tunneled, dialysis catheters should be routinely examined for bleeding, exit-site infections, tunnel infections, and potential externalization of the cuff. The intraluminal patency is indirectly examined while monitoring the access pressure on dialysis.

D. Maintenance. Infection is the most frequent reason for loss of a dialysis catheter. Antibiotic catheter locking has been shown to prevent infections in temporary or tunneled CVCs. Antibiotic-impregnated discs, placed at the exit site, are effective at reducing the incidence of exit-site infections. Prevention of intracatheter thrombosis with the use of anticoagulants is also another way to maintain an optimally functioning CVC. Heparin is the oldest anticoagulant in use, although the concern of increased risk of bleeding after the heparin catheter lock is released into the systemic circulation, is increasingly being recognized and has prompted a search for alternatives. Sodium citrate, an effective anticoagulant, is also known to possess some antiseptic properties.

E. Troubleshooting. The breaking down of intracatheter thrombus in the absence of infection or malpositioning is acceptable as part of maintenance needed to keep CVCs in use. One to 2 mg of Alteplase left indwelling within the catheter lumen for 30 minutes to 2 hours is successful in ~60% to 70% of cases. Recurrences of catheter thrombosis should prompt investigation for a malposition or kink in the CVC. The diagnosis can be confirmed with the use of an x-ray and/or intracatheter contrast imaging and is generally managed with rewiring and CVC replacement. Maintenance may be required to fibrin sheaths stemming from the catheter tip; if it is a temporary CVC, management involves removal and replacement but if it is a tunneled CVC, management includes angiography with possible angioplasty prior to replacement.

IV. PERITONEAL DIALYSIS

A. Suitable Candidates/Creation. The major determinant of suitability of a patient for peritoneal dialysis is an adequate peritoneum determined primarily by the abdominal surgical history of the patient.

B. Timing of Creation to Usability. The transition time to create a usable access is immediate to 2 months: immediate for "Urgent Start PD" and 6 to 8 weeks is the traditional time required for healing to lessens the chances for PD fluid leakages.

C. Examination. Examination of the peritoneal dialysis catheter site starts with inspection, with the examiner wearing a facial mask to reduce contamination. Redness around the exit site may be concerning for infection, or less commonly, for an allergic response to the catheter. Presence of discharge at the exit site suggests an active infectious process. The next phase of the examination involves palpation over the skin/subcutaneous tissue overlying the tunneled catheter. Induration upon palpation is suggestive of subcutaneous tissue involvement, which may further define the cause of an overlying erythema/redness. Tenderness along the tunneled part of the peritoneal catheter is highly suggestive of an associated tunnel infection that is an absolute indication to remove the catheter, which contrasts with the more conservative management of an exit-site infection. Point-of-care ultrasound (POCUS) examination allows for detection of fluid collection(s) and the definition of the affected tissue plane(s).

D. Maintenance. Maintenance of PD access/catheter after placement include prevention of exit-site infection, subcutaneous tunnel infection, and peritoneal cavity infection otherwise known as PD-associated peritonitis; others include dialysate leaks and PD access outflow failure. Prevention of exit-site infection is typically done using daily application of gentamicin or mupirocin antibiotic ointment. Ensuring proper PD placement techniques including sharp but tight skin exit of PD catheter during placement without skin suturing avoids exit-site and/or subcutaneous tunnel infections in the immediate postplacement period.

   1. Troubleshooting. PD cycler machines also incorporate some flow sensor mechanism for screening of low PD fluid flow which, if persistent, is an indication for further evaluation(s) including the use of contrast-enhanced imaging studies including interventional radiology guided interventions, or computer axial tomographic scans (CAT-Scan).

V. SUGGESTED READINGS

Asif A, Byers P, Gadalean F, et al. Peritoneal dialysis underutilization: the impact of an interventional nephrology peritoneal dialysis access program. *Semin Dial*. 2003;16(3):266–227.

Asif A, Leon C, Orozco-Vargas LC, et al. Accuracy of physical examination in the detection of arteriovenous graft stenosis. *Clin J Am Soc Nephrol*. 2007;2(6):1191–1194.

Beathard G. *Physical Examination: The Forgotten Tool*. Lippincott Williams & Wilkins; 2002.

Interventional Nephrology: In: Asif A, Agarwal AK, Yevzlin AS, et al., eds. Full Mcgraw-Hill Medical, First edition, 2012.

Lok CE, Huber TS, Lee T, et al. *KDOQI Clinical Practice Guidelines for Vascular Access*: 2019 Update.

Renal Transplantation

46

The Evaluation for Kidney Transplantation

Winfred W. Williams

When compared to dialysis, a kidney transplant (KT) offers a better quality of life, eliminates the need for repetitive volume and electrolyte removal and the associated complications and reduces the risk of infection from vascular or peritoneal access. It increases survival and the sense of control, independence, and well-being and allows resumption of a less restrictive lifestyle. It restores physiologic regulation of vitamin D, erythropoietin, volume homeostasis, and waste product elimination for which a well-functioning KT is far superior to any dialysis modality. The nephrologist must identify those candidates who show the greatest promise to complete the extensive testing required to meet selection criteria and who can be expected to enjoy a successful KT operation and outcome.

I. **WHAT ARE THE REQUIREMENTS?** Patients undergoing transplantation are classified into the following categories:
- Ideal candidates
- Candidates with no identifiable contraindications to KT
- Patients with relative contraindications who are considered high-risk KT recipients
- Patients who would be considered poor or marginal KT candidates
- Patients with absolute contraindications to KT

II. **AGE.** Presently, 70% of KT recipients are >55. Chronologic age limits are less important than "physiologic" age.

III. **ETIOLOGY OF END-STAGE KIDNEY DISEASE.** Although virtually no cause of end-stage kidney disease (ESKD) presently excludes individuals from receiving a KT, some etiologies entail a higher risk of kidney loss. Thus, some cases of primary focal glomerulosclerosis have a high and rapid rate of recurrence and progression to allograft failure while IgA nephropathy has a high rate of histologic recurrence (depending on the report, rates vary between approximately 20% and 60%) but generally a low rate of graft failure. Dense deposit disease, formerly classified as a subgroup of membranoproliferative glomerulonephritis, has a high rate of histologic recurrence and associated renal allograft failure. As a final selected example, Black patients with sickle cell disease can be very challenging to bring to transplantation. Recently, more of them have undergone a kidney transplant, but there is often allograft damage from sickling or thrombotic microangiopathy that limits graft survival. Late-generation immunosuppression is very effective at preventing immunologically mediated recurrent disease and protecting an allograft from acute kidney rejection. One-year graft survival rates now exceed 90% to 95% with deceased or live donors.

IV. PRETRANSPLANT SCREENING PROTOCOLS

A. Timing of Referral. The United Network for Organ Sharing (UNOS) states that patients are eligible for listing on the national KT waitlist once the estimated GFR is <20 mL/min/m². Referral can be initiated by a primary care physician, a nephrologist, or dialysis center, or even patient self-referral. CMS guidelines require referral for kidney transplantation upon initiation of dialysis. Ideally, referral should begin at an eGFR closer to <30 cc/min/1.73 m² to permit full transplant evaluation (which is labor-intensive) and timely preparation for dialytic renal replacement therapy, and to explore the potential of live kidney donors.

B. A Multidisciplinary Team Approach. It is the rule in many transplant centers to provide a comprehensive education about kidney transplantation and a methodical and comprehensive candidate evaluation.

C. The Transplant Center Team. The transplant center team is generally comprised of:
- Transplant coordinator
- Social worker
- Dietician
- Financial coordinator
- Transplant nephrologist or transplant specialized nurse practitioner (CNP) or physician assistant (PA)
- Transplant surgeon
- Others: transplant pharmacist, transplant psychiatrist

V. THE TRANSPLANT EVALUATION (SEE E-TABLE 46-1)

A. Patient History and Physical Examination. This entails a comprehensive medical history and physical examination and a focus on relevant factors such as bruits over the carotid arteries, heart murmurs or gallops, or diminished pulses in the lower extremities that all require further vascular interrogation. The objective of the physical examination is to discern whether a patient is a reasonable surgical risk and will benefit from the allocation of the scarce resource of a renal allograft. We alluded to the challenges of a patient with sickle disease. Similarly, by history, a young woman with a history of lupus nephritis and a lupus anticoagulant leading to thrombotic complications would need to undergo a formal hematologic evaluation to rule out hypercoagulability, which could be a threat to KT viability and necessitate anticoagulation at the time of KT.

VI. SELECTED ISSUES IN KIDNEY TRANSPLANT EVALUATION

A. Cardiac Clearance (See e-Table 46-2). All KT candidates undergo cardiac clearance to detect serious conditions that may require cardiac catheterization. These include moderate-to-severe valvular stenosis or regurgitation, a right ventricular systolic pressure >50 mm/Hg, a cardiac stress test with significant wall motion abnormalities, or ischemia by ECG or imaging. Cardiac catheterization revealing significant uncorrectable coronary disease would argue against proceeding with transplant. Chronic, unexplained chest pain or dyspnea also would likely rule out a candidate.

B. Surgical Clearance. Preoperative surgical evaluation is another requirement. Iliac vascular clearance is required to ensure that kidney transplantation is safe and technically feasible; this is generally done by abdominopelvic CT imaging of the vessels.

C. Cancer Screening and History of Prior Cancer Diagnosis. Most patients with an active cancer diagnosis would be excluded as a KT candidate until a remission was achieved and the appropriate waiting period after initial cancer diagnosis had elapsed. For most cancers, a period of 2 years from the time of remission is required, but recently this period has come into question and the duration of waiting time hinges largely on the type of cancer the patient has. Standard, primary care-based cancer screening, age and gender appropriate, is required. As an example, all candidates age >45 years or with a significant family history of colon cancer generally would be required to have a colonoscopy within 10 years of transplant. A cancer diagnosis within 10 years, except for nonmelanoma skin cancer, requires written clearance from an oncologist because of the high risk of cancer recurrence during immunosuppression.

D. Infectious Disease Considerations. Candidates with untreatable infections are not candidates for KT as their infections may worsen or become life-threatening under immunosuppression. Patients who test positive for HIV, have a positive history of TB, syphilis, strongyloides, schistosomiasis, or Chagas disease must undergo clearance from a transplant infectious disease specialist. Patients with an active chronic infection, such as refractory osteomyelitis, are not suitable candidates. Surveillance and screening are recommended for patients born in, or with extensive travel histories to areas endemic to certain diseases, including the Ohio and Mississippi River Valleys for exposure to Histoplasmosis.

These are selected examples of the many variables under consideration in the process for screening and selection for KT.

E. Psychosocial History and Profile. Transplant candidates cannot have active psychosis, major psychiatric illness, nor be actively abusing drugs. Candidates should have a robust social support network for the postoperative period. Those with a significant psychological problem would be counseled and referred for further evaluation.

In summary, the process of selection for a KT is extensive and involves a multidisciplinary team-based approach. The patient must satisfy many screening criteria; this includes adequate financial support (insurance coverage) to effectively manage the expense of hospitalization and immunosuppressant medications. Any known condition which is unlikely to improve with a KT or which renders KT unsafe or futile, including but not limited to cancer, untreatable chronic infection, heart or lung disease, bleeding or clotting disorders, psychiatric or neurologic illness, morbid obesity, severe vascular disease, or other advanced organ system disease, usually would eliminate the patient's candidacy. However, each patient is a valued individual and receives a careful evaluation tailored to lead to the best chance of success. The overarching objective is to support patients through the myriad of testing with the full intent of helping them achieve their goal of kidney transplantation.

VII. SUGGESTED READING

Wolfe RA, Ashby VB, Milford EL, et al. Comparison of mortality in all patients on dialysis, patients on dialysis awaiting transplantation, and recipients of a first cadaveric transplant. *N Engl J Med.* 1999;341(23):1725–1730.

Medical Complications Following Kidney Transplantation

Winfred W. Williams

Kidney transplant (KT) is widely considered the ideal treatment for end-stage kidney disease (ESKD), but it comes with the inherent risks associated with immune system suppression that can cause metabolic, cardiac, infectious, and neoplastic disease complications. Posttransplant infectious diseases will not be covered in this chapter.

I. DEATH WITH A FUNCTIONING KIDNEY TRANSPLANT—CARDIOVASCULAR MORBIDITY AND MORTALITY. Although cardiovascular disease (CVD) in ESKD is reduced to one-third after a KT, it remains the leading cause of premature patient and allograft loss. The CVD encountered includes coronary artery disease, heart failure, valvular heart disease, arrhythmias, and pulmonary hypertension. Remarkably, the commonest cause of kidney graft loss is death with a functioning allograft. The CVD mortality for KT recipients aged 25 to 34 years is increased by 10-fold. This is not explained by pre- or posttransplant diabetes, hypertension, or dyslipidemia. Atherosclerotic event-free survival is worse for those with multiple histocompatibility mismatches. Prophylaxis against cytomegalovirus (CMV) can mitigate CVD death with a functioning allograft. Assiduous attention to the management of CVD risk factors is essential in the transplant population.

II. POSTTRANSPLANT HYPERTENSION. Hypertension occurs in 60% to 80% of KT patients despite restoration of volume regulation by a well-functioning kidney allograft. Posttransplant hypertension is commoner in patients with pre-existing hypertension, older age, African-American race, male gender, higher BMI, diabetes, and left ventricular hypertrophy, while donor factors include deceased donor kidney transplant, older age, atherosclerotic renal vascular disease and hypertension. Immunosuppression, corticosteroids, and calcineurin inhibitors (CNIs) often provoke high blood pressure. Tacrolimus and cyclosporine cause renal vasoconstriction and renin release. Prednisone has both mineralo- and glucocorticoid effects leading to distal nephron salt and water retention potentiating hypertension.

Posttransplant renal artery stenosis (TRAS) should be suspected when blood pressure increases abruptly or becomes resistant to therapy. Patients requiring a high-dose, multidrug, antihypertensive regimen should be interrogated for TRAS. Deteriorating KT function may cause hypertension from impaired volume and salt excretion. Poorly controlled blood pressure results in diminished KT survival. KDIGO recommends a blood pressure target of <130/80 mm Hg. The FAVORIT trial reported that although a higher systolic BP was strongly associated with increased risk of CVD and all-cause mortality, a diastolic blood pressure (DBP) ≤70 mm Hg was associated with increased CVD and mortality. This suggests that high pulse pressure may be a culprit.

Treatment of hypertension generally includes calcium channel blockers (CCBs) followed by β and α-blockers or combined α/β-blockers. CCBs can cause proteinuria and hyperfiltration and diltiazem, verapamil, and nifedipine increase CNI levels, potentiating nephrotoxicity. Angiotensin-converting enzyme inhibitors (ACEIs) and angiotensin receptor blockers (ARBs) should be avoided in the immediate posttransplant period when CNIs are being introduced since CNIs constrict the afferent arteriole while ACEI/ARBs relax the efferent arteriole thereby reducing intraglomerular pressure and GFR. Where ACEI/ARB therapy is indicated, as in diabetes and proteinuric CKD, they may be introduced after about 3 to 6 months, when the dose of CNI therapy has been reduced to low maintenance dosing. One retrospective study of older KT patients with diabetes and a mean SCr of >1.3 mg/dL reported no reduction in CVD deaths at 1 year with ACEI-ARB treatment. The advantages of ACEI/ARBs include limiting proteinuria and, perhaps, diminishing fibrosis, while the disadvantages include the trade-off of a lower GFR (an expected outcome to efferent arteriolar relaxation) and hyperkalemia.

III. METABOLIC SYNDROME AFTER TRANSPLANTATION. Both cyclosporine and tacrolimus may cause metabolic syndrome from reactive oxygen species. The metabolic syndrome is defined by any three of the following:

- Abdominal obesity with a waist circumference in men >40 inches and in women >35 inches.
- Serum triglycerides (TGs) ≥150 mg/dL or drug treatment for elevated TGs.
- Serum high-density lipoprotein cholesterol <40 mg/dL in men and <50 mg/dL in women or drug treatment to raise high-density lipoprotein cholesterol.
- Blood pressure ≥130/85 mm Hg or drug treatment for elevated blood pressure.
- Fasting plasma glucose ≥100 mg/dL or drug treatment for elevated blood glucose

IV. POSTTRANSPLANT DYSLIPIDEMIA. More than 80% of KT patients have a raised cholesterol and 90% to 97% have an elevated LDL-cholesterol. Immunosuppression (IS) is a major driver. Glucocorticoids stimulate hepatic very low–density lipoprotein (VLDL) synthesis and downregulate LDL receptors. Cyclosporin A (CsA) inhibits hepatic bile acid 26-hydroxylase, thereby decreasing bile acid synthesis from cholesterol and reducing the subsequent transport of cholesterol into the bile and the intestine.

Mammalian target of rapamycin (mTOR) inhibitors cause profound dyslipidemia and increase TGs. Sirolimus and everolimus block insulin-stimulated lipoprotein lipase thereby reducing catabolism of apoB100-containing lipoproteins. Rapamycin increases TGs and cholesterol.

The Assessment of Lescol in Renal Transplantation (ALERT) study randomized 2,106 KT patients to fluvastatin versus placebo. Despite the expected statin-induced lowering of LDL, adverse cardiac events still occurred over the 5 years of the trial. However, an extension study of patients in the fluvastatin arm reported a significant reduction in cardiac death or nonfatal myocardial infarction. The KDIGO guidelines recommend treating all adult KT patients with a statin regardless of LDL concentration. We establish baseline lipid data 4 to 6 weeks after transplantation and repeat fasting lipids every 4 to 8 weeks until goal lipid levels are accomplished, and every 6 to 12 months thereafter. We treat

T A B L E 47.1	Risk factors for posttransplant diabetes mellitus	
Nonmodifiable	**Potentially modifiable**	**Modifiable**
Increased age >45 y	Hepatitis C virus	Obesity (BMI ≥30)
Obesity (BMI ≥30 kg/m²)	Cytomegalovirus	LDL cholesterol
African-American or Hispanic ethnicity	Pretransplant IGT/IFG	IS (steroids, tacrolimus, cyclosporine, sirolimus)
History of gestational diabetes	Proteinuria	Vitamin D deficiency
Family history of diabetes mellitus	Hypomagnesemia	
History of metabolic syndrome		
Prior transplant glucose-intolerance		
HLA mismatches		
Acute rejection history		
Deceased male donor		
Genetic polymorphisms		

Adapted from Feingold KR, Anawalt B, Boyce A, et al., eds. *Endotext* [Internet]. MDText.com, Inc.; 2000.

most patients with statins and combination therapy where indicated. Therapy should begin with the recommended starting doses but, because of the concern for rhabdomyolysis and myopathy when statins are combined with CNIs, we begin with very judicious, generally low statin dosing, sometimes on alternate days. Inhibition of cholesterol uptake with ezetimibe is a valuable addition. KDIGO recommends against the use of fibrates in combination with statins because of the risk of rhabdomyolysis. There may be benefit from statin therapy for atherosclerotic vascular disease and endothelial function and a reduction in KT vasculopathy and carotid remodeling.

V. POSTTRANSPLANT DIABETES MELLITUS. Posttransplant diabetes mellitus (PTDM) is a common complication of KT that occurs in 10% to 15% of nondiabetic KT recipients by 6 months but the prevalence has decreased recently. The risk factors are shown in Table 47.1.

Most PTDM is secondary to immunosuppressive (IS) medication. More than 90% of KT recipients in the United States receive a CNI in a three-drug regimen, namely tacrolimus plus a mycophenolate acid antimetabolite derivative (Myfortic or CellCept) and an oral steroid (prednisone in the United States). Tacrolimus is a major cause of PTDM by suppressing insulin synthesis. Maintenance corticosteroids add 30% to this risk but studies have shown that preemptive or rapid steroid withdrawal can precipitate renal allograft rejection.

VI. IMMUNOSUPPRESSIVE AGENTS AND RISK OF PTDM. Glucocorticoid-induced hyperglycemia entails dose-dependent enhanced hepatic gluconeogenesis and curtailed insulin-dependent peripheral glucose uptake. Transient hyperglycemia often accompanies initiation of high-dose pulse intravenous methylprednisolone. Most patients are treated with high-dose oral steroid therapy per protocol until a stable lower maintenance steroid dose is achieved.

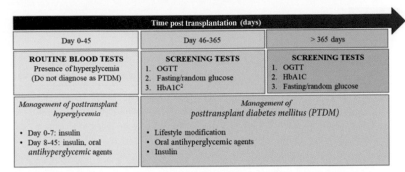

FIGURE 47.1: Screening, Diagnosis, and Management Recommendations for PTDM. (Reproduced from Feingold KR, Anawalt B, Boyce A, et al., eds. *Endotext* [Internet]. MDText.com, Inc.; 2000.)

Cyclosporine and especially tacrolimus increase the risk of PTDM by islet cell toxicity, which may be reversible. Belatacept causes a lower rate of PTDM than CNIs.

m-TOR inhibitors cause PTDM by pancreatic β-islet cell toxicity and decreased insulin sensitivity that is exacerbated by combination with CNIs. Azathioprine, the mycophenolic acid derivatives, and belatacept do not appear to have diabetogenic effects.

VII. HYPOMAGNESEMIA. Hypomagnesemia, often due to CNI-mediated renal tubular "leakage," is common after KT and is associated with PTDM. However, Mg^{2+} repletion is not a major therapeutic strategy (Figure 47.1).

KDIGO guidelines recommend measuring a fasting plasma glucose level weekly for 4 weeks, then at 3 and 6 months and then annually. PTDM should not be diagnosed within the first 6 weeks after KT since plasma glucose levels are often elevated during establishment of IS dosing.

VIII. DIAGNOSIS OF PTDM—LIST OF ADA CRITERIA FOR THE GENERAL POPULATION
- Symptoms of diabetes plus random plasma glucose ≥200 mg/dL
- Fasting plasma glucose ≥126 mg/dL
- Two-hour plasma glucose ≥200 mg/dL during an oral glucose tolerance test (OGTT)
- HbA1c ≥6.5%, after the first 3 months posttransplant

A1c alone has low sensitivity. PTDM patients should be monitored quarterly.

IX. TREATMENT GUIDELINES FOR PTDM. Usual life-style modifications include diet and exercise to minimize weight gain. Pharmacologic therapy begins with an oral hypoglycemic medication. Table 47.2 lists approved hypoglycemic drugs for use in patients with PTDM and their modes of action.

The use of hypoglycemic drugs based on the level of kidney function (eGFR/CKD stage) is reviewed in Table 47.3. SGLT-2 inhibitors have not yet been subject to rigorous clinical trial in KT recipients and are not currently recommended.

X. IMMUNOSUPPRESSION AND PTDM. Immunologic risk should guide selection of the IS agent with consideration for the potential for PTDM (Figure 47.2). Since African Americans have a higher risk for PTDM, their first choice CNI might be cyclosporine, or a belatacept-based IS regimen in selected patients.

DPP-4, dipeptidyl peptidase-4; GIR, gastric inhibitory polypeptide; GLP-1, glucagon-like peptide-1; NPH, neutral protamine hagedorn; PPAR, peroxisome proliferator–activated receptor; PTDM, posttransplant diabetes mellitus.
From Jenssen T, Hartmann A. Emerging treatments for post-transplantation diabetes mellitus. *Nat Rev Nephrol.* 2015;11(8):465–477. doi:10.1038/nrneph.2015.59

Drug class	Drugs	Main mechanisms of action	Risk of hypoglycemia
Sulfonylureas	Glimepiride, glipizide, glibenclamide	Increases insulin secretion by blocking β-cell K^+-ATPase	Yes
Glinides	Repaglinide, nateglinide	Similar action to sulfonylureas but exhibit a shorter half-life	Yes
Biguanides	Metformin	Decreases glucose production in liver and increases glucose uptake in muscle	No
Glitazones (PPAR-γ activators)	Pioglitazone	Increases insulin sensitivity in muscle, fat, and liver cells	No
DPP-4 inhibitors	Sitagliptin, vildagliptin	Inhibits degradation and increases endogenous levels of GLP-1 and GIP	No
Insulin	Insulin NPH, glargine, detemir, short-acting insulin and analogues	Insulin-receptor–stimulated glucose disposal and reduced glucose production	Yes

TABLE 47.2 Approved hypoglycemic drugs for use in PTDM

XI. POSTTRANSPLANT BONE MARROW DISORDERS. The prevalence of posttransplant anemia (PTA) is 20% to 40%. Predisposing factors include ESKD and suppressed erythropoietin prior to KT, bleeding from anastomotic leaks, anemia associated with major surgery, infection, and drug effects. Opportunistic infections with CMV and parvovirus B19 (PVB19) cause erythropoietin-resistant anemia. Parvovirus generally causes time-limited hemolytic anemia and CMV causes generalized bone marrow suppression. Immunosuppression with sirolimus, CellCept, Myfortic, and azathioprine can cause bone marrow suppression. ACEIs and ARBs are prescribed commonly to treat posttransplant erythrocytosis. Acute rejection can suppress red-cell production due to inflammation. Thrombotic microangiopathy (TMA) is associated hemolytic anemia and can be complications of the mTOR inhibitors, sirolimus and everolimus, but more commonly with CNIs. Finally, anemia may be a preceding symptom of malignancy, the risk of which is increased after transplantation.

XII. DIAGNOSTIC APPROACH TO POSTTRANSPLANT ANEMIA. It is imperative to check and replace iron stores (especially in preemptively transplanted patients), folic acid and vitamin B12, and to assess the reticulocyte count. Iron deficiency and

TABLE 47.3 Use of hypoglycemic drugs in PTDM and impaired renal function

Drug class	eGFR 60–90 mL/min/1.73 m²	eGFR 30–59 mL/min/1.73 m²	eGFR 15–30 mL/min/1.73 m²	eGFR <15 mL/min/1.73 m²
Sulfonylureas	Used without dose adjustment	Used with or without dose adjustment; caution for hypoglycemia	Not generally recommended due to risk of hypoglycemia	Not generally recommended due to risk of hypoglycemia
Glinides	Used without dose adjustment	Used without dose adjustment	Should not be used	Should not be used
Biguanides	Used without dose adjustment	Used with or without dose adjustment[a]	Should not be used	Should not be used
Glitazones (PPAR-γ activators)	Used without dose adjustment	Used without dose adjustment	Used with or without dose adjustment	Should not be used
DPP-4 inhibitors	Used without dose adjustment	Used with or without dose adjustment	Used with or without dose adjustment	Used with or without dose adjustment
GLP-1 analogs[b]	Not studied in PTDM	Not studied in PTDM	Not studied in PTDM	Not studied in PTDM
SGLT2 inhibitors[c]	Not studied in PTDM	Not studied in PTDM	Not studied in PTDM	Not studied in PTDM
Insulin	Used without dose adjustment	Used with or without dose adjustment; caution for hypoglycemia	Used with or without dose adjustment; caution for hypoglycemia	Used with or without dose adjustment; caution for hypoglycemia

[a]Not approved in the United States for patients with GFR <60 mL/min/1.73 m².

[b]Have been used safely in patients with type 2 diabetes and GFR >30 mL/min/1.73 m²; no documentation in PTDM.

[c]Reduced glucose-lowering effect at GFRs <60 mL/min/1.73 m²; no documentation in PTDM.

DPP-4, dipeptidyl peptidase-4; eGFR, estimated glomerular filtration rate; GLP-1, glucagon-like peptide-1; PPAR, peroxisome proliferator–activated receptors; PTDM, posttransplant diabetes mellitus; SGLT2, sodium-glucose–linked transporter 2.

From Jenssen T, Hartmann A. Emerging treatments for post-transplantation diabetes mellitus. *Nat Rev Nephrol.* 2015;11(8):465–477. doi:10.1038/nrneph.2015.59

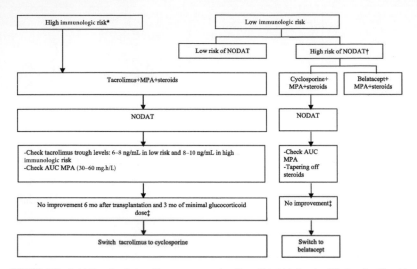

FIGURE 47.2: Guidelines for choice of immunosuppression. (From Ghisdal L, Bouchta NB, Broeders N, et al. Conversion from tacrolimus to cyclosporine A for new-onset diabetes after transplantation: a single-centre experience in renal transplanted patients and review of the literature. *Transpl Int*. 2008;21:146–151.)

transferrin saturation <20% are the most common findings in the anemia of ESKD that can carry over into the immediate postoperative transplant period.

XIII. THERAPY OF POSTTRANSPLANT ANEMIA. Adjustment of IS and/or prophylactic antibiotic/antiviral therapy may be indicated. Mycophenolic acid causes dose-dependent bone marrow depression. Erythropoietin and/or ESA agents may be used as adjunctive therapy, especially during highly bone marrow toxic regimens, for example, sirolimus in combination with mycophenolate mofetil (MMF). Iron replacement is essential for those with a low transferrin saturation and often requires intravenous iron transfusion.

XIV. POSTTRANSPLANT ERYTHROCYTOSIS. The etiology is not clear. It is reflected by increases in hemoglobin and hematocrit of >16.5 to 18 g/dL and 50% to 54%, respectively. These thresholds can be adjusted for gender. The prevalence of posttransplant erythrocytosis (PTE) is 8% to 15% of patients. The risk factors are shown in Table 47.4.

PTE most often occurs in patients with retained native kidneys or polycystic kidney disease. The serum EPO levels are elevated relative to the increased Hgb levels. Other hematopoietic factors may enhance the sensitivity to EPO. Activation of the renin–angiotensin system increases the growth of erythroid precursors, stimulates EPO secretion, and induces hypoxia-inducible factors that promote the production of EPO and iron metabolism.

PTE occurs 8 to 24 months after KT. Some patients experience headache, lethargy, and malaise and 10% to 30% develop arterial or venous thromboembolic events with a 1% to 2% mortality with thrombosis of digital or branchial arteries, thrombophlebitis, stroke, or pulmonary embolus.

The diagnosis of PTE should be suspected in KT recipient with hemoglobin >17 g/dL and/or hematocrit >51% for more than 2 to 3 months. Secondary

T A B L E 47.4	Risk factors for posttransplant erythropoiesis

- Male sex
- Rejection-free post KT
- Retained native kidneys
- Preserved GFR
- Transplant renal artery stenosis

- Hypertension
- Diuretic use
- Diabetes
- Long duration dialysis
- Smoking

From Vlahakos DV, Marathias KP, Agroyannis B, Madias NE. Posttransplant erythrocytosis. *Kidney Int.* 2003;63(4):1187–1194.

causes of erythrocytosis from malignancy should be evaluated to exclude renal cell and hepatocellular carcinoma.

The goal of management is to lower the Hgb. When critically high, the removal of 1 to 2 units of blood is indicated. The first-line pharmacologic treatment entails an ACE inhibitor or an ARB where responses are usually apparent in 2 to 4 weeks. Finally, patients who smoke cigarettes require smoking cessation strategies.

XV. LEUKOPENIA. A decrease in white blood cells is common after KT especially when high-dose IS is used. Bone marrow suppressants include mycophenolate acid and its derivatives, the combination of allopurinol and azathioprine, valcyte and Bactrim (used as prophylactic antimicrobials) and thymoglobulin. Infections are a longer-term complication and may be facilitated by the fall in white blood cell count. Viruses that occur opportunistically include EBV, CMV, and parvovirus B19 and are common in the immunosuppressed host. A survey for opportunistic infection often requires assays for viral copy number for EBV and CMV, and serologic testing for parvovirus.

We try to avoid major adjustments in IS based on changes in white cell count. Granulocyte colony–stimulating factor (G-CSF) is often given with good results and little risk of inducing rejection.

XVI. THROMBOCYTOPENIA. Thrombocytopenia, in the early posttransplant period, is usually caused by thymoglobulin. In later periods, other drugs are often implicated. A careful drug survey is indicated. The differential diagnosis includes a fall in platelets with CNI-induced TMA that would necessitate a change in IS but can also occur with mTOR inhibitors.

XVII. POSTTRANSPLANT MALIGNANCY. The attenuation of normal immune surveillance that occurs with IS increases the risk for neoplastic complications in transplant recipients. IS interferes with antitumor surveillance and antiviral suppression. Many cancers may be secondary to EBV, human papillomavirus, hepatitis B and C viruses, and human herpesvirus 8. Posttransplant malignancies are the third most common cause of death among KT recipients.

A large survey reported that cancer incidence increased slightly among dialysis patients (standardized incidence ratio [SIR] = 1.35) but increased markedly at 25 anatomic sites after transplant with an SIR = 3.27. Most of the cancers were associated with a viral-mediated etiology. The role of IS was emphasized in this large registry series.

XVIII. POSTTRANSPLANT LYMPHOPROLIFERATIVE DISORDER. Posttransplant lymphoproliferative disorder (PTLD) is the commonest posttransplant malignancy in children and the commonest cause of cancer-related posttransplant mortality. It typically occurs in the first 12 months after KT. PTLD includes an early lesion with plasma cell hyperplasia that mimics infectious mononucleosis, a polymorphic PTLD that entails polyclonal or monoclonal lymphoid infiltrates and malignant transformation, and a monomorphic PTLD with monoclonal phenotype of the B-, T-, or NK-cell lineage. Most PTLDs are of B-cell lineage. Their risk factors include transplantation of EBV-positive donors into naïve recipients (EBV D+/R), young age, potent IS and the net cumulative IS dose, anti-lymphocyte induction therapy (especially thymoglobulin), and CMV infection.

PCR monitoring for EBV is essential in the setting of EBV D+/R− KT recipients. The viral load begins to increase progressively by 4 to 16 weeks prior to clinically manifested PTLDs. For this D+/R− donor–recipient pair, we monitor PCR viral copy number for EBV monthly for 6 months and at 2-month intervals through 12 to 18 months.

The first step in management is a reduction of IS dose with consideration of adding the CD20 monoclonal antibody, rituximab. Our initial approach is to cut CNI-based IS by 50%, discontinue the antimetabolites MMF and azathioprine but to continue prednisone. These decisions require consideration of tumor burden and patient preferences regarding the risk of allograft injury—acute rejection— and return to dialysis. Many centers favor R-CHOP that includes rituximab, cyclophosphamide, doxorubicin, vincristine, and prednisone. Patients whose tumors are CD20 negative are treated with chemotherapy that consists of CHOP alone. Radiotherapy can be considered. These are only broad, general guidelines and require the expert guidance of oncologic consultants.

XIX. SKIN CANCERS. Skin cancers are the most prevalent solid organ tumors in KT recipients who are 65 to 250 times more likely to develop squamous cell carcinomas, and 6 to 16 times more likely to develop basal cell carcinomas. Skin cancers account for nearly 40% of malignancies in organ transplant recipients, with a rate of 50% in white recipients and approximately 6% in non-white recipients. There may be direct oncogenic effects from azathioprine and cyclosporine since CNIs and azathioprine impair the repair of UV-radiation–induced DNA damage. Azathioprine has been associated with an increased risk of squamous cell, melanoma, and Merkel cell carcinoma. KT recipients are more likely to develop multiple and aggressive tumors on sun-exposed areas. The lower legs are a common site for Kaposi sarcoma.

Other, often aggressive cancers encountered in KT recipients include cervical, vulvar, anal, and colorectal cancers. Renal cell carcinomas have a 15-fold increased incidence in KT recipients. Risk factors include prior RCC, acquired cystic disease, tuberous sclerosis, and analgesic nephropathy.

Medical Reimbursement and Economics of Nephrology

SECTION XI

Medical Reimbursement and Economic Impact

48

Medical Reimbursement and the Economics of Nephrology Practice

Behnaz Haddadi-Sahneh, Robert J. Rubin

In 1972, the United States passed Public Law 92–603 that provided coverage for end-stage kidney disease (ESKD) to all Americans with little debate or analysis. Importantly, no limits were placed on the payments made under the ESKD program. In 1974, there were 10,300 patients receiving care at a cost of $241 million. In 2019, there were 746,557 prevalent patients with ESKD representing <1% of Medicare patients but accounting for 7.2% of Medicare costs.

I. **DIALYSIS**. Initially, hospital-based hemodialysis was paid on a reasonable cost basis while independent facilities were paid on a reasonable charge basis. Both systems had a payment ceiling of $138 per treatment. Hospitals were able to receive an increase through an exceptions process, increasing their average rate to $159 per treatment. Home dialysis was also paid on a reasonable cost basis. In 1983, a dialysis-specific prospective rate (composite rate) was established which included all costs associated with dialysis. From time to time, Congress reduced the composite until 1989, when the average composite rate for independent units was about $54 in 1974 dollars – an almost two thirds reduction. In 1989, the first erythropoietin-stimulating agent (ESA) was approved for use in anemic dialysis patients. Dialysis units were paid separately for it, and there was a fixed price of $40 for <10,000 units initially. This was quickly changed to a specific price per 1,000 units due to concern that dialysis providers were charging the $40 but giving substantially less than 10,000 units and making "windfall" profits. Over time, separately billable drugs included vitamin D analogs and iron as well as ESAs which made up 84% of the total were increasing. Congress, in an effort to improve provider efficiency, required Medicare to establish a prospective payment system for dialysis services (Bundle) that "bundled" all separately billable items such as drugs (both intravenous and oral) and laboratory services with the composite into one rate. Subsequently, Congress postponed the inclusion of oral only drugs until 2025. The theory is that by providing a fixed price, the government was incentivizing efficient providers by letting them keep the difference between the cost of providing care and the government set price. To ensure that providers did not cut costs at the expense of patient care, a Quality Incentive Program (QIP) was put into place and was linked to provider payments.

Each year the Centers for Medicare and Medicaid Services (CMS) publishes their proposed rules and payments (notice of proposed rulemaking [NPRM]) in the summer, and after receiving public comments, they publish the rules that

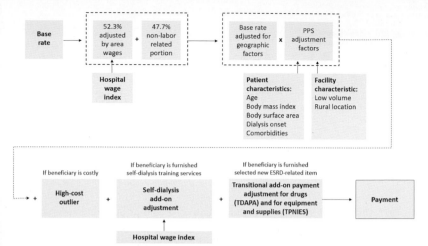

FIGURE 48.1: Dialysis prospective payment system. TDAPA, transitional drug add-on payment adjustment; TPNIES, transitional add-on payment adjustment for new and innovative equipment and supplies. This figure represents the dialysis prospective system for beneficiaries 18 and older. For beneficiaries under 18: (1) the base rate, adjusted for geographic factors, is multiplied by patient case-mix characteristics and dialysis method; (2) the low-volume adjustment and rural factors do not apply; and (3) the outlier payment policy and add-on for self-dialysis training do apply. The payment rate may be reduced by up to 2 percent for facilities that do not achieve or make progress toward specified quality measures. (Medicare payment advisory.)

will govern the Bundle for the next calendar year (Fig. 48.1). The following is an example of the proposed 2021 payment per hemodialysis treatment. The base rate is divided into labor costs (52.3%) and nonlabor costs (47.7%). The labor costs are adjusted by an index that is based on the location of the facility and the base rate is then adjusted for "budget neutrality" to ensure that wage index adjustments do not increase or decrease total payments. In 2021, calcimimetics will be added to the Bundle and so the payment will increase by $12.06 (regardless of whether a patient gets a calcimimetic). Finally, the government recognizes that the cost of providing the service increases each year (these inputs are called the market basket) which is offset by providers becoming more efficient (productivity adjustment), which in 2021 is proposed to be 2.2% and 0.4% respectively. These result in a base rate of $255.59 (239.01*.998652 = $239.01) +12.06 = 251.07*(2.2 − 0.4) = $255.59. In addition, the base rate is adjusted for facilities that only do a small number of dialyses a year, as well as rural facilities, and certain patient factors that have been shown to increase treatment costs namely, age (18 to 44, 45 to 59, 60 to 69, 70 to 79, and 80+), body mass index, body surface area, first 4 months on dialysis as well as a list of acute and chronic morbidities. CMS also realized that they needed to foster innovation, so there are two additional add on programs. The first is the transitional drug add-on payment adjustment (TDAPA). Under TDAPA, a payment adjustment, in addition to the base rate, pays facilities for certain new dialysis drugs and biologics, including biosimilars that the Food and Drug Administration (FDA) approved on or after January 1, 2020.

These drugs fall into one of the eleven functional categories of products that have been included in the end-stage renal disease (ESRD) prospective payment bundle since 2011. The TDAPA does not apply to new generic drugs and certain other drugs. The TDAPA will apply for 2 years, with payment set at each drug's average sales price (ASP) or average wholesale price (AWP) if an ASP does not exist. After 2 years, CMS will include the drug in the prospective payment system (PPS) payment bundle without any change to the base rate. The second is the transitional add-on payment for new and innovative equipment and supplies (TPINES). Under the TPNIES policy, CMS includes a payment adjustment in addition to the base rate that pays facilities separately for certain new and innovative renal dialysis equipment and supplies under the ESRD PPS. ESRD-related equipment or supplies will be eligible for the TPNIES if the item is new (granted marketing authorization by the FDA on or after January 1, 2020 and within 3 years from the date of FDA approval), is commercially available, has applied for a Healthcare Common Procedure Coding System billing code, is not a capital-related asset, and is truly innovative (meeting the substantial clinical improvement criteria that have been established by CMS for other programs). Specifically, CMS considers a technology innovative if it represents an advance that substantially improves, relative to technologies previously available, the diagnosis or treatment of Medicare beneficiaries. The TPNIES will apply for two calendar years, thereafter, the product will be included in the PPS payment bundle without any change to the base rate. The TPNIES payment will be based on 65% of the price established by the Medicare administrative contractors using information from sources that include the invoice amount, facility charges for the item net of discounts and rebates, and payment amounts determined by other payers. CMS's most recent proposal will provide the TPNIES for eligible new and innovative capital-related assets that are home dialysis machines when used in the home. They would limit the payment for new and innovative dialysis machines to those used for home dialysis for an individual in order to further incentivize the use of home dialysis. Currently, in-center and home dialysis are paid the same rate. There is also an additional payment for self-dialysis training. CMS pays for up to 15 peritoneal dialysis training sessions and 25 sessions for hemodialysis.

II. OUTLIER POLICY. In any prospective payment system, there will be instances where the costs of a particular treatment session will be significantly greater than the payment amount. Each year CMS sets a threshold amount and pays 80% of the cost above that amount. CMS is supposed to set the threshold so that outlier payments equal 1% of the total payment to facilities. However, they have consistently fallen short of that mark. CMS adjusts the base rate by age and dialysis modality for children under 18.

III. QUALITY INCENTIVE PROGRAM (QIP). To ensure that Medicare beneficiaries are receiving quality care within the bundled payment system, CMS instituted a QIP. A facility's payment may be reduced by up to 2% if it fails to meet or make progress toward achieving quality goals. Each year (performance year) the goals are set and the penalties are then applied 2 years later (payment year) after CMS has analyzed the data. In 2019, of the 6,800 facilities with a QIP performance score, 73% had no payment reduction, 18% had their Medicare outpatient dialysis payments reduced by 0.5%, 6% had payments reduced by 1.0%, 2% of facilities had payments reduced by 1.5%, and 1% of facilities had payments reduced by the maximum, 2%. Outcome measures for 2020 payment year include: dialysis adequacy, vascular access (use of fistulas and catheters), unplanned hospital readmissions in a 30-day period, transfusions, proportion of patients with hypercalcemia (an indicator of the quality of bone and mineral metabolism management), number of positive blood cultures, qualitative patient satisfaction surveys, and hospitalizations. Process measures include the following:

- The number of months for which facilities report all required data elements associated with:
  - the ultrafiltration rate for hemodialysis patients;
  - National Healthcare Safety Network dialysis event data to the Centers for Disease Control and Prevention (CDC);
  - dosage of ESAs, hemoglobin, or hematocrit levels;
  - the percent of patients screened for depression; and
  - serum phosphorous levels.
- The number of facility staff who had a timely influenza immunization.
- The percentage of patients who have documented pain assessments as well as a follow-up plan if pain is present.

The weights and scoring for these measures are published prior to the performance year and have changed over time.

IV. PHYSICIAN PAYMENT.

Since 1992, physicians have been under a national physician fee schedule (PFS). The PFS establishes three national relative value units (RVUs) that are each adjusted for geographic variations in costs (Fig. 48.2). The first RVU is a measure of *clinical work* and reflects the time, effort, stress, and skill required to provide the service. The second is the *practice expense* RVU and is a measure of costs to hire staff, and to rent an office and supplies necessary for a particular service. The final RVU is the cost of *professional liability insurance* associated with the service. The RVUs are aggregated and multiplied by a conversion factor (CF) to determine a payment. Medicare, in general, pays 80% of this amount and the beneficiary is responsible for the remaining 20%. If physicians provide services in a "health professional shortage area" (HPSA)

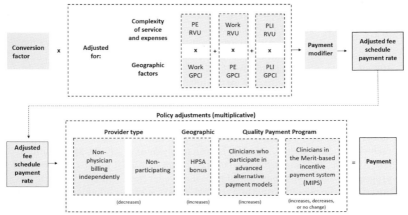

FIGURE 48.2: Physician payment system. RVU, relative value unit; GPCI, geographic practice cost index; PE, practice expense; PLI, professional liability insurance; HPSA, heath professional shortage area. Clinicians who participate in advanced alternative payment models receive an incentive payment of 5 percent of their professional service payments. Clinicians in MIPS receive a positive or negative payment adjustment (or no change) based on their performance in four areas: quality, resource use, advancing care information, and clinical practice improvement. (Medicare payment advisory.)

Medicare provides a 10% bonus to encourage physicians to go to these areas. Beginning in 2019, there was a quality adjuster for physicians in advanced alternative payment models or in the Merit-based Incentive Payment System (MIPS). Under MIPS, physicians can receive an increase, decrease, or no change based on their performance in quality measures, resource use, clinical practice improvement, and care information (electronic medical records). These criteria and scoring are set forth annually in a process like that described for dialysis above.

Nephrologists are paid a monthly capitation fee based on the number of times they see their outpatient dialysis patients in a month. There are separate payment amounts for seeing a patient four times, two or three times, and one time. For 2021, CMS has proposed to increase the value of these codes by 29%, 27%, and 13%, respectively. CMS is also proposing to increase the value of the monthly home dialysis visit by 27%. Nephrologists also bill evaluation and management (E and M) codes when they see patients in their office. While all E and M codes show a proposed value increase for 2021, because of the decrease in the CF, only established patient visits will have an increase in the amount paid. These examples show the importance of both parts of the payment equation, the RVUs as well as the CF (whose formula is set by law).

V. THE FUTURE. On July 10, 2019, the President of the United States signed an order to launch an initiative *Advancing American Kidney Health* (AAKH). The three main goals were to decrease the number of Americans developing kidney failure by 25% by 2030, have 80% of new ESKD patients either receive a preemptive transplant or have dialysis at home, and to double the number of kidneys available for transplant by 2030. One of the tools CMS will use to accomplish these goals are various payment methods that reward and/or punish providers for meeting these goals.

The End-Stage Renal Disease Treatment Choices (ETC) model is mandatory and will involve 30% of beneficiaries, their associated dialysis facilities, and "managing clinicians." There will be two types of payment adjustments. The first is a positive for home dialysis and home dialysis services. The second, which applies to both facilities and clinicians, can be either positive or negative and is based on home dialysis rate and transplant waitlist rate as well as living donor transplant rate. These adjustments increase over time. Interestingly, CMS expects to save $23 million over 5 years—so it seems that they expect the decreases to be greater than the increases. The second set of payment models are voluntary and seek to accomplish the AAKH goal of increasing transplant and home dialysis while decreasing the number of Americans developing ESKD. These models include patients with chronic kidney disease (CKD) stage 4 and 5 as well as dialysis and transplant patients. There are two distinct types of models in this set. The *Kidney Care First* model, which capitates payment for the patients and rewards or punishes providers based on performance-based measures, and the *Comprehensive Kidney Care Contracting* model with three variants based on the degree of risk the participants are willing to take relative to the total cost of care. The global variant allows the provider to assume 100% of the risk. If successful, this would achieve the goal that Medicare has been aiming for over the last 40 years of shifting payment risk to providers while monitoring the quality of care for its beneficiaries. It also allows providers to practice medicine efficiently and reap the financial rewards (or suffer the consequences if they cannot).

VI. SUGGESTED READINGS

Medicare Payment Advisory Commission. Payment *Basics, Outpatient Dialysis Services Payment System.* 2020 http://medpac.gov/docs/default-source/payment-basics/medpac_payment_basics_20_dialysis_final_sec.pdf?sfvrsn=0.

Medicare Payment Advisory Commission. *Payment basics, physician and other health professional payment system.* 2020 http://medpac.gov/docs/default-source/payment-basics/medpac_payment_basics_20_physician_final_sec.pdf?sfvrsn=0.

Rettig RA, Levinsky NG, eds. *Kidney Failure and the Federal Government.* National Academy Press; 1991.

Rubin RJ. Epidemiology of end stage renal disease and implications for public policy. *Pub Health Rep.* 1984;99(5):492–498.

Note: Page number followed by f and t indicates figure and table respectively.